PRAISE FOR
MASTERING STOCKS AND BROTHS

"*Mastering Stocks and Broths* is the most thorough book on the subject I've come across. Rachael Mamane's writing is as beautiful, thoughtful, and caring as her approach to food, the table, and her stocks. And I love the intriguing recipes that she has interspersed throughout the book. If one really used this book, one would emerge a truly excellent cook and, I dare say, person. Here is to deep passion and thoroughness. Kudos!"

—DEBORAH MADISON, author of
Vegetable Literacy and *In My Kitchen*

"If you have ever tried to imagine the most definitive encyclopedia on stocks, sauces, and broths, here it is. *Mastering Stocks and Broths* is wildly practical and comprehensive. Everyone who aspires to see health germinate from their kitchen needs to follow Mamane's lead. I can't imagine a single question unanswered in this marvelous book."

—JOEL SALATIN, Polyface Farm;
author of *You Can Farm*

"Rachael Mamane takes stock making to a whole new level in *Mastering Stocks and Broths*, from making a basic stock to the many ways of thickening and flavoring this fundamental ingredient into delicious sauces, gravies, soups, and stews. This book deserves a place in the kitchen of all serious—and not so serious—cooks."

—SALLY FALLON MORELL, president,
The Weston A. Price Foundation

"Equal parts inspiration and encyclopedia, this fabulous book will be reached for again and again. It truly does contain everything you need to know to let broths and stocks enrich your kitchen with nutrition, flavor, and depth. Mamane's recipes are truly irresistible, and the science and history she weaves throughout add multilayered meanings to the guidance she provides, inviting you on an adventure with each dish she offers."

—JESSICA PRENTICE, author of *Full Moon Feast;*
cofounder, Three Stone Hearth

"It's always been my preference to surround myself with people who are willing to go deep. I'm not really interested in making time for anyone else. By *deep*, I mean people who work and study hard, people who aren't afraid to ask questions, people whose enthusiasm for experimentation never wavers, people who, above all else, are willing to sacrifice for the sweet pleasure of slowly obtained mastery. I especially like to read books written by those people. Rachael Mamane is one of those people. In this remarkable tome, she manages to write about bones and broth and stock on four very different levels at once: the spiritual, the symbolic, the technical, and the practical. Maybe I should throw in the political, too. Read this book. Like Rachael's stocks and broths, it will heal you. It will also bring you into the deep."

—CAMAS DAVIS, butcher; writer;
owner, Portland Meat Collective

MASTERING
STOCKS AND
BROTHS

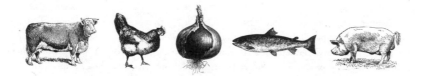

A COMPREHENSIVE CULINARY APPROACH
USING TRADITIONAL TECHNIQUES
AND NO-WASTE METHODS

RACHAEL S. MAMANE

CHELSEA GREEN PUBLISHING
WHITE RIVER JUNCTION, VERMONT

Project Manager: Patricia Stone
Developmental Editor: Makenna Goodman
Copy Editor: Mary Reilly
Proofreader: Laura Jorstad
Indexer: Shana Milkie
Designer: Melissa Jacobson

Printed in the United States of America.
First printing May 2017.
10 9 8 7 6 5 4 3 2 1   17 18 19 20 21

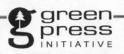

Chelsea Green Publishing is committed to preserving
ancient forests and natural resources. We elected to print
this title on 100-percent postconsumer recycled paper,
processed chlorine-free. As a result, for this printing, we
have saved:

103 Trees (40' tall and 6-8" diameter)
46 Million BTUs of Total Energy
8,840 Pounds of Greenhouse Gases
47,942 Gallons of Wastewater
3,209 Pounds of Solid Waste

Chelsea Green Publishing made this paper choice because
we and our printer, Thomson-Shore, Inc., are members
of the Green Press Initiative, a nonprofit program
dedicated to supporting authors, publishers, and suppliers
in their efforts to reduce their use of fiber obtained
from endangered forests. For more information, visit:
www.greenpressinitiative.org.

Environmental impact estimates were made using the Environmental Defense Paper Calculator.
For more information visit: www.papercalculator.org.

Our Commitment to Green Publishing

Chelsea Green sees publishing as a tool for cultural change and ecological stewardship. We strive to align
our book manufacturing practices with our editorial mission and to reduce the impact of our business
enterprise in the environment. We print our books and catalogs on chlorine-free recycled paper, using
vegetable-based inks whenever possible. This book may cost slightly more because it was printed on paper
that contains recycled fiber, and we hope you'll agree that it's worth it. Chelsea Green is a member of the
Green Press Initiative (www.greenpressinitiative.org), a nonprofit coalition of publishers, manufacturers,
and authors working to protect the world's endangered forests and conserve natural resources. *Mastering
Stocks and Broths* was printed on paper supplied by Thomson-Shore that contains 100% postconsumer
recycled fiber.

Library of Congress Cataloging-in-Publication Data
Names: Mamane, Rachael, 1975– author.
Title: Mastering stocks and broths : a comprehensive culinary approach using
    traditional techniques and no- waste methods / Rachael Mamane.
Description: White River Junction, Vermont : Chelsea Green Publishing, [2017]
    | Includes bibliographical references and index.
Identifiers: LCCN 2016059355| ISBN 9781603586566 (hardcover) | ISBN 9781603586573 (ebook)
Subjects: LCSH: Stocks (Cooking). | Cooking. | LCGFT: Cookbooks.
Classification: LCC TX819.S8 M36 2017 | DDC 641.81/3—dc23
LC record available at https://lccn.loc.gov/2016059355

Chelsea Green Publishing
85 North Main Street, Suite 120
White River Junction, VT 05001
(802) 295-6300
www.chelseagreen.com

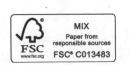

MIX
Paper from
responsible sources
FSC® C013483

*For Ema, who taught me how to cook with affection,
and without words*

CONTENTS

FOREWORD

There is an extraordinary nature to something that is one of a kind, and the allure to uniqueness is undeniable. There are certain qualities that can set our senses in motion unlike anything else—whether it is the sensual experience of eating an oyster or the swirling sensations of deep love. Pleasure from uniqueness engulfs us so much that the determination to rekindle that experience can become an obsession.

At the heart of our lifelong venture to encounter these unique experiences is the recognition of how truly exquisite it can be to experience a genuine, irreplicable moment of time and place. And there may be no better way to engage all the senses in such an experience then through food.

Harvesting food from soil is exactly that: the preservation of a moment. Vegetables that reflect a region, weather, the soil they thrived in; animals that roam freely, subsist on the flora around them, and contain traces of it all in their flesh. There is a beautiful realization when one stops trying to *replicate* a flavor and so experiences authentic *terroir*—the taste of place—through food.

In the food world, uniqueness is a conundrum. Chefs design menus around dishes that aim for the unique, in both flavor and artistic appeal. And yet the success of the restaurant is so often determined upon replication, night after night, dish after dish.

The quest for consistency underpins success in every facet of food and agriculture. Industrialized meat is produced in a manner so that each carcass conforms and is processed exactly like the one that came before it. (Robots are now often used, automating the butchery of our modern meat.) Variation, both in genetics and flavor, is the enemy to the bottom line of high-volume meat processing.

The "ugly" fruit and vegetable movement—saving and using food deemed aesthetically or structurally unacceptable in the conventional marketplace—challenges the need for surface "perfection" in produce and calls into question whether the food's aesthetic perfection even translates to superior flavor. It's no wonder that food waste is a hotbed issue in the culinary world right now. (Rachael Mamane is right: Save the scraps. Make stock.)

The struggle to shape nature for commercial expectations—seeking year-round consistency in availability and systems for producing meat and produce—is manifesting in disastrous ways when it comes to our physical and mental wellbeing. Food sustains us, and if it can't flourish, neither will we. Industrial food systems are not nourishing, regardless of how "much" food is produced.

The dramatic shifts in the food system toward automation, volume, and speed have transpired almost without notice to most of the masses. In meat, tenderness has beat out flavor as the winning characteristic of a wonderful cut. Animals are being slaughtered at younger and younger ages as carcass growth increases by unnatural forces through subtherapeutic antibiotics. Sadly, animal confinement facilitates tenderness in meat; but feedlots and grain-based diets produce a diluted and considerably less dynamic flavor than can come from pasture-based operations. These are the conditions that expedite industrial meat production and provide "melt in your mouth" meats. I'm pro-*chewing*, however. I don't want meat that just melts in my mouth; I want deeply nutritious meat that serves my body well. Research shows that toothsome qualities in meat combined with incredible flavor produce more pleasurable responses in consumers.

Few people realize that the growing conditions that promote tenderness in meat are in complete opposition to those that produce flavor. Flavor is produced during the animal's life (what it eats, how it was raised); tenderness we can deal with during preparation. You can never reverse-engineer flavor into a cut.

Flavor comes from muscles that are active; animals that roam, root, and forage for their food. Animals on pasture eat what's around them, and diversity of flavor comes from diversity in diet. Allowing animals to mature provides opportunities for more compounds to develop in their tissue, equating to a greater flavor profile on our plates. Suddenly you are tasting an expression of the environment that animal lived in.

We celebrate inconsistency in other areas of food. Cheese and wine are two areas in which terroir is exalted. Year to year, the seasons provide shifting weather patterns, and—depending on where the farm is located—soil composition, minerality, and other attributes to the land affect the flavor profile of the products emerging from the farm. We can do this with meat and produce as well. In fact, when we start prioritizing flavor as the top tier quality of food, we will begin unraveling these industrial and commodified structures.

The societal pendulum may continue to swing towards speed, uniformity, and excess, but there are people out there who resist with all their might and offer a new way forward. Rachael Mamane is one of those unique people. She doesn't give a shit about the status quo. She'll show up to a farm slaughter in a black pencil skirt and matching high-heel boots—and still get dirty. She upends odds; she smartly persists; she'll write a book on the most underappreciated ingredient in your kitchen—what for many amounts to just cloudy water—that will make you want to cook the way you live.

That Mamane chose to make stocks her mission won't shock anyone who knows her; she's a connector, happy to be behind-the-scenes. Stocks are the backbone to cuisine, truly a foundational ingredient but one that has been so watered down in recent decades.

The idea of stock is so simple it's beguiling: hot water left to simmer with ingredients that may often end up in a compost pile. Patience is key. As Mamane clearly states throughout this incredible and well-researched tome, applying simple techniques transforms thrift in the kitchen to deliciousness beyond expectation. (Don't worry—those techniques are all laid out exceptionally and with detail.)

This book's layout emulates the role of stocks in a kitchen: foundational skills mastered first; delicious results built upon them later. She reminds us again and again that the potential of a dish is only so great as the quality of the ingredients—a message echoed from kitchens over many generations—and stocks are no different. Quality ingredients come from farms with a holistic view on preservation of resources and restorative management.

Don't be fooled by the title of the first section, "The Basics of Stocks and Broths." The information shared by Mamane here is anything but basic as she delves deep into areas of history and cultural significance of stocks and broths, reminding us that when we cook we share a deep connection with generations past and the origin of cultural cuisines that were built on a concept of resourcefulness and utility. A properly made stock has the power to change the course of one's appreciation for the hidden forces in the world around us. Water, bones, heat, and time.

In times past (and still in some regions of this world left unspoiled by the seduction of modern excesses), bounties were preserved through techniques passed hand-to-hand for generations. Waste was low, and you coaxed the most out of that which was available when it was available. "Waste not, want not" as a motto perished decades ago amidst the rise of "Flaunt more, want more."

I see a new reality on the horizon. Earnest chefs around the world are connecting to form a mesh network with the tensile strength to resist the pressures of industrialized agriculture's doomed promises of a bountiful future. Pastured meats are starting to be recognized for their geographic, genetic, and dietary diversity; produce and livestock seasonality is helping to support local communities and reconnect consumers to the food that sustains them; solutions for looming environmental catastrophes are being found in traditional and regenerative agriculture practices.

Mastering Stocks and Broths calls for us to aspire towards *succulence*. Indeed, our greatest food memories will be rooted in delicious flavor. This book is a cookbook, a manifesto, and a deeply practical guide for maximizing memory potential in every dish you make. And once we, as a nation, begin to recognize and demand extraordinary flavor in our food, we will, quite literally, change the modern world.

—**ADAM DANFORTH**, butcher; author of
Butchering Poultry, Rabbit, Lamb, Goat, and Pork

FAMILIAL STOCK: MY FOUNDATION

A ripple in the Sephardic Jewish community came to my attention over a recent meal with my aunt and uncle. The food was simple—an array of prepared salads and fresh fish—while the meal was significant. I was there to celebrate their blissful retirement—a graduation from long-held service to worldwide adventure, the spark in their eyes vibrant with possibility. Our plan was to daydream about the future over a homemade meal—glasses clinking and forks scraping, an audible invitation to relax and reconnect.

Reunions in my family are rare, and yet the celebration of food is constant. Taking cue from tradition, seven salads were served situated around the table, glistening with ingredients that spoke of the Mediterranean. We carried custom from heritage—gingerly nibbling from small plates of eggplant, peppers, olives, and more, a signature welcome for an honored guest—while threading bites with inquisitive dialogue. "Where will you travel? Ooh, is this the salad your mother used to make?" This tactic at once succeeds in evoking distant memories—flavors meld to remind us of the past while conversation firmly roots us in the present. It is true: The only family discussions I remember, vividly and in color, are the ones that took place around the dining room table.

It came as no surprise when the conversation shifted from them to me. Just as we sample from plate to plate, so does the focus move from person to person. What did amaze was the shift from familial to cultural inquiry; no longer were the questions about my business, my relationships, or the city I called home. Rather, my uncle delivered the twist in the form of an invitation: Would I be interested in dual citizenship with Spain? As if inviting me to fully embrace their retirement, I came to learn that Spain was offering automatic citizenship to descendants of Jews who were exiled in 1492, and my name was on a list.

———

Some of my earliest childhood memories include walking into my grandmother's foreign kitchen and taking in rich smells that spoke of her spending days behind the stove. My family would travel from America to Israel to visit with our larger family abroad, and it was these trips that spawned curiosity about my heritage and shaped my interest in food, poorly at first. It would be a long time before my relationship with diet was about sustenance over comfort, efficiency over excess.

I was a plump child, and my grandmother knew I had a thing for fast food. She would emulate America in her modest home, welcoming me to her foreign land with bottomless batches of homemade french fries, placating my misguided adoration of McDonald's. In her home, it was familial love that turned a blind eye to my unhealthy diet, and there that I could accept myself as she accepted me. I slept on a small cot on the porch, fat and happy, and felt the richest of children, surrounded by the affection of distant relatives.

I remember the irregular placement of ingredients strewn about her kitchen. And the background conversation, spoken in English so she wouldn't understand: "She leaves those things out? Doesn't she throw *anything* away?" My father would explain without detail that butter and eggs were kept at room temperature in his culture, and little went unused in her kitchen. It wasn't until years later that terms like *mise en place* came into my lexicon and an education about *smen*, the pungent aged butter of Morocco: a level of organization beyond adolescent comprehension and a smell entirely off-putting to a child's nose. These moments were the seed of my interest in slow cooking.

My father has deep childhood memories associated with food. He left Morocco at an early age and seemed only to look back with longing when reminiscing about its distinctive cuisine. It came as a surprise to him, my chasing his heritage through an understanding of gastronomy. After all, my grandmother and I didn't speak the same language; the innate connection was a curious one. But even now, I can call him to speak of *brik* or *b'stilla*—cuisine acting as a cultural bridge—and hear in his voice the warm recollection of his youth.

I know now that my drive to learn about nutrition and nourishment comes from this feeling of being disconnected from family. An endless education about food fills in the cracks created by time and distance: I have become a passionate home cook with deep nostalgia for a lost heritage, and my hunger for connection has prompted the development of a rich community. This search has led to meaningful introductions of like-minded folks—a global family of professional chefs and food lovers who are on a similar journey, those who share a desire to revive past generations through culinary celebration. What used to be an unhealthy excuse to eat in excess has become an obsession about efficiency, an endeavor to make more with less, perhaps as a way to welcome additional people to the table. Deconstructing a recipe links me to tradition, and feeding those around me makes them feel like kinfolk.

Since learning about Spain's apology to my ancestors, I realize that a personal reconciliation awaits me: a life spent searching for family, wading through murky details, assigning meaning through the connectedness of food, and arriving full circle. I am now the recipient of an invitation to make a home where my grandmother was born. Stocks, like heritage, are at the core—bones, a literal translation of a solid foundation.

ACKNOWLEDGMENTS

Laughter. This would be my response had anyone told me that a brief conversation on the subway would turn into a six-year-long adventure, untethered from corporate structure and in pursuit of social entrepreneurship. That my tiny bouillon business would culminate in the written word. Or that the people in my life would be immeasurably supportive of this wild journey. This book is the reflection of friends and family, colleagues and community. Without them, it would not be possible.

At the core of my appreciation for food is my grandmother. Is it silly to believe her spirit speaks to me from the pot? Perhaps so, and yet it was in her actions that I see my own—an innate comprehension that feeding the ones around us also feeds our souls.

Family, at times, confounds—I'm the baby, after all. And yet not even geographic distance interferes with their endless support of my unscripted lifestyle. My father, too, teaches through action: His commitment to kin and ancestry was instilled at an early age, the oldest of many siblings, now apparent in the way he takes care of his own. (My father is also the first person to have eaten bone marrow in front of me. I thought it was gross at the time.) My mother showed me, also through influence, how to lean into the unknown; to embrace life as it comes.

Jim, my companion and best friend, witnessed the everyday details. To watch me write a book while lifting a principled business, and all the ups and downs that go with it, is perhaps the most noble of actions. It is with immense satisfaction (and a little surprise) that he is still here, by my side. He is my rock.

Whether by fate or chance, I am honored to call Ben Giardullo a business partner. There is no one like him: His brain calculates at an incredible speed and his actions inspire the people around him. He sees what is possible where others see barriers. In a few short years, I have watched him grow multiple businesses, all with a social mission intact, while also growing himself and a family. His belief in Brooklyn Bouillon endures; he will be at the center of its success.

The day my editor Makenna Goodman reached out is the day a new world revealed itself. We became pen pals for a year before a contract was official. In this time, she revealed herself to be a true champion for the book, the publisher, and me. Her approach to the trade is objective, intelligent, and reliable, while her demeanor is warm, merciful, and affable. She inspired the book to life and walked me through the process with absolute grace. My gratitude extends to Fern Bradley, who fielded moments of doubt with kindness and patience, as well as the entirety of Chelsea Green Publishing, whose vision for a better food system aligns with my own. I couldn't ask for a better publisher.

Now like an older, wiser sister, Holley Atkinson adopted me early upon my entry to New York City. She is a magnet to many in the food systems community, and I am lucky to have her in my life. All will agree: Holley is genuine, generous, and so much fun to be around. Her review of the book was as influential as it was efficient. She is a true powerhouse.

There are many chefs, butchers, and cooks to thank, too. Kate Hill, *maman* to butchers across the globe, is always available to answer questions. She acts on her belief that word-of-mouth dialogue preserves knowledge across generations. More than just one of the girls, Maurine Jernigan Fischel is a fierce business-woman and a passionate cook whose love for food and culture has led to an adventurous life; we encourage our respective escapades (and delicious indulgences) from afar. Camas Davis and Cathy Barrow, authors who share interest in building community around the table, provided encouragement and tips along the way. My appreciation goes further to all the women in Grrls Meat Camp, an international collective of empowered women in the meat industry.

When I first expressed my desire to participate in a harvest, Adam Danforth did not hesitate to include me. His education about humane butchery still informs my approach to buying and consuming meat. Bryan Mayer, too, has shared his dedication to the trade. Both are butchers who teach by example and whose humanity for all beings is apparent in their work.

Farmers have also been supportive of this process. Jonathan White of Bobolink Dairy is to thank for his quick-draw scientific knowledge; Andrew Chiappinelli of Grazin' guided me through a tough ethical decision. Lee and Georgia Ranney of Kinderhook Farms were incredibly gracious when the business was finding its place. Without their dedication to responsible farming and land management, Brooklyn Bouillon would not exist.

Jesse Hirsch, notable journalist, offered a grounded perspective on the writing experience. Hank Shaw, author and educator, made sense of the publishing industry. Kelsey Kinser, chef and friend, was always around to field frustrations and laugh about the details. Michael Lashutka, a top-notch home cook, and Felipe Ribeiro, a writer whose voice is strong, offered incredible feedback and a safe place for the final push. Jessica and Joelle, who shared a kitchen in the valley, always knew when it was time to take a beer break. And, last but not least, my Butcher Bears were never short of wit and charm; a source of comedic relief for the thrust toward completion.

As a small business owner, I am always amazed when formal organizations show their support. These associations include Stone Barns Center for Food and Agriculture, GRACE Communications Foundation, The Livestock Conservancy, and Monterey Bay Aquarium. Over the course of three summers, Stewardship Farms actively shared my vision for minimizing waste, and Mount Tremper Arts provided artistic sanctuary from proposal to completion.

Combined, these are the ingredients that make a solid foundation. I am forever grateful.

INTRODUCTION

Indeed, stock is everything in cooking. Without it, nothing can be done. If one's stock is good, what remains of the work is easy; if, on the other hand, it is bad or merely mediocre, it is quite hopeless to expect anything approaching a satisfactory meal.

—Auguste Escoffier, *The Escoffier Cookbook and Guide to the Fine Art of Cookery*

It seems the culinary start for many passionate cooks has origins with a grandmother. Perhaps it's the trigger of comfort associated with compelling smells that waft from a kitchen, knowing that a provider of nourishment resides within. For many, as with myself, it is the indirect influence of this maternal constancy that lands us in a kitchen; a profession that chooses us without regard for institutional education. The kitchen is one of the few places where patience comes with ease—despite shortened fingernails (an early lesson with chef knives!)—and it is within this discipline that trial and error serves as a syllabus. Patience is also a knowing guide when breaking down a recipe to its base elements—finding appreciation not only on the palate but also from its pedigree.

Today the requisite need for formal culinary training is in question: The industry is ripe with talent driven by commitment and passion to the trade, and yet the long hours and low pay are forcing many cooks out of the kitchen. Amidst economic decline and corporate greed in the early part of this century, many young professionals—in Brooklyn, NY, and other burgeoning urban food hubs around the country—decided to abandon their formal careers and embrace artisanal trade. These chefs and purveyors are pioneers of local industry; they understand the value of small farmers and are paving the path for emerging artisans across the country.

As far as my education in the culinary world goes, I am not a studied chef in the traditional sense. I took the course of a liberal arts degree and focused on the sciences, though it soon became apparent that my passion is in food—everything about it—from how it grows to how it is distributed, how it lands on the plate, and how it appeals to all senses. On the heels of finishing pre-med requirements,

I turned my first apartment into a laboratory for making chocolate—windows sealed, humidity identified, thermostat adjusted—my tiny galley kitchen replete with a salvaged marble slab. This was perhaps not the medical career my father was hoping for.

Though the true test and testimony to my dedication to the culinary arts was when I went in search of an entire baby lamb many years after graduation. The purpose of this exercise was to gain insight into the life of a small farmer and to learn how to break down an animal in my home kitchen. Curiously, the idea of hosting a dinner party with the bounty was an afterthought. It was also a seminal text—*The French Laundry Cookbook* by Thomas Keller—that solidified my interest in exploring a deeper, more technical relationship with food. Why? Well, Chef Keller teaches by example. His ability to be mindful about source and playful with ingredients, writing for an audience at large, stands as a reason for his influence on professional and home cooks in America over the past two decades.

Keller's recipe for a degustation of baby lamb was one of the first I followed as a narrative. First, he said, locate a farmer who will sell you the whole animal. And so I did, with comedic ignorance, inquiring of my favorite farmer, George Page of Sea Breeze Farm on Vashon Island, WA, with no regard for when lambs were harvested or how they were butchered. "Isn't a lamb already a baby?" I asked. The definition of *lamb*, after all, is "young sheep"; it was curious to me that chefs at the time were in search of ever-younger animals. (This trend is changing in some circles; humane butchers are now advocating appreciation for older animals.) As it turns out, a baby lamb refers to the meat of a sheep that is six to ten weeks old, whereas spring lamb is from a sheep from five to six months of age. Luckily, George saw my spirited request as an encouraging sign of a healing customer base, and he accommodated in his requisite salty manner—three months later, we transferred a partially butchered lamb—older than baby and younger than spring—from the back of his pickup and into my car in the back alley of Seattle's Pike Place Market.

Following Chef Keller's recipe from source to plate was the beginning of my education in whole animal cooking and how I discovered the importance of stocks. I found immense satisfaction in deconstructing an animal into its parts; cooking each part in a way that correlated to how the live animal used its anatomy; and patiently making use of the entire animal until all parts were presented for consumption. In his recipe, nothing went to waste. While I spent more money on a whole lamb than I did for a month of groceries, the lamb provided nourishment for much longer.

After my dish was presented—pressed breast acting as base to saddle, rack, and leg; seared kidney teetering on top and the sauce as paint on plate—tidbits of the animal still remained. The additional *farce* was transformed into *merguez*; the remaining meat into *rillettes*. The bones were used first for a quick sauce, and then for a lengthier classic stock.

A greater misnomer in culinary terminology might not exist than when describing the quickness in making this "quick" sauce. A quick sauce builds on existing stocks, usually chicken and veal, and relies on roasting bones and vegetables to bring out flavor, followed by iterative deglazing, reduction, and clarification. The dumbing down of its name is intended to distinguish a sauce, made in small batches on the same day, from a classic stock, made in big batches over several days and reserved for future use. It takes several hours of simmering alone to arrive at the first extraction and multiple rounds of straining to achieve a sauce without particles.[1] To the home cook, this method hardly qualifies as expeditious. But to a passionate and patient one it can be the beginning of a love affair with process, with tradition, and perhaps most importantly, with flavor.

The first time I made a quick sauce, the name duped me into placing it on my prep list almost too late for the intended guests. As it simmered, slowly, methodically, and unaware of my intimidation, I felt regret that this first exercise in degustation was not entirely successful, as though Chef Keller was chiding me in my imaginary professional kitchen, "What is a degustation without the sauce?" And then I remembered an important lesson taught to me by my father: Before any meal you serve, and especially those you might find stressful, stop half an hour before guests arrive, pour yourself a glass of wine, and remember: *It's just food*. Julia Child would at once be proud and appalled.

A Conversation Between Omnivores and Vegetarians

And let's not forget about vegetables! My ethos about using the whole of every-thing extends beyond the animal and well into alliums, nightshades, and really, almost anything green and edible.

Young and self-righteous, waiting for food to arrive to the dinner table, I was fourteen when I declared myself a vegetarian. For years, I wore this decision as a badge of honor; it was taking a stand for the animals and against factory farming, all of which was an act of rebellion in the eyes of my meat-loving family. And for years my father was in denial. A brief return home from college would always be met with my favorite childhood dish—an intensely yellow chicken stew built with bright, bold spices (see Seared Moroccan Chicken, page 172, for

Grass is, in fact, the base layer of the global food system. It continually converts massive quantities of solar energy into food for grazing animals. Grasses and herbivores, working together, are the indispensable intermediaries between humans and the energy of the sun.[2]

—NICOLETTE HAHN NIMAN, *Defending Beef: The Case for Sustainable Meat Production*

a recipe adaptation)—simmering on the stove. But I refused to eat it, much to my father's dismay.

Yes, I was staunch, and remained dedicated for over a decade. It wasn't until my mid-twenties when an athletic boyfriend influenced a change of heart. An expert rock climber, Vance taught me how to eat for fuel: We would meet in Seattle on Friday nights and drive six hours north to Squamish in British Columbia or six hours south to Smith Rock in Oregon, a near-weekly quest for physical adventure. Two seasons of this lifestyle, amidst a poorly planned vegetarian diet, and my body started craving meat.

Still, to this day, my diet is mostly plant-based. My belief system has not wavered, only transformed into an education about eating meat mindfully. And perhaps now more than ever, my perspective aligns with a collective of individual choices; together we must stand to influence a misguided industrial agricultural system. It seems omnivores and vegetarians are sitting at the same table, with a clearer vision of shared values—a common belief that responsible stewardship of land and animal is the right step toward an improved food system.

A few years ago, butcher Adam Danforth, now the recipient of a James Beard award for his manuals on humane butchering, invited me to join him and a few novice friends to harvest goats at a farm in the Hudson Valley. We knew each other from the bustling food scene in New York City: Adam took an early interest in my company, Brooklyn Bouillon, and was always available for questions about his trade. He was conducting research for his first book and offered the day as an introduction to slaughter—guiding the experience through his holistic narrative. Upon arriving to the farm and meeting the animals, Adam gave us an overview of procedure and outlined the importance of a "clean kill." He advised us to let our bodies respond to the experience without suppressing emotion. This was an important consideration when deciding which role to accept: We learned that presence of mind is key when slaughtering an animal in a humane way. The moment of death happens when skill is applied to minimize discomfort and make certain use of an animal's life.

Among those in attendance was Adam's doula for his firstborn child. She was a magical presence—mindful in her actions and visibly moved by the experience. The beginning of life is at the core of her work, and she wanted to understand purposeful death in the rawness that slaughter demands. I was impressed by her bravery, an active participant in conduct that was contrary to her profession. She sat on the sidelines as we applied bolt gun to head and knife to throat, and just as I was stunned into teary-eyed submission from my participation, she stepped in to assist with the remainder of the procedure.

My first harvest hit me hard. It was in Adam's humane guidance, his doula's perspective on the cycle of life, and my desire for education that I was given a holistic view into animal welfare. This process has since guided me in the way I buy and consume meat.

There is deep satisfaction in using the whole of everything, whether animal or vegetable. My first degustation and subsequently my first harvest taught me how to see value in the entire animal—how it is raised, harvested, prepared, and consumed. Working with all parts of the animal is an education in both anatomy and cooking. And through this experience I have gained a lens into the value of other ingredients. Now when I pick up a carrot, greens attached, I think, "What can I do with the carrot tops?" It is an innate appreciation for the whole that a farmer, butcher, and cook adopts as a holistic practitioner of food.

Today's responsible ranchers and butchers are crying out: "Eat less meat, eat better meat!"[3] Our mixed vegetable farmers are expanding the variety of their starts and finding more homes for "ugly" produce. Our butchers are encouraging us to buy lesser-used parts of the animal. And our chefs are teaching us how to cook the funky bits, the ugly chunks, and all parts in between.

My Business Brewing Bouillon

On the professional spectrum, I reside on the periphery of industry—I am neither a butcher nor a chef. I do not spend my days breaking down animals nor do I find myself in the weeds at a restaurant, toiling over a stove at the customer's request. Mostly I am a passionate home cook who cares about where my vegetables are grown, how the animals I eat are raised, and how the land is respected; particularly with a focus on the economy of making more out of less. For six years now, my little Jetta has taken me from farm to farm in search of bones and potentially wasted food, an ever-expanding exploration of how one person might support a healing industry.

Brooklyn Bouillon, my little, yet loud, stock company, came about on the subway. On the dreaded G train, I was riding home with a vegetarian friend after a tiring day of selling duck at Greenmarkets. "Hey, Jonathan, I have another idea." He had heard many before, having spent ten days with me on the road from Seattle to Brooklyn, where much of our traveling dialogue was about how our lives would be different in the city. "You might not like it. It has to do with meat . . . but the good kind." I told him what a farmer had told me about bones: that the cost of getting them from processor to farm to market and back again outweighed their current value; that many of them ended up in the incinerator. "What about using them for stock?" Instead of dismissive laughter or an explanation of his beliefs, Jonathan simply nodded approval, giggled, and said, "You could call it Brooklyn Bouillon." It was a half joke about all the attention the borough was getting for its emerging artisan culture. And, yet, it stuck.

We had arrived to the city only a few weeks prior and were settling into a new life. For me, it was a big change—I was consulting to Fortune 500s and tech start-ups while searching for a professional home within food systems. My decline in pay grade was steep, despite the hike in cost of living in New York. I begrudgingly called it "New York Math"—recognition that the move was about passion over profit, as many starving artists had done before us. I sat down and did some basic projections, preparing for my next discussion with a farmer friend, a self-made man who happened to know a thing or two about the world of finance.

Whether it was my spirited approach, or simply that I was willing to fund the pilot, Dan Gibson of Grazin' Angus Acres gave me a chance. I inquired with certifying agencies about the legitimacy of working with bones from small livestock farmers and received many confused responses. Some had asked before but no one had ever done it to scale. All I knew was that I had to start with USDA-certified bones. Dan's operation is the model by which farmers are inspired to continue farming: With a deep commitment to land and animal welfare, he offered an education with every exceptional cut, and consumers would come from afar to pay him well for his efforts. His short ribs were served at Chelsea Clinton's wedding![4] And his bones, yes, they were certified.

So, now I had bones. The next challenge was finding a commercial kitchen with an hourly rate that wouldn't negate the margin. Until recently, the classic incubator model was designed for caterers and pickle producers, not makers of long-simmering stocks. This step made me realize that producing demi-glace—a low-yielding reduction that takes days to produce—was out of the question. I would forge ahead with an abbreviated line of stocks, intended to highlight the significance of responsible farming and butchery.

A constant supply of Animal Welfare Approved beef bones would place Grass-Fed Beef Stock as our primary offering; supplemented with a three-season production of Pastured Chicken Stock; and highlighted by a Farm-Fresh

Vegetable Stock, featuring aromatics from a neighboring organic farm. The Sustainable Fish Fumet would come later, after the emergence of Community Supported Fisheries across the city.[5] No matter how many inspectors had to be convinced, I was adamant about placing the name of the farm on every label. Produced in small batches, the stock could then be sold by the farmer, a kind of double value-add from the source.

Next came getting the word out. In the beginning, many chefs—accustomed to making their own stocks—laughed at me; those who didn't, inquired about batch size. Farmers were skeptical at first, wondering if the consumer would ever find value in bones. Retailers were excited to make room on their freezer shelves; they knew broth in a box wasn't the real thing. Even techies showed interest, suggesting the category was ripe for disruption. Within three months of launching a website, I was approached by consumers and producers from five out of seven USDA regions, asking how I was doing it and whether or not it could be replicated elsewhere.

So focused on mission, rarely did anyone ask about flavor. It was as if the language of our grandmothers was distilled into one certainty: A healthy animal from good land and a fresh vegetable plucked from rich soil—looked after with care in the pot—will result in a delicious essence. There was not much marketing effort required. It was when Daniel Boulud's sommelier approached me for a sample that I knew this tiny business had a future. Little did I know the difficulties ahead: that much of our purpose would be in developing regional infrastructure, or that I would become a country girl.

Agribusiness in New York's Hudson Valley

From a market perspective, Brooklyn Bouillon arrived to the city five years too early and to the Hudson Valley three years too soon. When we launched in 2010, consumers were becoming aware of food waste and chefs were beginning to embrace nutrient-dense foods. The association of food and technology was emerging as a stand-alone industry, attracting financiers who were shifting attention from bytes to bites. Farmers and butchers were being hailed as rock stars of the industry.

Early attention to Brooklyn Bouillon came from organizations such as Slow Food and Slow Money, and while the numbers looked good on paper, there wasn't enough urban infrastructure to support the endeavor. Demand was enormous, and not only from within the city—support poured in from all over the country despite our commitment to remain local.

THE LIFE OF BONES

Bones, a symbol of strength and a mark of permanence, harness an interesting place in history. In prehistoric times, bones were formed to make tools and weapons, such as shovels, axes, and knives. Bones acted as building material, used alongside hide, stone, metal, and clay; they were also considered a fuel source.[6] A popular art medium, bone carvings were featured in religious ceremonies and fashioned into adornments. The oldest known instrument is the bone flute: Three of the earliest varieties were discovered in a European cave, made from the wing bones of a vulture and a mute swan and ivory from the woolly mammoth.[7]

In ancient China a writing system was applied to bones, called *oracle bones*, used for divination purposes.[8] "Will it rain?" asks a king. "Will there be misfortune?" pleads another. To this day, prophecy is found in the wishbones of fowl—from chicken to wild turkey—a tradition that started with the Etruscans, to be adopted by the Romans, and learned by the English.[9]

The Maori people once turned whale bones into fishing hooks, called *hei matau*—some functional for catching fish, others treasured as family heirlooms—and now rely on cattle bones to continue the practice. *Scrimshaw* refers to tools and art also made from the bone of whales; detailed engravings performed by sailors who were unable to work when the seas did not cooperate.[10] The International Convention on Whaling has put a stop to these practices in their traditional form.

Of particular significance to this text is the use of bones in medicine. A symbol of Chinese culture, dating back to 100 CE, fossils of dead animals, called *dragon bones*, were combined with oyster shells for a sedative effect, intended to "settle uprising yang."[11] Many centuries later, osteopathy was founded on the belief that health is related to strength of the musculoskeletal system; bone broth is often prescribed to inhibit infection and reduce joint pain.

Over the ages, bones have formed the little things, too—like needles, buttons, and beads, as well as playthings, like dice and poker chips. It seems the symbolism of bones withstands the test of time: Skulls still adorn walls, a show of strength and valor.

But what happens to the animal bones of modern-day farmers and fisherman?

Here is a glimpse into the world of food safety: After an animal is processed, bones are often sent to be rendered into inedible products. Other certified methods of removal are burial, incineration, composting, anaerobic digestion, and exotic animal feeding.[12] While some of these methods are worthwhile, disposal is the last stop for bones; there are other uses, too, including pet food and fertilizer.

One step shy of incineration, *bone char* is the product of burning cow bones in a low-oxygen vessel to produce activated carbon. A method widely used in the States in the 1940s and still employed in developing countries around the world, the tricalcium phosphate found in bone char removes fluoride and metal ions from water.[13] Until recently, bone char was used to remove color in the refinement of sugar, though associated costs and social concerns have impacted the method: It now relies on activated carbon or ion-exchange resins to achieve the same effect. Black pigment for artistic applications is also a product of bone char. The pigment called *ivory black*, once made with ivory and now a synonym for *bone black*, can be seen in the works of, say, Rembrandt and Picasso. *Dippel's Oil*, the organic material that developed from melting bones, was used as chemical warfare during World War II. This oil made water from enemy wells undrinkable—an attack made acceptable by Geneva Protocol because it was not lethal.[14]

Although most uses of bone char are now out of practice, some regenerative farmers are producing biochar from bones as an ingredient for fertilizer. Rancher Mike Callicrate worked with a retort manufacturer to develop a system that renders biochar from bones instead of wood; it is rich in phosphorous and calcium and adds carbon to the soil. The end product is ground and sold in buckets to be blended with compost and other nutrient-rich organic materials from the farm.[15] Below is the compositional data on a bag of Callicrate Cattle Co. Bone Char:

CALLICRATE CATTLE CO.
Bone-Char Bag

35.87% – Phosphorous
33.17% – Calcium
00.86% – Potassium
00.77% – Iodium
00.75% – Sulfur
00.71% – Magnesium
00.30% – Nitrogen

The counter to bone char is *bone ash*, a white powder achieved by calcifying bones to maintain cellular structure. Bone ash is also used as a fertilizer; however, the color variation affords it other applications. Bone ash is accountable for about half the raw material in *bone china*—stark white porcelain largely produced in the United Kingdom.[16] With a high thermal stability, bone ash also acts as a powder coating for metal equipment and as molding around furnace floors.

Bones charred for fuel have recently made an appearance in high-end restaurants around the country. Dan Barber, renowned chef of Blue Hill and Blue Hill at Stone Barns, features dishes grilled on charcoal made from the bones of livestock and shells from shellfish. The ash from this process has even been used on aged cheese. One journalist quips about the phenomenon:

> *Interestingly, unlike other initiatives that return chefs to the land, there's no real historical precedent for the burning of animal bones for the sake of cooking. In North America, the Aleut and Tlingit tribes both used bones and tallow for heating when wood was scarce; New York City's earliest days saw oyster shells being burnt to produce lime; and in the 1830s, the U.S. adopted a French technique of using crushed, pyrolyzed animal skeletons to refine sugar, which became the industry standard. But apparently, nobody had the notion to, say, grill pork over its own carbonized bones.*[17]

Other applications are more readily known, including *bone meal* made from ground bones and *gelatin* rendered from collagen-rich bones, both of which have a unique list of applications. Instructions on how to produce bone charcoal, bone meal, and gelatin in a home kitchen are included in this book (see "Recipes Using Spent Bones," page 352).

INTRODUCTION

Any investor worth his weight in bones will tell you that infrastructure comes before fulfillment. Sure, it makes sense now, but at the time, I figured Brooklyn Bouillon was just a project. So I plugged along, working twenty-two hour shifts in an incubator kitchen and managing distribution on my own. With very little working capital, I had no means to pay for an assistant, and I refused to take on an intern without an ability to provide fair compensation. Very quickly, demand exceeded my ability to supply—both an honor to bear and a terrible reality to face. Customers who believed in the power of bone broth would bring me before and after pictures to illustrate the visibility of their skin improvements. When we would sell out, I would offer tips to disheartened customers on how to make small batches at home. It was satisfying saying yes to small shops and no to big retailers, and yet frustrating to turn down opportunity for growth.

Back then I didn't have the vocabulary to approach investors or the will to ask for funds from a crowd. Instead, I sought an executive position with a food-tech company, relying on the risk of return for the potential to grow my brand. On call 24/7, at the whim of a ruthless CEO and his demanding clients, I was often called in at all hours of the night to troubleshoot a problem. This approach lasted the whole of a year: Our tireless efforts helped effect the company's acquisition, and I was shown the door at the last hour, effectively losing my share in the company. For a split second, my financial value would have clocked in over a half million dollars, enough to kick-start Brooklyn Bouillon and then some.

It was around this time that a land investor directed my attention to the Hudson Valley. The valley brought to a city girl's mind images of rolling hills dotted with hay bales, apple picking in fall, and swimming holes kept secret by locals. I had only ever visited to gather bones from farmers, knowing little of the culture that existed from tiny town to tinier township along the Hudson River. And yet, abject from rejection and depleted of funds, the idea of being closer to farm partners while saving on rent seemed sound for both the business and me.

At the same time, we were receiving high-profile attention from reputable media outlets. A brief but personal exchange with Florence Fabricant led to a shout-out in a Valentine's Day issue of the *New York Times*. Photographers started showing up at my loft to document the process, and bloggers across the city were hailing the product. The most significant show of support, however, came from Liza de Guia, a powerhouse filmmaker with a penchant for story-telling, when she offered to produce a documentary for her *Food Curated* series. To this day, the acknowledgment we receive from this grassroots endeavor is generous; her expansive audience, mostly home cooks and fellow artisans, is genuinely interested in the stories of farmers, chefs, and producers. It seemed an odd time to move amidst all the accolades, and yet in hindsight, our start in the city helped secure the brand, and it was time to transition to the valley in search of infrastructure.

Despite the beauty of the Hudson Valley, living there requires a hardy constitution. Winters are often bitter and long; snow blankets farmland while townships tuck in for the season. Near the end of my first Hudson Valley winter, when friends on the West Coast started acknowledging signs of spring, I was shivering at home—unprepared for the cost of heating, the valley still cold and quiet. And yet spring and summer and fall in the valley are glorious, the legends of vibrant green rolling hills, plentiful orchards, and secret swimming holes all true!

The economy of the valley is as strict as its seasons, and it leans on the big city for support. Sort of an unwritten contract: The valley brings the best of its bounty as long as city-goers pay a good price. It's not uncommon to see a dearth of, say, foraged ramps at upriver markets at a time when they run rampant throughout the city. And it was here, in the small town of Hudson, where I hoped to grow a business built on principle and with limited resources.

I arrived to the valley with dreams of going big—owning a facility that would attract more farmers and make use of their excess harvests. With the move came an introduction to Benjamin Giardullo, the financial brain of our operation. Looking at what I had cobbled together, Ben developed projection after projection and together we identified rebound strategies. And while we were doing this, the consumer value of quality bones tripled, almost overnight, as bone broths started getting national attention. With each price hike in our supply, Ben went back to the financial drawing board.

Over the course of our research, we discovered that bones mostly stop at the slaughterhouse with the prime pieces continuing on with the farmer. As with any commodity, the increased demand for bones gave farmers a reason to haul them to market and a motive for processors to further their product offerings. The market was catching on to what we knew all along—that a scalable category for higher-quality stocks existed—and what a relief! It meant the people who cared for the animal could now acknowledge its full value; that the prime cuts were no longer all that mattered—and gave us room to think on a larger scale.

As a value-added producer, we were forced to question our relevance. With our commitment to farmers and the land, as well as a desire to stay local, the

The United Nations estimates 600 million tons of food is wasted every year—after harvest, during processing and distribution—*before* it reaches consumers.[18]

trend appeared to be great for regional farmers and bad for the small-batch stock business. The value of bones, direct from the farmer, quadrupled in as many years. Our initial value peaked in marketing overreach: The brand helped guide home cooks to freezer shelves in search of a better product, even if our product wasn't there in large supply. Consumer choice demanded transparency and big brands, once trusted, were experiencing a decline in sales. And while those farmers, processors, butchers, and chefs were making use of the basic infrastructure we were after, the search convinced us that a need for regional infrastructure still exists on a larger scale. The reason goes beyond stocks.

It turns out that spent bones and produce seconds have many uses outside the kitchen. We developed a way to make multiple products out of one batch of materials—a bone factory of sorts—all ending in compostable bone char. With a regional facility, we will be able to honor farm requests for participation while maintaining a commitment to the home cook.

Some days it feels as though Brooklyn Bouillon has accepted Sally Fallon Morell's charge of creating a *"brothal* in every town,"[19] at least for my area. Our social intention is to be part of a larger conversation about wasted food; our goal is to continue innovating ways to extend a harvest that will feed more people. It might take another five years, or the work of a lifetime, but the present tastes delicious and the future looks bright.

This Book's Intention

In recent times, my culinary library has become increasingly populated with titles that work in favor of my gut. Books that have succeeded in turning *fat* and *fermentation*—topics once taboo or misunderstood—into popular interest for home cooks. This wasn't a conscious effort. Somehow fat has become sexy and alluring; fermentation, a geek's endeavor on par with what home brewing was a couple of decades past. As a culture that once feared the egg on account of high cholesterol, we now celebrate it as a virtuous staple in the kitchen—one versatile ingredient that boasts quality protein, good fats, and all nine essential amino acids. Collectively these books guide us on healthy pleasures: responsible hedonism at its finest.

Similarly, the intention of this book is to align culinary stocks and nutritive broths with this health-driven theme—from the no-waste perspective of a farmer, who springs food from soil; a butcher, who appreciates the whole animal; and a chef, who treats ingredients as a holistic and artistic medium. More than a century of research and development informs us that stocks are venerable ingredients and broths are good for the soul. Therefore, in this book, I offer information on the practical benefits of animal and vegetable stocks alongside detailed methodology on how to develop, store, and use them in your home kitchen. The completed dishes begin with the foundation of an origin stock and place a playful emphasis on the importance of zero waste. Measurements for larger batches of stocks are also included for the chef who wants to introduce a *saucier* to his format or for the ambitious home cook who has freezer space to spare.

This book goes beyond making stock from the carcass of a store-bought roast chicken; rather, it appeals to the serious home cook who sources carefully and lets nothing go to waste.

Use this book when you find yourself wondering about practical kitchen matters—what to do with a stockpile of bones in your freezer or how to make vegetables go further—or if you are intrigued by culinary curiosities, such as what glue and Jell-O have in common, or how veal was once prepared in the medieval style of sturgeon.

A good stock takes time. This is part of the pleasure—simmering one is meditative and meaningful, if you allow yourself the occasion. Building a stock often happens in the background of most kitchens—a smell that permeates a residence, a gentle warmth that emits from the pot. My hope is that you use this book as inspiration to start from scratch, to find relaxation in the kitchen, to nourish your bones, and to connect with loved ones over good home cooking.

How to Use This Book

This book is divided into two parts: The first part is a narrative that explores the definition, history, nutrition, and science of stocks and broths; the second part is a practical guide to producing and using culinary stocks and nutritive broths. Read the first section if you are intrigued by how food history and nutritional research inform modern-day food and farming infrastructure. You will learn about the best regenerative practices for land animals, sea creatures, and ground plants. Consult the second part when you are ready to cook.

The recipes in this book all begin with a good foundation; from a splash of stock to develop flavor in the pan to the infusion of meat, vegetables, and aromatics for a satisfying broth. The practical part of this book encourages you to think like a butcher and act like a chef. Meat dishes often employ uncommon parts of an animal, such as veal sweetbreads or beef heart; vegetables are highlighted as main ingredients, sometimes cut to effect a toothsome quality usually found in meat. While some of the dishes come together quickly, most require patience. It is my belief that a cook who has time for a proper stock will also have the fortitude for slow cookery.

Vegetable stocks also create a stellar and often unique foundation. This book uses the essential basis of stock making to explore flavor extraction in vegetables—starting with type and extending into variety and application. For instance, you'll find an entire section on tomatoes—stocks made from red, green, and heirloom varieties, another transformed by roasting tomatoes over fire. The same approach is applied to onions, garlic, squash, and other produce. The idea here is vegetables—and the soil from which they emerge—deserve the same honor and respect as animals.

In addition to the basics of stocks and broths, the recipes herein endeavor to reduce waste in a home kitchen. Fats rendered and reserved from a stock appear throughout the text, and ingredients often discarded in contemporary recipes are given purpose. In those instances when an ingredient doesn't fit into a recipe, you will find tips on how to make use of it elsewhere. And please don't throw away spent bones! An entire section is devoted to making bone meal, dog food, even charcoal.

PART ONE

The Basics of Stocks and Broths

While food at its core is simply calories that fuel and nourish us, the essence of it seems also to fall on a spectrum. On one side, food is diminished into fast junk, that which feeds us on the go; on the other, food is elevated to chef-quality works of art, that which we photograph to document our status. Nevertheless, there is a sound philosophy emerging from somewhere within this spectrum that confirms what my father taught me. Take care with your food, honor it, and realize its true purpose: It does fuel and sustain us; it also brings people together. Food is the stuff of family.

Similarly, our comprehension of stocks seems to lie within this same continuum. Both chefs and home cooks agree that stocks are the foundation of good cooking, and yet what is available on the market is often full of unnecessary salt, sugar, and oil. When average consumers walk into a supermarket, they head to the aisle of cans and boxes, rarely questioning why they aren't looking in a cold case instead. And when chefs succeed in opening their own restaurant, they are occasionally forced to cut corners, limited by time or space, and settle for an expedited solution within a commercial base.

Sometimes what is beautiful is not deeply nutritious, and yet popular science has a way of influencing our belief system. The history of commercial stocks is a curious one—connected to fears of famine, the needs of soldiers, and ultimately, the birth of processed foods. And yet it is no surprise that broth, with the comfort a steaming bowl instills, has adapted itself throughout the ages and across cultures as a nutritional fix. These introductory chapters dig deep into the story of stocks and broths—how they evolved from the work of landowner to food scientist, innkeeper to hotel chef, and ultimately to a provident endeavor of home cooks. What little science exists is explored in detail, intended to elucidate why tried-and-true home cooking is important to health and happiness.

If you ever have a chance to visit a grass-fed cattle farm, I encourage you to do so. The farm will smell richly of healthy grass, and if harvested with the welfare of the animal in mind, so will the meat, once processed. Cows and chickens live in unison—the cows grazing on grass, followed by the chickens reviving the pasture, as they both rotate across the land. The bones are the structural integrity of an animal; a healthy animal will provide healthy bones. For a small vegetable farmer, the types of crops on display help tell the story of the land where they reside. It is all connected—from the soil to the bowl. The latter part of this section explains the significance of quality sourcing and serves as encouragement for supporting your local economy whenever possible. As simple as it sounds, this purchasing principle will ensure quality in your kitchen, and ultimately, your health.

From here, a comprehension about the foundation of good cooking becomes a matter that is mostly practical and a little scientific. This section concludes with a detailed review of how to set up your kitchen for building, and cooking with, stocks and broths. It explains the structural design of a stockpot; the equipment required to develop an elegant and functional base; and outlines a few staple ingredients that will make a difference in your cooking. The basic science of stocks and broths is deconstructed into steps—nuanced ones that explain why a gentle simmer yields the clearest stock, and complex ones that provide instruction on how to guarantee excellence in the pot. With the comprehensive awareness of history and nutrition and the practical knowledge of logistics and science, the fundamental activity of making stocks and broths will become an intuitive part of your time in the kitchen.

CHAPTER ONE

The Importance of Stocks and Broths

For more than a century, the importance of a good stock has been over-shadowed by convenience. The bouillon cube was commercialized in the early twentieth century as a synthetic alternative to authentic meat extract or homemade beef tea. Inexpensive to produce and stable at room temperature, the dehydrated cube would yield a higher profit and travel longer distances than its liquid counterpart. Until the end of this century, stock recipes were mainly showcased in professional texts to be used as reference by chefs; for home cooks, basic recipes were relegated to the introduction or appendix of a cookbook.

Other than the longtime teachings of Sally Fallon Morell, co-founder of the Weston A. Price Foundation, and recent chef-converts, such as Marco Canora, we haven't seen sipping broths as a focal point since Victorian times. Stocks, even if deferred to the back matter of a cookbook, have always garnered attention from chefs—from the work of Richard Olney more than thirty years ago to Thomas Keller and other renowned food professionals today. In an article published by the foundation, Fallon says:

> *What America needs is healthy fast food and the only way to provide this is to put* brothals *in every town, independently owned brothals that provide the basic ingredient for soups and sauces and stews. And brothals will come when Americans recognize that the food industry has prostituted itself to short cuts and huge profits, shortcuts that cheat consumers of the nutrients they should get in their food and profits that skew the economy towards*

industrialization in farming and food processing. Until our diners and
carryouts become places that produce real food, Americans can make broth
in their own kitchens. It's the easy way to produce meals that are both
nutritious and delicious—and to acquire the reputation of an excellent
cook.[1] *(emphasis added)*

She did well to predict this trend. As if taking cues from the Great Depression, our society is showing a greater interest in cooking, a way to save money in a challenging economy. Shoppers continue to express a desire to know where their food comes from; farmers, butchers, and chefs are being heralded as heroes. In restaurants where it used to be bad etiquette to take home leftovers, it is now encouraged to waste nothing.

Despite the hardship on jobs and wages across many trades, the specialty food industry grows year over year,[2] and our DIY curiosity is leading trends in homesteading—from turning beautified lawns into food-rich gardens, to raising backyard chickens for personal egg and meat consumption. Here, too, we begin to see the emergence of broth-based restaurants and product companies that make use of bones and vegetables from local farms—perchance, the *brothals* of Fallon's image. Now you have a better chance of finding quality ready-made stocks where they belong—in the refrigerator or freezer—and from a trusted source.

These days, passionate home cooks and responsible chefs have something in common: a shared belief that the excellence of a dish is directly related to the quality of its foundation. To a farmer, stocks reflect the health of their harvest: Bones are the structural component that connects land to animal. The value of stock to a butcher is that nothing goes to waste: Using bones honors the entire animal. A chef employs stocks not only to enhance the dish, but also to break down tougher cuts of meat; even a baker can use stock to develop a starter. To a nutritionist, stocks promote digestive health, among other restorative merits. Stocks make your pantry go further and are satisfying to consume.

The Etymology of Stock and Broth: A Culinary Distinction

There is much modern-day confusion about the difference between stock and broth. Culinary definitions vary from commercial interpretations. Nutritionists base their distinction on nutrient density of gelatin and mineral content rendered from bones. To further confuse you, chefs often use the terms interchangeably. Sir Balthazar Gerbier's proverb, "Too many cooks spoil the broth," seems appropriate here.

To understand the difference, you must start with a *fond*, the French culinary term for foundation. To the French, stocks are considered *le fond de cuisine*— the essence of ingredients diffused in water, to be used as a building block for cooking. A fond can start with bones and water in a stockpot or develop into a sauce when crusty bits of meat and juice on the surface of a pan are loosened by deglazing with water, stock, or wine. Stock, then, is the foundation by which a broth—the collection of ingredients suspended in stock—is built.

Let's dig a little deeper into the etymology of stocks and broths. The word *stock* is of Germanic origin, meaning "trunk" in Old English. Similarly, *stock* is commonly used to reference shipbuilding materials and has evolved to have many related meanings around the idea of supplies and foundation.[3] A word-smith can have fun with the word *stock*, illustrating its use across many industries, from finance to firearms, finding all roots in the strength of a foundation.

While stocks have presumably been around since the discovery of fire, their first codified use for culinary application was in the eighteenth century when sauces were categorized within the classic French system. *Stock* was used as a general term to refer to the foundation of cooking: the use of basic materials to bring harmony and balance to a dish. Stocks were intended to be a fundamental ingredient, full of bones and clarified in advance of building soups and stews, used for braising meats and generally adding character to dishes that appeal to the eye. Georges Auguste Escoffier, often referred to as the father of modern French cookery, said of sauce made from stock: The *partie capitale* of cuisine![4]

By contrast, *broth* is a more specific term with Germanic roots going back to 1000 CE. *Broth* is related to the Old English words *bru*, or *brew*, and refers to a substance that is prepared by boiling.[5] From its earliest documentation, a broth could be vegetable or animal; by the seventeenth century, it was largely associated with a meat base. Traditionally, broth contains more meat than bones and is simmered for a shorter period of time before getting strained and seasoned. Today this definition extends to extracting the essence from vegetables, not only bones. The goal is to develop a light, flavorful liquid that is served as a part of the dish itself. Think of broth as the enhanced liquid in your bowl.

Similarly, the French word *bouillon* means "liquid in which something has boiled." Credit for the invention of bouillon is given to the Duke of Godfrey, who was said to have developed a clear, flavorful soup in his castle in Bouillon, Belgium. It wasn't until the early twentieth century that bouillon was processed into a granulated cube.

The Italians use the term *en brodo*, literally "in broth," to describe dishes that use an animal or vegetable stock as its own broth. Tortellini is often seen *en brodo*. Matzah ball soup can be considered the Jewish version of *en brodo*, using chicken stock as the base by which to float the matzah balls.

Other examples of broth include Vietnamese *pho* and Japanese *dashi*, two highly aromatic bases upon which to add meat or fish, vegetables, and herbs. Another popular Japanese broth is ramen: It develops a complex flavor by first simmering kelp and mushrooms, and then boiling pork belly and pork bones— all in the same batch of water. The goal here is to extract flavor from the seaweed and mushrooms (without introducing bitterness), followed by a session with meat and bones over higher heat to instill loads of taste and texture into the liquid. This type of broth is less about clarity and more about flavor.

Over the years and across many cultures, nutritionists have taken cues from Jewish mothers, Chinese acupuncturists, and Victorian tea parties to examine the healing properties of bone broths. The word *restaurant*, meaning "to restore to a former state," derives from a fortifying meat-based elixir that was served in French establishments of the same name. A bone broth, then, is an animal stock that uses collagen-rich bones and simmers for an extended time to maximize gelatin extraction into the liquid.

Bone broth is built similarly to traditional stock but differs in a few ways: 1. Bones are always meaty and full of collagen. 2. Bones might be soaked in vinegar before simmering, a step believed by some to aid the leaching of minerals. 3. Bones are simmered longer than a stock. This process ensures a healthy rendering of gelatin in the liquid, which can differ from a traditional stock in the quantity absorbed by, and clarity of, the final liquid. A nutritionist also cares less about clearness of liquid and more about concentration of nutrients.

Fallon and her partners have written extensively about bone broths. Their assessment goes beyond the common cross-cultural belief that chicken soup is soothing for colds: Gelatin is known to easily absorb into the body and aid digestion. Bone marrow contains cells that might assist building immunity and repairing wounds. Cartilage, the connective tissue found in beef knuckles and chicken feet, is believed to fortify joints.[6] Compared with store-bought stocks, there is no question that a homemade stock or broth is more nutritious. Still, there is research to be done on the potential benefits of bone broths. This book evaluates factors, such as time and temperature in a stockpot, that affect the composition of stocks and broths.

Conversationally, it is easy to refer to stock (the foundation) and broth (the composite liquid) as the same; after all, the distinction is technical and lends itself to overlap in the kitchen. In this book, stock is approached from its use in a professional kitchen using French culinary technique: It reflects the steps a chef takes to produce a clarified essence. Broth, when referenced on its own, is reserved for finished dishes. A few recipes highlight different methods to develop stocks and broths from around the world, all preceded by an explanation of their distinction. On the other hand, bone broth is approached from the nutritionist's perspective and refers to a stock that is customized to extract as much gelatin from the bones and mineral content from other source ingredients as possible, but without losing culinary integrity.

About Commercial Stock and Broth

While the government does not distinguish between stock and broth, manufacturers do, using the USDA definitions of processed additives as a guide. Most commercial stocks do not use bones as an ingredient, relying on meat-based extracts and other additives to emulate meaty flavors.

The USDA requires a ratio of 135 parts water to only 1 part animal for broth manufacturers.[7] This means that less than one ounce of meat for each gallon of water is used to make a batch of commercial broth.[8] By contrast, the recipes in this book use around four pounds of meaty bones for every gallon of water.

On food labels, both *stock* and *broth* refer to the percentage concentration of protein to water in the container, or the Moisture-Protein Ratio (MPR), as defined by the USDA. Broth is typically used to name the product—what you will find on the front of the box or can—and stock is listed as an ingredient. Here, *stock* refers to a higher concentration of protein to water, about 67 parts water to 1 part beef. Additional ingredients—such as beef extract, beef powder, beef fat, and yeast extract—are used to enhance flavor and protein content. In short, with so little meat—and no bones—used as the foundation, commercial stocks require additional substances to *approximate* the viscosity and nutrition seen in homemade stocks.

Let's take an older carton of popular commercial beef broth as an example. Before average consumers showed an interest in the content of their food, many manufacturers would list ingredients according to their scientific names. Cartons would often start with beef stock, which contains the highest MPR, and continue with salt, which stabilizes the broth for storage at room temperature. The ingredients listed and defined on page 10 are a collection of glutamates, by-products, colorants, and stabilizers that give this broth a beefy profile. These ingredients still exist on the market and are often obfuscated by names that sound less foreign.

THE SIGNIFICANCE OF COLLAGEN AND GELATIN

Whether stock, broth, or bone broth, the body that develops from animal varieties is attributed to connective tissue found in bones. Connective tissue is rich in collagen—a strong, fibrous protein that converts to gelatin when heat is applied in a moist environment. A sign of healthy gelatin content in well-developed stock is a pronounced jelly-like jiggle that becomes apparent during the chilling process. A seasoned stock maker will be able to tell when a warm batch is ready—extraction is indicated by a subtle increase in viscosity and an almost silken texture of the composite liquid.

Collagen derives from the Greek word *kola*, or glue—a reference to the early process of boiling skin and sinew, mostly from horses, to produce a fibrous adhesive. Use of this glue dates back over 8,000 years, its various applications recently discovered on artifacts in a cave in Israel—a protective coating on fabric, utensils, and ritual objects. The Egyptians later used collagen as a binder for paintings, and Native Americans applied it in the production of bows.[9] Collagen now holds many significant applications in medical science, including bone grafts, tissue regeneration, joint mobility, and wound care. It also serves as a tool for reconstructive and cosmetic surgery, and can be found as an ingredient in many beauty products.

When making an animal stock, the connective tissue in bone slowly breaks down in heated liquid, affecting a reaction within water, known as *hydrolysis*. This denaturation process renders collagen into gelatin—a colorless, flavorless edible with notable gelling properties and varied application.[10] Heat is what drives the speed of hydrolysis; this is why making stock in a pressure cooker quickly yields a gelatinous result (see chapter 15, "Simplified Methods," page 363). Nevertheless, you can produce a stock or broth that is thick with gelatin, high in protein and apparent with trace minerals by holding the liquid in a steady state—just hot enough to render gelatin and cool enough to preserve heat-sensitive compounds. This process is how most of the stocks and broths in this text are developed.

Originating from the Latin *gelatus*, meaning "frozen," *gelatin* has evolved to refer to the transformation of a liquid into a solid. *Gelata*, or "congealed," more closely resembles the modern-day purpose of gelatin in the kitchen, which arrived to the commercial market in the early nineteenth century. The British instilled a patent in the mid-1800s that held governance over the production of gelatin in sheets or strips, known as *leaf gelatin*. In 1890, Charles Knox disrupted the market by releasing the first pre-granulated commercial gelatin, noted for its ease of measurement and quick dissolution.[11] Prior to these events, cooks used calves' feet to impart a gelatinous result in both sweet and savory recipes.

Commercially, gelatin is made predominantly from skins, hides, and bones of porcine or bovine species.[12] There are rare instances when skins from piscine and avian species are used instead. Gelatin extracted from the swim bladders of warm-water fish is called *isinglass* and is known to possess stronger gelling properties than extractions from cold-water fish.[13] The production of most gelatin involves an iterative process of soaking skins in either an acid or alkaline treatment to break down connective tissues, and then extracting gelatin through dissolution in hot water. First extractions are the highest in quality—clear, light, mild, and sturdy. The extraction is then filtered, concentrated, formed into leaves, dried, and sometimes ground.

Gelatin, a mixture of peptides and proteins, is known for its strength. In 1925 Oscar Bloom patented an instrument that measures gel strength, called a *gelometer*, and established the *Bloom Scale*, the industry standard for assessing molecular weight of gelatin. There is much trade fuss over the classification of strength in retail varieties—most brands do not include bloom strength and refer instead to a color classification. Only a few select brands state the origin or quality of their source ingredients. Thus, this book relies on pre-standardized methods—simply rendering bones from a known source into gelatin—to achieve and assess gelling properties.

As a binding agent, gelatin is what gives stock and broth a rich mouthfeel and silken texture. In cooking, gelatin is applied to thicken or stabilize food—a key ingredient across sweets and savories, from Bavarian cream to soup dumplings. Without gelatin, there would be no marshmallows (see chapter 13, "Desserts," page 320)! Other uses for gelatin include gels for theatrical lighting, slippery capsules for pharmaceuticals, color blocks for printmaking, implantable medical devices, even a ballistic medium for testing ammunition.

The composition of gelatin is about 99 percent protein. When it comes to dietary nutrition, however, gelatin is considered an incomplete protein because it lacks certain essential amino acids.[14] When hydrolyzed and concentrated into a supplemental form, gelatin is beneficial to skin, hair, nails, and teeth.[15] It contains chondroitin, which has shown some scientific instances of improving arthritis and other degenerative joint conditions.[16]

TABLE 1.1. Amino Acid Content in Gelatin

Amino Acid	Percentage Content in Gelatin
Proline and Hydroxyproline*	30
Glycine*	27
Glutamic Acid†	12
Alanine†	9
Arginine*	8
Aspartic Acid†	6
Other Amino Acids	8

* Conditionally nonessential amino acid
† Nonessential amino acid

There is limited research that suggests gelatin can aid in the repair of intestinal damage, referred to as *leaky gut syndrome* by some practitioners. Rich in glycine, gelatin has been shown to promote stomach digestion and liver detoxification. The list goes on—findings go further to show that gelatin can help you sleep, lessen sensitivity to tannins, and reduce the impact of methionine from meat consumption.

Some manufacturers market a product labeled *vegetable gelatin*, which is neither vegetable nor gelatin. Instead, it is a plant-based hydrocolloid, such as agar-agar and carrageenan (gathered from seaweed), pectin (found in citrus fruits), and *konjac* (found in a tropical perennial plant of the same name). This is good news for those who hold religious or cultural beliefs that restrict the consumption of animal-based gelatin. Many of the vegetable stocks in this book use kelp, a type of edible seaweed, to infuse body, flavor, and nutrients into the final liquid.

COMMERCIAL BEEF BROTH INGREDIENTS

Beef Stock, Salt, Yeast Extract, Beef Fat, Monosodium Glutamate, Flavoring, Caramel Color, Autolyzed Yeast Extract, Disodium Inosinate, Disodium Guanylate, Beef Extract.

YEAST EXTRACT, OR AUTOLYZED YEAST EXTRACT

This ingredient is a glutamate that lends umami, the fifth taste, without being as simple as regular salt. The process of autolysis—when yeast cells automatically break up after they die—deconstructs proteins into simpler compounds. The remaining extract is a mixture of protein, fats, vitamins, minerals, and naturally occurring monosodium glutamate. Yeast extract is a low-cost way to enhance flavor and is found in many processed foods.

BEEF FAT

The USDA considers this ingredient to be a by-product of beef. Like yeast extract, it is also rich in glutamates and nucleotides. As a secondary product, this kind of beef fat is not tallow, the nutritious fat rendered from marrow bones in a traditionally simmered stock. Instead, it is a glutamate that sounds like an unprocessed ingredient, narrowly masked within the definition regulated by the government.

MONOSODIUM GLUTAMATE (MSG)

MSG is the most common form of glutamate found in processed foods. While some labels are transparent about the use of MSG, be aware that many manufacturers rely on other glutamate-rich ingredients to avoid labeling it on the package. Some people claim that MSG causes migraine headaches; while advocates, including well-known chefs, tout that glutamates occur naturally and are harmless. Regardless of your position, MSG is an additive here instead of a naturally occurring by-product of the manufacturing process.

DISODIUM INOSINATE AND DISODIUM GUANYLATE

These are additives that are often used in conjunction with MSG to enhance flavor. When they appear on the package—even if MSG is not listed—it is a good indication that glutamates are an additive within the product.

BEEF EXTRACT

This term is an ingredient that the USDA refers to as a mixture made from boiling consecutive batches of meat in the same cooking liquid until it yields 75 percent solids to 25 percent moisture. The extract is made from highly processed meat, such as corned beef or related by-products, and is likely where most of the protein content comes from in commercial broths.

Ingredients will always vary by brand, and many current labels will not actively list some of these ingredients. As more consumers show an interest in how products are made, many large manufacturers have begun to edit lists of ingredients: an effort to disguise how heavily processed the final product must be in order to withstand distribution and maintain affordability. This is another reason why it is so important to know the source of your food.

In developing my business, I saw how challenging it is to manage the bottom line while delivering the highest-quality stocks possible. The process of producing slow-simmering stocks for a large consumer audience requires a lot of time and patience: Quality bones are pricey. This challenge is one of the reasons we have remained focused on our local audience, so that we can maintain quality without compromising integrity. It's no surprise that what we see on the shelves of supermarkets relies on techniques that extend savory flavors without using traditional time and materials. Buyer beware!

The Versatility of Stock and Broth

One of my favorite examples of how to maximize a stock is through the double simmering of chicken in Twice-Cooked Chicken and Braised Leek Soup (page 171). This recipe illustrates how stocks add body and flavor to a dish while using the whole animal. It requires a few basic ingredients and mostly unattended time to produce. One small batch feeds a family of four, likely with leftovers, and the carcass of the second chicken can be used to make another batch of stock.

Moroccan women say that semolina is magic. Paula Wolfert, author of *The Food of Morocco*, agrees: "There's a side to everyone where they believe in magic. Like couscous—it doubles, triples, quadruples each time you steam it. It's always enough food to feed everyone. That's magic." I feel the same about making stocks at home. Begin with a whole animal or an entire vegetable, break it down into its respective parts, and extend its life through the cooking process. One chicken provides meat, stock and broth; two chickens provide double the meat and four times the stock and broth. Magic!

Most home cooks think of using stocks to make soup or stew, and while this is an agreeable way to use them, it is only the beginning. Stocks offer a versatility in the kitchen—from developing the foundation of a dish to finishing one. Here are a few ways you can employ stocks and broths:

BASTING

Basting is a slow-cooking technique that produces a succulent texture in roasted meat or vegetables. It is achieved by brushing or spooning a liquid—such as stock, pan drippings, or melted fat—over the ingredients while cooking in the oven or on the stovetop. Aged Rib Steak (page 136) and Spatchcocked Bourbon Red Turkey (page 186) are recipes that use basting to add moisture to the dish.

BOILING

Boiling refers to the temperature at which liquid turns to steam—water boils at 212°F (100°C) (at sea level). Beans and grains can be boiled in stock, such as Three Fennel Cassoulet (page 160), or a combination of stock and ingredients can be boiled to produce a flavorful broth, mostly in Asian cookery, as in Ox Bone Soup (page 130). This text recommends simmering—which generally occurs at 200°F (93°C)—an unfinished stock; however, once the solids are strained and the liquid is clarified, gently boiling stock as a cooking liquid is a common practice.

BRAISING

Braising is another slow-cooking method that uses dry, and then, moist heat to break down tough cuts of meat, fish, or vegetables. The main ingredient is first seared over high heat, and then simmered in a moderate amount of liquid. During the simmering stage, the cooking vessel is covered, and the liquid gently conducts heat to the food. The braising liquid is often strained and reduced as a sauce for the dish, or can be used as a compound stock for another dish. Examples of braising are found in Milk-Braised Lamb Neck (page 142) and Choucroute Garnie (page 163).

CODDLING

Coddling is a technique where food is cooked slowly in liquid held just below the boiling point. The word derives from *caudle*, a warm drink intended for the ill. Coddled eggs are a common example of the method, where the eggs are cracked into a ramekin and cooked over a water bath. Dublin Coddle is an Irish dish made from leftovers—traditionally layers of barley, rashers or bacon, potatoes, and onions, covered in bouillon, sealed, and cooked for many hours.

DEVILING

Deviling refers to foods that are cooked with hot spices or condiments. The term originated as a noun in the eighteenth century, a reference to highly seasoned dishes and the Devil himself, and evolved into a verb by the nineteenth century. Deviling has also come to apply to potted meats, such as the classic Underwood Deviled Ham, which holds the oldest existing trademark in the United States. See the recipe for Deviled Bones on page 352.

GLAZING

Glazing derives from the Middle English for "glass" and indicates a glossy coating applied to the surface of food. Aspic, a type of savory glaze made from stock and gelatin, plays a prominent role in Moulard Duck Galantine (page 197). *Glace de viande*, a French term for "meat glaze," refers to stock that is reduced to a syrup. It serves as the foundation for many sauces. Alternatively, *deglazing* refers to the addition of liquid to a hot pan to loosen the fond, another building block for sauce. This method is referenced in numerous recipes throughout the book. Deglazing the pan is an essential step when building the foundation for Grand Seafood Paella (page 316).

POACHING

Poaching is a method where delicate food, such as eggs or fish, is simmered in liquid held just below the boiling point. The liquid can be stock, milk, wine, or water. Foods can even be poached in oil held at about 200°F (93°C). A poached egg is cooked either without its shell or in its shell—a small hole poked into the shell to prevent cracking—in simmering water or stock, to yield an egg that holds its structure. The goal is to gently cook the egg whites while sustaining a runny yolk. A delicious example is Yellow Split Pea Cakes with Poached Duck Eggs (page 285). Poaching fish in stock, as in Sea Bream à la Nage (page 224), preserves moisture without adding fat.

SOPPING

Sopping is a term used to describe dipping a piece of bread or toast in liquid, commonly referred to in medieval cookery. More of a dish than a technique, the word *sop* also shares etymology with *soup* and appears in the Bible in this context. A contemporary interpretation of a sop is seen in Vegetarian French Onion Soup (page 256).

STEWING

Stewing refers to a preparation of meat and/or vegetables that are submerged and cooked slowly in simmering liquid. Ingredients are cut into small, uniform pieces and immersed in the cooking liquid, making this technique distinctly different from the large cuts and moderate amount of liquid associated with braising. A classic example of a stew is Traditional Plum Pottage (page 141).

REDUCING

Reducing is the process of distilling flavor from, and altering texture in, a liquid through evaporation. As a stock reduces, those components that have the highest boiling point remain in the liquid, creating a thickened structure with concentrated flavor. A demi-glace is a type of reduction, as illustrated in Farmhouse Rooster Coq au Vin (page 174), as are pan sauces and gastriques.

———

Regardless of origin—whether simmering in a restaurant kettle or on a home stove—stocks are a significant component to any kitchen. The commercial importance of collagen and gelatin is telling, even beyond its versatile application in cooking. The next two chapters explore the history and composition of stocks and broths, and reveal how their commercial chronology around the globe helped shape popular beliefs about their nutritional value. The story of this culinary staple is a fascinating look into how cultures endeavor to make the most of their resources. Stocks and broths, both delicious to eat and efficient to make, are an endless source of creation in the kitchen and comfort in the bowl.

CHAPTER TWO

The Fundamentals of Stocks and Broths

For a cook, perhaps a more notable achievement than technical proficiency is a sense of intuition in the kitchen—the agility to move from task to task without much thought, an integral understanding of space and material sufficient as a guide. Learning the significance of and science behind a good foundation expands culinary range. In my kitchen, the stovetop is rarely bare of a simmering stock; the back-right corner of the range is always reserved for a stockpot. The practice of rinsing bones, chopping vegetables, and filling a pot full of water becomes a part of every day, often a morning ritual as common as brewing coffee.

To nurture this intuitive sense, it is important to understand the fundamental stock types and their derivatives. These stocks are designed by food group and cover all types of animals and vegetables; knowing the differences among them will help develop an informed approach to cooking. From here, crafting sophisticated broths and sauces will become second nature—a little spice here, a longer reduction there—an act that you perform perhaps while another stock is simmering in the background.

The stocks, broths, and sauces reviewed in this chapter mostly abide by classic French technique. This is one of many philosophies about how to develop flavor, intended to be an introduction to an everlasting education about the essence of cooking. Every culture has its own cuisine; some borrow from others, others are uniquely their own. This chapter ends with an overview of some of my favorite stocks and broths from around the world.

The Fundamental Stocks

At the highest level, classic culinary stocks can be categorized into four types: meat, poultry, fish, and vegetable. The French refer to stocks as the fond, or base, by which the foundation of a dish is developed. From here, technique determines the depth of flavor and color your stock will exhibit: The decision to blanch or roast bones, or sauté or roast vegetables, establishes the purpose of the stock in your final dishes—whether to be prominent or to blend in the background. All stocks have the addition of *mirepoix* and other aromatics in common, which mellows the forward flavors of the main ingredient and brings a stock to a balanced state. As you become proficient with the technique, considering the purpose of the stock before making it will become an ingrained part of the process.

After a stock is made, you can adjust its clarity and concentration to achieve other fundamental states. We'll review the main stock types below, as well as their derivatives, before digging deep into each category in subsequent chapters.

WHITE STOCK

A white stock, or *fond blanc*, is light in color and silky in texture. It is made by cleaning bones to remove impurities without adding color. Sometimes bones are clean enough to require only a thorough rinse, though most bones need to be blanched to achieve purity. The bones often used are full of collagen—such as veal bones for a white veal stock or supplemental chicken feet for a white chicken stock—and result in a gelatinous finish. A mirepoix of common vegetables—either raw, or lightly sautéed—is introduced to the liquid in order to maintain a delicate hue in the finished stock.

Due to their light color, white stocks are commonly used as a neutral cooking component. They can blend with, rather than overpower, the ingredients of a

QUICK TIPS FOR WHITE STOCK

- A white stock is made from washed or blanched bones.
- The aromatics are raw or lightly sautéed.
- The finished stock is light in color and silky in texture.
- It is intended to be used as a neutral cooking component.
- It should blend into the background of the dish.
- White stocks made with meat or poultry tend toward a lengthy simmering time, depending on the size of the bones.
- Also known as fond blanc; referred to as basic stock throughout this book.

dish, allowing a main ingredient to remain the feature. White stocks are also great for adding liquid to, or finishing a dish; a splash of a gelatinous stock will bring ingredients together in the pan, making it ideal for risotto or other grain dishes. With their silken texture, white stocks are an excellent foundation for soups or other dishes where a well-developed broth is essential. White stocks also make an ideal poaching liquid, which can be stored after use as a compound stock, also known as a double stock.

In classic French texts, *fond blanc* typically refers to poultry stocks, but has come to mean any stock made with ingredients that have not been roasted for color, including all types of animals and vegetables. As such, you will find many white stock variations in the chapters devoted to meat and vegetables (chapters 8 and 11, respectively). Throughout the book, this type of stock is referred to as a basic stock and serves as the introductory stock recipe for each category.

BROWN STOCK

A brown stock, or *fond brun*, is rich in color—ranging from a golden brown to a deep mahogany—and full in body. It is made by roasting bones, and often vegetables, which add a caramelized flavor to the stock. For some brown stocks, tomato paste is roasted with the bones or folded into the stock to brighten the hue and further develop texture. In the case of lamb and duck stocks, the vegetables are sautéed instead of roasted; this variation prevents the liquid from becoming too dark.

With their rich, dark shade, brown stocks are intended to guide the flavor and texture of a dish. They can be featured in a stew or served as a rich soup base, where the broth is a main ingredient. Roasted stocks are often used for braising meat and vegetables; the braising liquid can be strained and reduced at the end to make a velvety sauce

QUICK TIPS FOR BROWN STOCK

- A brown stock is made from roasted bones.
- The aromatics are roasted or sautéed.
- The finished stock is rich in color, from dark brown to mahogany, and viscous in texture.
- It often includes tomato paste to brighten its hue and develop its texture.
- It is intended to anchor a dish, as a rich foundation or as a braising liquid.
- Brown stocks made with meat or poultry tend toward a lengthy simmering time, depending on the size of the bones.
- Also known as fond brun; referred to as roasted stock throughout this book.

for the dish. This reduction step applies to brown stocks as well, not just braising liquids: After straining, the stock can be significantly reduced to make a *glace de viande*, or meat glaze. This process further concentrates flavor—it's reduced about eight to ten times, and a little goes a long way. A small scoop is the ideal base for gravies and sauces.

In classic French texts, *fond brun* most commonly refers to veal stocks, but has come to mean any stock made with ingredients that have been roasted for color. As with white stocks, this expansion includes all manner of animals and vegetables. Throughout the book, this type of stock is referred to as a roasted stock and their recipes come after the basic stocks within each category.

FISH STOCK

Similar to all animal-based stocks, fish stock is made by simmering meaty fish bones that have been leached, blanched, or roasted with aromatics. Fish bones, however, impart a unique quality to liquid—both piscine and briny—unlike the characteristics gleaned from any land animal. The French refer to fish stock as *fumet*, which commonly contains white wine and is reduced to concentrate the flavors. Stocks made from shellfish are also included in this category.

Classically, fish stock is made from the bones of neutral flatfish, such as halibut, flounder, or sole, and comes together in the pot in less than an hour. Any more time, and the stock will develop a bitter taste. In contemporary cooking, it is acceptable to use the bones from white bony fish, such as snapper, grouper, and cod. These varieties can withstand a longer simmering time, and the cartilage in the bones breaks down to develop a gelatinous base. I enjoy incorporating monkfish tail for its delicate flavor and adding a small amount of skate wing or fish collars when a thick-bodied stock is the goal. Fish heads can also be used, provided the eyes and gills are removed before use.

Aromatics play a versatile role in the making of fish stock. The buttery flavor and texture of leeks softens the intensity of the piscine flavor. Sometimes carrots are omitted from the aromatic base, in order to preserve a neutral color in the stock; parsnips can be a flavorful substitute that won't alter the hue. Fennel is a superb match with seafood and is regularly featured in stock recipes. At times, it is further highlighted in finished dishes with a splash of an anise-based spirit. Similarly, tarragon, an herb with a subtle licorice aroma, lends itself well to shellfish stocks.

As a general rule, fish stock should not be made with oily fish, such as mackerel or salmon, due to their pungency. Nevertheless, some dishes, such as noodle stews fortified with flavorful aromatics like star anise and lemongrass, will benefit from the intensely flavored broth these types of fish produce. This book does not review strong fish stocks; use your discretion when bones from oily fish are at hand.

Stocks made from shellfish are rarely included in classic texts; likely because the foundation is most often built from the liquid inside the shell, not from the shell itself. Still, shellfish, such as mussels, clams, and oysters, are not only flavorful, but also good for their environment. These types of shellfish filter algae from their aquatic atmosphere, which cleans the water and improves habitat for other marine life. The stocks made from their essence are concentrated and powerful, imparting unique brininess to food—a flavor that is specific to their territory. These stocks are individually showcased in this book. As a decadent alternative to shrimp stock, which is not covered here due to global exploitation of stock and labor, a base made with lobster shells is offered.

QUICK TIPS FOR FISH STOCK

- A fish stock is made from meaty fish bones and fish heads, most often from white, non-oily fish. Bones can be leached, blanched, or roasted.
- The aromatics are lightly sautéed or roasted. Sometimes carrots are omitted; parsnips can be used instead.
- The finished stock is light in color and gelatinous in texture.
- Stocks made from shellfish fit within this category. Mussels, clams, and oysters should be alive when extracting their liquor; lobster shells can be used after the meat is removed.
- Seafood stocks are intended for recipes with fish or shellfish—as a base for chowders, as a poaching liquid for fish, or as an aspic for terrines.
- Fish and shellfish stocks tend toward a short simmering time, due to the size of fish bones and short cooking time of shellfish.
- Also known as *fumet*, which commonly uses white wine and can be reduced for concentration.

Fish and shellfish stocks possess a delicate body that is often laden with natural umami. Their bases are intended for recipes that incorporate some element of the sea or the water from which they are harvested—from dainty broths to thick chowders. Fish stock also works well as a poaching liquid, thereby developing a compound stock, which can be reduced to a sauce, or frozen for later use. When chilled, a properly made fish stock will congeal like jelly and serves as an excellent aspic for seafood terrines. Fish and shellfish stock also match well with pork stock or dairy whey, working together to develop a mellow, yet complex, foundation.

VEGETABLE STOCK

Vegetable stock is made by simmering raw or roasted vegetables with herbs and spices to develop a foundation that is light in flavor and body. It can be made with a mixture of vegetables, similar to those found in animal stocks, or it can feature one main ingredient, such as mushrooms or tomatoes, with other vegetables blending into the background.

In a pot of simmering water, vegetables break down more quickly than bones do, and therefore require less simmering time than animal-based stocks. Some recipes call for chopping the vegetables in a food processor before adding them to the pot. This step increases the surface area of vegetables to liquid and further expedites the extraction process. Since bones are not used to make a vegetable stock, the liquid does not contain gelatin and is therefore very fluid. Sometimes seaweed is added to incorporate body where animal gelatin is not wanted.

Vegetable stocks can be used in place of many meat-based stocks. For instance, the earthiness of a mushroom stock is a nice replacement for the meatiness of a beef stock. Similarly, a light winter squash stock will add a savory nuttiness to food and is a fine replacement for chicken stock. Still, stocks made with vegetables stand on their own—they can be made in less than an hour, offer endless variation and versatility, and enhance the flavor and texture of food better than water alone. Since there is no binding protein in vegetable stock, it loses its flavor quickly; it should be used within two days of making or frozen for later use.

QUICK TIPS FOR VEGETABLE STOCK

- A vegetable stock is made from a mixture of raw or roasted vegetables and herbs and spices.
- It may feature one vegetable while other aromatics blend into the background.
- Sometimes vegetables are finely chopped before simmering to increase surface area in the pot and decrease cooking time.
- The finished stock is bright in color and fluid in texture.
- Vegetable stocks may be used in place of animal-based stocks; however, there is no gelatin in vegetable stocks. Seaweed, such as kelp, can be added for body.
- Vegetable stocks tend toward a short simmering time, since vegetables break down quickly in simmering water.

REMOUILLAGE

A *remouillage* is a secondary stock made from bones that have already been simmered to make a primary stock. In French, the word *remouillage* means "rewetting"—here, a reference to the bones being submerged in water twice. It is also known as a second stock. A remouillage is a sophisticated way to get the most from high-quality bones without compromising the clarity of a foundation.

The second extraction is weaker than the first and rarely used on its own. Classically, both extractions are married and reduced to create a silky, complex finish. This method is often applied to veal bones due to their significant collagen content. The double extraction slowly converts collagen into gelatin, and the net effect of combining strong and weak stocks is a smooth, neutral foundation. The recipe for Two-Day Veal Stock (page 111) illustrates how to make and wed a remouillage. In some cases, the combined stocks are reduced further to make a glaze.

This technique is effective in converting a significant amount of collagen, packed tightly within the protein matrix of bones, into gelatin. As such, I incorporate a remouillage into the method for making concentrated bone broths. This allows an increased simmering time without compromising the quality of the extraction.

The secondary extraction can also be used in place of water in dishes, where a splash of diluted stock adds more value than the neutrality of water. An unwed remouillage is an excellent and efficient base for quick soups and as a braising or poaching liquid, which then evolves into a compound stock.

DEMI-GLACE

A demi-glace is a rich base made by combining and reducing brown stock and Espagnole sauce, a basic brown sauce, otherwise known as one of Escoffier's classic mother sauces. A demi-glace, or "half glaze," comes from the French word *glace*, which means "icing" or "glaze"; here, it refers to the glossy coating that a demi-glace develops when poured over meat or presented as a plated sauce. A classic demi-glace employs veal

QUICK TIPS FOR REMOUILLAGE

- A remouillage is made from bones that have already been simmered to make a stock.
- The stronger primary and weaker secondary extractions are often married to create a smooth, balanced stock.
- A remouillage is classically made from veal bones, which contain a large amount of collagen, but now applies to any bone that is run through twice.
- The method gently converts collagen into gelatin without clouding the stock, making it an excellent technique for bone broths.
- The secondary stock is also great as a flavor agent and textural enhancer in place of water.
- It can be used as a braising or poaching liquid, which then makes it a compound stock.
- *Remouillage* means "rewetting" in French; also known as a second stock.

for the brown stock, though it is now widely accepted to use a brown stock made from beef and poultry.

An important though subtle distinction: Demi-glace is not a type of glace de viande, or meat glaze. To be classified as a demi-glace, a brown stock must be combined with a basic brown sauce before the reduction. A demi-glace is reduced only by half of its original liquid, whereas a glace de viande is reduced eight to ten times from its original state. Nevertheless, it is common to see small amounts of demi-glace referenced in contemporary cookbooks where glace de viande should be; in small quantities, this substitution is acceptable. This deviation from the original recipe was introduced by Julia Child, who published a recipe for Semi-Demi-Glace. Her shortcut combines two quarts of brown stock with two tablespoons of red wine and slowly reduces it to a cup, excluding the Espagnole sauce altogether.

QUICK TIPS
FOR DEMI-GLACE

- A demi-glace is made from equal parts brown stock and classic brown sauce, known as Espagnole, and then reduced by one-third to one-half.
- It is different from a glace de viande, which is a brown stock reduced to a glaze, though they can act as substitutes in small quantities.
- Demi-glace serves as a foundation for many sauces, or it can be diluted to make a stock.
- Use a demi-glace when a recipe calls for a generic base. Homemade is always preferred, since commercial versions are often made with hydrogenated oils and stabilizers.
- A demi-glace requires more time to make than a stock, but it lasts a long time in the freezer, doesn't require defrosting for immediate use, and is used sparingly.
- *Demi-glace* means "half glaze" in French, which derives from *glace*, to mean "icing" or "glaze."

If you see a recipe that calls for a quarter cup or more of demi-glace, rest assured that the author intends for demi-glace to be used.

Demi-glace is the foundation for many sauces: You can simply whisk in a tablespoon of demi-glace while deglazing a pan with water or wine. If a dish requires additional flavor, folding in a scoop of demi-glace will add umami without overpowering other ingredients. It is also an excellent way to fix a bland stock or broth. Alternatively, should you find yourself with a container of demi-glace but no stock on hand, you can develop a simple stock by diluting 1 part demi-glace in 4 parts warm filtered water. Use demi-glace in any recipe that calls for a base—homemade is always preferable here, as commercial options are laden with hydrogenated oils and stabilizers.

Making a batch of demi-glace requires time and patience—even more than when making a basic stock; however, the result is a deeply developed base that will enhance your cooking for many meals to come. Due to its thick consistency, demi-glace freezes exceptionally well. I recommend storing it in a small container with a wide lid, perhaps in the doorway of your freezer. When you need a scoop, you can easily dip a warm spoon into the frozen demi-glace to scoop out enough for immediate cooking.

CONSOMMÉ

Consommé is a type of pure, flavorful soup or broth that has been clarified. It is a delicate offering, served hot or cold, and is considered to be a notable achievement for a chef. *Consommé* means "complete" in French, a stock that is brought to a perfect state in both appearance and taste.

The classic method for making consommé involves stirring a mixture of ground meat, egg whites, mirepoix, and aromatics into a stock and simmering until the mixture develops a raft on the surface. This raft is a protein matrix that captures impurities from the stock. It is left to simmer for an hour before ladling and straining, and results in a crystal-clear liquid. The clarified stock can be passed through a coffee filter to capture any fine particles; it can also be refrigerated to easily collect any remaining fat that congeals at the surface. Sometimes egg whites and crushed eggshells are used in place of the ground meat.

A *double consommé* refers to a consommé that has been reduced for concentrated flavor and texture. It can be achieved by

QUICK TIPS FOR CONSOMMÉ

- A consommé is a soup or broth that has been clarified. A double consommé is a clarified soup that has been reduced by half.
- It is traditionally made by simmering a protein raft in a prepared stock. The raft acts as a filtration network at the surface and captures impurities from the liquid.
- The protein raft can be made with a slurry of ground meat, egg whites, and mirepoix, or simply egg whites and crushed eggshells.
- A traditionally made consommé is clear, silky, and flavorful. When chilled, it can be used as an aspic to seal terrines or preserve fatty meats.
- A contemporary method, popular in molecular gastronomy, creates a consommé through gelatin filtration, which results in a clear, light-bodied broth.
- *Consommé* means "complete" in French, a stock that is perfect in flavor and appearance. Chefs consider consommé to be a sophisticated culinary achievement.

doubling the quantity of meat to form the raft; reducing a consommé by half; or executing a raft on an already prepared consommé.

Due to the high protein content, a classically prepared consommé, and especially a double consommé, will exhibit gelatinous properties when chilled. A chilled consommé can be used as an *aspic*, or meat jelly, to seal a terrine or preserve fatty meats. Throughout history, a properly gelled consommé was often sugared instead of salted and matched with fruits to make a sweet jelly—a clear predecessor to contemporary gelatin desserts. Tomatoes also form the foundation for a popular chilled consommé, a variation that produces clarity without gel.

A consommé prepared with a raft requires a high quantity of meat—often double the amount of meat to the yield of finished soup—and can therefore be wasteful. Amidst the rise of molecular gastronomy, *New York Times* writer and food scientist Harold McGee popularized a revised method for producing a consommé, called gelatin filtration. This clever technique removes small particles from a gelatinous stock. It is first frozen and then slowly thawed and passed through a filter into a receiving vessel. The gelatin and particles remain in the filter, producing a stock with pristine clarity and clean flavors. This type of consommé does not have the same mouthfeel as its traditional counterpart due to the complete loss of gelatin. Nevertheless, because it requires no heat, some cooks apply this method to ingredients that are not stocks, such as fruit juice or even brown butter, adding gelatin before freezing and then refining a clear, flavorful consommé variant.

BROTH

Broth is a categorical derivative of stock, made by adding ingredients that go beyond the essence of its foundation. It can be seen as a fortified stock, enhanced with additional meat, aromatics, herbs, and spices. Broth is a developed part of the dish as opposed to a building block. A broth can be the defining component of a recipe, as illustrated in Sea Bream à la Nage (page 224), where the poached fish "swims" in its broth on the plate. The process of building a broth invites unlimited creativity in the kitchen: It can be bold and flavorful, subtle and nuanced, or somewhere in between.

Technically, *broth* also refers to a stock made with meat instead of bones. Since meat does not contain binding agents, such as collagen, it requires less simmering time than bones to extract its essence. As such, broths made with meat and no bones remain fluid due to the lack of gelatin content. An excellent example of a simple homemade broth is Classic Beef Tea (page 327), where a chunk of beef is steeped in hot water. Though the USDA does not make a distinction between stock and broth, commercial containers labeled as broth are commonly made with trimmings from processed meats.

BONE BROTH

Bone broths have recently emerged as a stand-alone category, referring to a gelatin-dense stock that is sipped like a broth. The goal of a bone broth is to render as much collagen into gelatin as possible in the simmering liquid, and also extract trace minerals.

There are many recipes for bone broth, and guidelines often contradict culinary intuition, such as length of time cooking and what constitutes a spent ingredient. Nevertheless, most bone broth recipes have three things in common: 1. They use meaty bones from parts of the animal that are rich in collagen. 2. Bones might be soaked in vinegar before simmering. 3. The mixture is simmered longer than a traditional stock. As such, the final broth is viscous, and according to some recipes, might be cloudy instead of clear.

With a few minor adjustments, bone broths can be nutritious and flavorful, as well as technically deft. In this book, I employ a remouillage to extract gelatin while maintaining clarity of the liquid. Bones should never crumble or cook to the

QUICK TIPS FOR BROTH

- A broth is a fortified stock that acts as a main component of a finished dish.
- Technically, a broth is also a stock made with meat instead of bones. It has less gelatin than stocks made with bones.
- A broth is fluid and flavorful, often holding additional meat, aromatics, herbs, and spices.
- Commercial broths are made with trimmings from processed meats. Homemade broths are more nutritious than those found in a box or can.

QUICK TIPS FOR BONE BROTH

- A bone broth is a hybrid of stock and broth, made from meaty bones and often sipped like a beverage. It can also be used for cooking.
- The goal of a bone broth is to extract as much gelatin and trace minerals from the bones as possible.
- There are many recipe variations for bone broths; however, they all use meaty bones, often include a vinegar soak, and simmer for a longer period than regular stocks.
- This book employs a remouillage to extract maximum gelatin from bones while maintaining clarity in the liquid.
- A vinegar soak is optional yet not recommended. Research has shown it is not effective in bringing collagen and minerals to the surface.
- Sourcing quality bones from humanely raised animals is required to make a nutritious bone broth. This conscientious approach should be applied when making any stock or broth.

STORING YOUR STOCKS FOR LATER USE

I like to think of my freezer as a well-supplied pantry: Shelves are lined with containers of stocks, reductions, soups, and stews, waiting to be defrosted for further development or simply reheated for a quick meal. Based on the needs of the moment, I will reach for containers of varying size: A scoop of veal demi-glace dissolves into the base of a quick sauce, a pint container of chicken stock produces soup in minutes, and a quart container of vegetable stock becomes dinner for a week. When a freezer is filled with a variety of stocks and broths, the versatility of your kitchen reveals itself—you can spend an hour making one meal or days producing delicacies for a special affair. With your foundation at the ready, half the work is already done.

The types of stocks to keep on hand can be categorized into primary and secondary categories: Staple stocks, such as basic chicken or roasted vegetable, are used with frequency, whereas ancillary varieties, such as roasted duck or aged garlic, are used less often. My freezer always has large containers of Basic Chicken Stock (page 166), Roasted Beef Stock (page 125), Basic Fish Fumet (page 213), and Basic Vegetable Stock (page 245). If room permits, I hold reduced quantities of Two-Day Veal Stock (page 111), Roasted Lamb Stock (page 140), and Smoked Pork Stock (page 153)—all of which add a unique character to dishes, sort of a secret flavor arsenal that will instantly elevate your home cooking. My kitchen makes use of many vegetable stocks as well; however, because they come together fast *and* lose their flavor quickly, I tend to reserve freezer space for stocks that require a lot of time to develop. When vegetable stocks reach the freezer, they typically feature a highly seasonal ingredient, such as heirloom tomatoes—a foundation to keep on hand for the colder months, an extension of your pantry and the seasons.

Assess your cold storage space, both refrigerator and freezer, before making a variety of stocks. Stocks and broths made with meat or poultry will keep well in your refrigerator for a few days; the gelatin from bones acts as a mild preserving agent. Those made with seafood or vegetables have a shorter shelf life—about two days in the refrigerator before they go bad or lose flavor. Stocks and broths keep well in the freezer—up to six months and sometimes longer in quart containers—before they develop freezer burn. If you prefer to use glass instead of plastic, you must fill the containers with

point where they cloud the stock. Time in the pot is determined by size of the bones—for instance, a chicken bone broth requires less simmering time than a beef bone broth. The vinegar soak is optional, as research has shown it does little to coax collagen and leach minerals from the bones before simmering. Recipes are also provided for those animals whose bones are dense with collagen and whose flavor imparts a pleasant "savoriness" on the palate—beef, pork, chicken, turkey, rabbit, and fish. An emphasis on quality sourcing is placed throughout the book—the nutritive properties of a well-made bone broth (or any stock or broth, for that matter) will reflect the health of the animal from which it derives.

cooled stock, maintaining enough headspace for the stocks to expand as they get colder, and freeze first *without* lids. Once frozen, you can seal the jars with lids. This initial freezing step prevents the glass from breaking in your freezer.

You can also freeze stocks in ice cube trays, either popping out the frozen cubes and storing in freezer bags, or simply wrapping the trays as the storage container itself. Due to exposed surface area, the cubes will develop freezer burn quicker than stocks stored in larger containers. The benefit, however, is single-use servings—in this format, stock becomes a staple you can reach for as intuitively as a pat of butter. This storage method works especially well for heavily concentrated stocks—gelatinous reductions that save space in the freezer and dilute well in the pan.

In addition to how much cold storage you have available, your eating habits will provide guidance when deciding how to stock your freezer. If you find yourself roasting chicken or duck often, for instance, then it is easier to store roasted bones and keep poultry stocks on hand. One ancillary benefit of participating in a meat share—where whole animals are collectively purchased and distributed among members—is that stocks store more efficiently than bones do. Seasonal ingredients, such as heirloom turkey or summer lobster, might encourage you to store a large batch of turkey stock or a small quantity of shellfish stock. To ensure a gelatinous quality to my bone-based stocks, I always keep chicken feet, cow knuckles, and skate wing in my freezer.

If you are cooking with frozen stocks or regularly sipping bone broths, try to plan ahead: Transfer containers from the freezer to the refrigerator the night before you intend to cook. Alternatively, you can place the containers in a cold-water bath until defrosted, or if you are in a particular rush, you can quick-thaw the stock in a hot-water bath to help expedite the process. See "Guidelines for Making Stocks and Broths," page 88, for more about defrosting methods.

For longer-term storage, consider making Soup Cubes (page 335), the modern-day equivalent of portable soup (page 41). Simply remove a cube from cold storage and reconstitute with water, fortifying with meat, vegetables, and grains as you wish. If you have limited freezer space, or are planning an outdoor adventure, you can make Dehydrated Bouillon (page 337), a dried mixture made of homemade broth, fresh vegetables, and spices—a much better alternative to commercial bouillon cubes.

Stocks Around the World

Cultures around the world have their own interpretation of stocks and broths— rich bowls of compound liquids that speak to origin and environment, independent of influence from the French or British. My historical exploration tells only part of the story. And yet to survey the global history of stocks and broths—country by country—would provide enough content for another book. For now, we'll acknowledge a few formative foundations specific to cultural identities around the world. Admittedly these are what inform my personal kitchen experience.

THE BASICS OF STOCKS AND BROTHS

CHINA: MASTER STOCK

In China, there exists the legend of stocks that have survived for hundreds of years, passed down through generations and nurtured as you would a bread culture. Called a *master stock*, this compound base begins with an aromatic broth—commonly spiced with soy sauce, rice wine, star anise, cassia bark, and more—and is used to poach or braise meats. The stock that results from this process is chilled or frozen for reuse, intended to develop a complexity of flavor with each subsequent simmer. In Southern China, the Cantonese term *lou mei* refers to any dish that is made by simmering meat, offal, tofu, or kelp in a master stock.

JAPAN: DASHI

Dashi is a simple yet elegant broth that serves as the foundation of Japanese cuisine. This broth is made by quickly and gently simmering *kombu*, a type

---

MASTER STOCK

ACTIVE TIME: 1 hour | **TOTAL TIME:** ½ day, including simmering and chilling |
YIELD: Makes about 2 quarts (1.9 liters)

---

2 quarts (1.9 L) Basic Chicken Stock (page 166)
   or Basic Vegetable Stock (page 245)
¾ cup (180 ml) tamari or light soy sauce
¾ cup (180 ml) Shaoxing wine
½ cup (110 g) palm sugar or light
   brown sugar
2 small shallots, minced

3 cloves garlic, sliced
3 slices galangal or ginger
6 dried shiitake mushrooms
2 dried chilies
3 whole pods star anise
2 sticks cinnamon, preferably Ceylon
½ teaspoon Szechuan peppercorns

Place all the ingredients in a stockpot. Turn the heat to medium-high, and slowly heat the liquid. When the liquid starts to ripple, before it breaks into a boil, lower the heat to medium and simmer to infuse the spices, about 30 minutes. Turn off the heat and rest the stock on the stove, about 15 minutes. Set a fine-mesh strainer over a container large enough to hold the liquid contents of the pot. Strain, cover, chill, and reserve until ready to use.

Use the stock as a braising liquid for meat. After each use, strain the stock and store it in the refrigerator for up to 3 days or in the freezer for up to 6 months.

of edible seaweed, with *katsuobushi*, fermented and dried skipjack tuna, to extract intense flavor into the liquid. Umami owes its identity to the glutamic acid found in dashi. This early-twentieth-century discovery came when Japanese chemist Kikunae Ikeda was sipping a dashi that was more intense than usual; curiosity led him to isolate the natural glutamates in kombu and later to patent an extraction process for monosodium glutamate.[1] Similarly, katsuobushi is rich in sodium inosinate, also a source of umami. See page 297 for a Dashi recipe.

ITALY: PESTAT DI FAGNANA

From the Roman blend of *stracciatella*, the world's first egg drop soup, to *minestra maritata*, a marriage not of vows but of vegetables in broth, Italy is rich with cultural references to soup built from stock. Yet, like many culinary discoveries in Italy, regional nuance reveals the best that local *terra* has to offer. One such instance exists in a small hilly region in Friuli, where agriculture dictates activity: Butchers preserve the autumn pig harvest in a soup base called *Pestat di Fagnana*. Pork fat is combined with a small dice of vegetables and a healthy addition of herbs and spices, stuffed in natural casings and ripened in a cool cellar, alongside salami and other fermented meats. Once cured, the casing is removed to release a dressing, which is packed in jars for use in the winter months. A dollop of *pestat* in a medium-hot pan yields rendered fat and slightly caramelized vegetables, ready for liquid to be added—a preserved bouillon that speaks of seasons past.

KOREA: OX BONE SOUP

In Korea, soup is often served as an entrée instead of an appetizer. Soups are categorized by type: *guk*, a thinner soup often eaten at home, and *tang*, a concentrated soup commonly found in restaurants. A popular restaurant dish, *seolleongtang*, is made by boiling meaty ox bones in water until the liquid turns cloudy and appears milky white—a technique that varies from most instruction in this book. This broth is served in a large bowl with steamed rice, seasoned with sea salt and scallions at the table, and often accompanied by kimchi and other flavorful ferments. Aside from being delicious, seolleongtang has a legendary history associated with the harvest sacrifices—known as *sŏnnongje* or "venerated farmer"—of the Joseon dynasty. It was King Sŏngjong who visited a sacrifice and decreed upon the people to develop dishes that would extend the food supply, among which was this bone soup.[2] See the Ox Bone Soup recipe on page 130.

MEXICO: SOPA DE LIMA

The staple crops of Mayan culture—corn, squash, beans, and chilies—remain prevalent in Mexican cuisine; a historical success story of how complementary cultivars can feed entire cultures. The Yucatan's *Sopa de Lima* incorporates two of the four—corn and chilies—with the wild turkeys and bitter limes introduced by Spanish conquistadores, to create the region's most popular soup. The key to the soup is bitter lime, a citrus fruit that grows with ease in the Yucatan, and adds a tang to an otherwise salty foundation. Over time, this soup has developed a strong association with the warmth of a grandmother's kitchen; a recipe handed down to youth through participation, rarely accompanied by weights and ratios of ingredients, and often served as a cure-all for the common cold, akin to the chicken soup of Jewish culture.

SOUTHEAST ASIA: FISH SAUCE

Though fish sauce serves largely as a condiment in modern cookery, its prevalence in classic Roman cooking, appearing in majority of recipes in the world's first documented recipe collection from the first century CE, lands it firmly in the class of culinary foundation. Perhaps passed from Europe to Asia along trade routes,[3] fish sauce is now a staple ingredient in many Southeast Asian cultures, including Vietnam, Myanmar, Cambodia, and Thailand, predominantly made from preserved anchovies and often used in place of salt. In Thai cooking, fish sauce is used sparingly to enhance many fish-based dishes, such as Tom Yum Soup, adding an undeniable pungency that concentrates some flavors and heightens others within the dish. The magic of fish sauce is that it can guide a dish, akin to a culinary stock, or blend into the framework, as would a balanced broth.

VIETNAM: PHO

The political climate of Vietnam shaped the origins of *pho*, its most widely known soup dish. Less than a century old, pho evolved alongside French unification with Vietnam. With the political and culinary influence of the French, the Vietnamese began to harvest cows otherwise used for land management, and with the introduction of meat, the French *pot au feu*, or "fire in the pot," evolved into Vietnamese pho. When the country split many years later, so did the varieties of the soup: *pho nam* became the dish of the South, where food was abundant, and *pho bac* became the counterpart of the North. Pho nam is known to be lavish—a heavily spiced broth, rich with a variety of meats, fish sauce, and fresh herbs. Yet it was the impoverished North that is credited with popularizing

FISH SAUCE

ACTIVE TIME: 1 hour | TOTAL TIME: 4 to 6 weeks, including fermentation |
YIELD: About 2 cups

---

1 pound (455 g) fresh sardines or anchovies
3 tablespoons sea salt
4 cloves garlic, minced
3 bay leaves

2 teaspoons black peppercorns
1 tablespoon lemon peel
2 tablespoons Basic Whey (page 303)
1½ cups (350 ml) filtered water, cold

Rinse the fish under cold water. Pat dry with a clean kitchen towel. Chop the fish into ½-inch (1.25 cm) pieces; smaller pieces will yield a greater extraction. Transfer the fish to a bowl and mix in the salt until well combined. Add the garlic, bay leaves, peppercorns, and lemon peel. Transfer the mixture to a mason jar, pressing down to release juices, and pour in the whey. Add enough filtered water to cover the fish mixture, leaving about 1 inch (2.5 cm) headspace in the jar. Cover tightly and leave at room temperature for 3 to 4 days.

Transfer to the refrigerator and ferment for at least 4 weeks and no more than 6 weeks. Line a fine-mesh strainer with cheesecloth and set over a medium bowl. Strain the fish through the strainer, reserving the solids for a second extraction if desired.

Store the liquid in small glass bottles, chilled, up to 6 months.

the dish, using the meat and bones not wanted by their French captors to create the simple beef, broth, and noodle bowl that is prevalent today.[4]

It is my hope that an education about the fundamental stocks encourages a lasting appreciation for slow cookery. Over time, the patience required could become a meditative action, an intuitive process that happens in the background of your kitchen. For many, the French technique of making stocks serves as a springboard into understanding how other cultures perceive a culinary foundation. The next chapter provides historical narrative about how stocks and broths came to be indispensable in the kitchen—starting in the Stone Age and arriving in the modern-day kitchen.

CHAPTER THREE

A Brief History of Stocks and Broths

It might be impossible to detail a complete lineage of stocks and broths—after all, every grandmother has her own version of chicken soup. What's in the stockpot tends toward ubiquity. To render the essence of animal and vegetable matter into a liquid requires three things: A heat source, a vessel, and clean water. Over the centuries, this simple culinary effort has evolved from primal and functional—stock simmered in pit ovens and condensed to pocket-sized coins—to refined and sophisticated—the clearest consommé an indication of culinary excellence. Bones have been reduced to glue, manufactured into Jell-O, and liquefied into broth for the infirm. Revealed within the story of stocks and broths is an example of history repeating itself: Bones, as a foundation, inspire innovation—whether a cube to be reconstituted or a thick soup that boasts restorative properties. The narrative of stocks and broths has always been about extending our food supply to feed more people.

Soup in the Stone Age

For most chefs, the history of stock and broth traces back only as far as Marie-Antoine Carême and Georges Auguste Escoffier—two notable chefs who systemized French cuisine in the early nineteenth and twentieth centuries, respectively. With the correct vessel and proper technique, the modern chef need not be bothered with who made the first bowl of soup. This task is left to the archaeologists who must not only think like a cook, but also an engineer, a geologist, and a physicist, as a means of decoding signs found across ancient landscape. If charred pottery is discovered among rubble, then the question is more about the vessel than its contents. "How did it withstand fire?" comes before "Did it contain soup?"

A recent discovery—perhaps the world's oldest piece of cookware—revealed this line of inquiry. Ofer Bar-Yosef, an archaeologist at Harvard University, unearthed 20,000-year-old pottery from a cave in China. While the pots show scorch marks—a visible sign of exposure to fire—it is doubtful that their organic contents will ever be known. Archaeological features suggest that nomadic foragers inhabited the cave, yet radiocarbon dating places the pottery ten millennia before the appearance of agriculture. The finding simply tells us containers that could withstand heat and water existed much earlier than originally thought.[1]

Thematic to an archaeologist's work—and to the origins of cooking—is this general curiosity: When was man first able to control fire? After all, all you need is a vessel and controlled heat to make a pot of broth. For many years, archaeologists on the hunt for artifacts would find piles of rocks covering sites intended for discovery. These fist-sized rocks were cracked, burnt, discarded—generally seen as a wall interfering with what may lie underneath.

It wasn't until three decades ago that an archaeologist suggested these rocks might also be signs of activity. Further digging, as it were, culminated in the modern belief that rocks were used as a heating element for pit ovens. Cracked rocks were heated over fire until red-hot, transferred to a pit, layered with food, and locked in with dirt for baking, or moist plants for steaming. Dry pits were intended for roasting meat; pits lined with hide held liquid. The process of heating and cooling the rocks would cause them to char and break into identifiable pieces over time.[2] A composite of this archaeological record places the first instance of hot-rock cooking over 25,000 years ago in Western Europe.

And yet with no hard evidence to complete the story, there is a belief that the means to boil was necessary even in the era of Neanderthals.[3] The argument is that our ancestors required a mechanism to render fat from animal bones; the fat was needed to temper a diet rich in lean animal protein. By suspending a waterproof container, using animal hide or perhaps even tree bark, over fire, liquid can be brought to a boil without burning the vessel. Any organic material used for this purpose would have since eroded, leaving no trace for archaeologists. The combination of meaty bones rendered in hot water, then, might date the first broth to about 46,000 years ago—as old as fossil teeth containing starch grains, recently discovered in Iraq.[4]

Further evidence of this methodology was seen much later in the historical preservation sites of American Indians. A more recent record informs us of process:

BLUEBERRY VENISON PEMMICAN

ACTIVE TIME: 1½ hours | **TOTAL TIME:** 1½ days (including dehydrating and resting) |
YIELD: About 12 servings

---

5 pounds (2.3 kg) venison, fat trimmed,
  partially frozen

4½ pounds (2 kg) beef fat, melted
1 cup (170 g) dried blueberries

Slice the venison across the grain into thin strips. Place in a single layer on drying sheets, if using a dehydrator, or on foil-lined sheet pans, if using an oven.

Set your dehydrator to the highest setting or your oven to its lowest setting. Dehydrate until the meat is dry throughout; strips should crack when bent. A dehydrator will take at least 8 hours and an oven will take about 6 hours. Rest the oven-dried meat at room temperature for a full day before grinding.

Assemble a meat grinder with the largest plate. Feed the dry meat into the grinder one strip at a time. Run the meat through a second time to achieve a uniform grind. The meat should appear fibrous and fluffy.

Weigh equal amounts of dried venison and beef fat. Place the beef fat in a saucepan and melt over low heat. Remove from the heat as soon as it has melted. Mix the meat and blueberries into the melted fat and stir to combine.

Using a spoon, transfer into tin molds or a cupcake pan and pack the mixture to remove as much air as possible. Set aside to harden. When set, pemmican can be wrapped and stored in a dark, dry place for many years.

Kill sites and processing areas varied, but typically bones were boiled in pits that had been dug with sticks, or tools fashioned from bones. Once the pit was dug, it was lined with a bison hide (furry side down), and filled with water, using bladders, or other containers. American Indians used rocks to crush the longer bones of the animal into pieces the size of potato chips or smaller. These were put into the water along with red-hot stones that were carried with sticks or antlers from a nearby fire. Heat from the stones caused the water to boil, liquefying the fats trapped in the bone matrix. These fats floated to the surface where they solidified as the water was allowed to cool. Finally, it [the fat] was skimmed off. Much of the grease was used to make pemmican; a mixture of pulverized jerky and dried berries, held together by the nutritious grease.[5]

While this doesn't put an actual date on the world's first bowl of soup, it informs us that broths have likely been around since long before our ancestors. We also begin to realize that the goals then were not so much different than today: a need for sustenance and a desire to waste nothing.

Sauce in Medieval Times

There is much that intrigues in the first collection of recipes ever documented: an expansive compendium assembled by a wealthy epicure, Marcus Gavius Apicius, in the first century CE. The many translations of *The Art of Cooking (De Re Coquinaria)* lend to a wild variance in interpretation and subtleties of language, in part because the recipes came from many sources, including Apicius's own elaborate nose-to-tail instruction. It wasn't until the late fourth or early fifth century that the recipes were formally compiled into numerous volumes.[6]

As the first thorough composition on cooking—about 500 recipes across ten books—there were no previous standards by which to write a recipe. The books are logically organized by focal ingredient, similar to the second part of this book—from meat to seafood to vegetables, and so on. Yet recipes are written for an advanced audience, guiding the reader only with general direction. Ingredients are embedded within the recipe, rarely with indication of quantity or ratio. Apicius was required reading for a confident cook of the era.

Nearly every recipe in the text includes a sauce, most of which were fermented, though the distinction between liquid and ferment was confused throughout history. The first translation—*Cookery and Dining in Imperial Rome*—completed by Joseph Dommers Vehling in 1936—separated these liquids by definition: liquamen and garum. *Liquamen* referred to any kind of liquid—whether stock or broth, savory or sweet—and leaned on the reader to determine which was best for the occasion. The translation instructs the reader to use the "best kind of broth" for the dish without any detailed explanation. Brine, too, fit within the category of liquamen.[7]

Garum, on the other hand, refers to a type of fermented fish sauce primarily used as a condiment to intensify a dish. A host of recipes were employed to manufacture garum, yet autolysis was always at the core of the process. The blood and intestines of fish, such as anchovies, sardines, and mackerel, were crushed and fermented in brine. Each batch was cured in the sun, a process that stimulates water osmosis and protein dissolution, in turn producing a clear liquid. Strained from the fermenting vessel, the liquor was bottled and graded for quality, leaving sediment—called *allec*—to be gathered as a secondary condiment. Garum, priced at a premium with tariff attached, was afforded by the upper class, often used as an ingredient in a recipe; while allec, with its thick texture-limiting application, was reserved for the poor.

Given its high cost, garum was commonly blended to make *oenogarum*—a dressing of wine, olive oil, vinegar, and other spices—and served tableside with every type of dish, from steamed seafood to boiled meat. Mixed with vinegar alone, it was called *oxygarum*; with honey, it was known as *mellogarum*. Indeed, if food was too salty,

What is called *liquamen* is thus made: the intestines of fish are thrown into a vessel, and are salted; and small fish, especially *atherinae*, or small mullets, or *maenae*, or *lycostomi*, or any small fish, are all salted in the same manner; and they are seasoned in the sun, and frequently turned; and when they have been seasoned in the heat, the *garum* is thus taken from them. A small basket of close texture is laid in the vessel filled with the small fish already mentioned, and the *garum* will flow in the basket; and they take up what has been percolated through the basket, which is called *liquamen*; and the remainder of the feculence is made into *allec*.

—*Geōponika: Agricultural pursuits, Vol. II*, translated from the Greek by Thomas Owen, 1806

honey was added to balance flavor. Diluted with water, *hydrogarum* was imbibed by the Roman legions. Fish sauce, too, was used as an ointment for many ailments:

> *Fish sauces also were used as an unguent in healing, both for humans and animals (Pliny, XXXI.96ff). Allec was said to cure scabies in sheep and also was a good antidote for the bite of a dog (or sea dragon). Garum heals burns, although the patient should not know that it is being used, and is especially efficacious for ulcers and the bites of crocodiles. The veterinary authors Pelagonius and Vegetius, writing in the fourth century AD and copying remedies from earlier sources, also recommend treatments using garum and liquamen.* [8]

As documented in the *Corpus Inscriptionum Latinarum IV*, liquamen and garum were considered two distinct liquids. Over the course of centuries, however, liquamen and garum became interchangeable. This is perhaps because Apicius's collection came from many sources and direct translations failed to achieve consistency across recipes. One academic writes:

> *The picture of fish sauce that emerges from the ancient literature is complex. The ancient writers who discuss these products do so without the precision we need and often contradict each other so that precise understanding of which sauce corresponds to which recipe, production process or name is less than clear.* [9]

A deeper assessment of who wrote the recipes and how they were compiled is necessary to truly understand the subtleties of the text. Luckily, by the fifth century, *garum* was the term of choice, strictly referring to fish sauce, and has since remained the prevailing reference. The contemporary fermented anchovy sauce of Campania, Italy, called *colatura di alici*, is considered a derivative of early garum.[10]

While garum is neither stock nor broth, its historical precedence is significant: Liquamen, a basic foundation in cookery, evolved into garum, a concentrated liquid to enhance the flavor of almost any dish. With fish being more prevalent than meat in ancient Rome, and an emphasis by Apicius on using the whole animal, it makes sense that garum was the condiment of choice.

So proficient was Apicius at whole animal cooking that a recipe might begin with what to feed an animal preceding its harvest. One recipe instructs the cook to treat the liver of sows as you would geese, stuffing with dried fruit, but not before giving the live animal honeyed wine just before slaughter. His recipes took care to waste nothing, going so far as to instruct on how to improve a broth:

> *If a broth has contracted a bad odor, place a vessel upside-down and fumigate it with laurel and cypress and before ventilating it, pour the broth in this vessel. If this does not help matters and if the taste is too pronounced, add honey and fresh spikenard to it; that will improve it.*[11]

Barring the modern-day difficulty of locating spikenard, an essential oil from the Himalayas, I don't recommend this method today. (Very simply, toss it if it smells off.) With his propensity for outlandish ingredients and far-reaching procedures, it seems appropriate that Apicius included a range of recipes that also assist digestion.

Apicius's dedication to gastronomy was significant: Upon losing his wealth, overwhelmed with debt and unable to continue a life of gluttony, he killed himself in despair. One historian refers to Apicius as the world's first celebrity chef, on account of his grand exit.[12]

Broth of the Explorers

This book would be incomplete without a nod to the dehydrated broth of history's most famous explorers. It took three centuries of sporadic documentation and various applications—from rations for soldiers to an energy elixir for male travelers—before it landed on the voyage of Lewis and Clark.

Portable soup—a type of dry gelatin with an indefinite shelf life—first appeared in the unpublished notes of Sir Hugh Plat, an English inventor and writer on agriculture, in the late sixteenth century. His recipe was simple: Reduce broth from the boiled feet or legs of six or eight cows until strong and stiff like jelly; air-dry on clean cloth; cut and powder with flour to prevent sticking. For a personal touch, the soup coins could be stamped for distinction. Produced only in winter months and stored in wooden boxes, portable soup would keep for years, making it an ideal "Victual of Warr," per Plat's description of his invention. He envisioned the use of his portable soup as rations for soldiers in the field and sailors out at sea.[13]

Plat knew a thing or two about cooking: He advised that the jelly should not be cooked with salt or sugar, else the flavors would concentrate in an undesirable manner in the pot. Instead, one could add rosewater for aroma and saffron for color, bread for sustenance, or isinglass for thickness. Only upon reconstitution would the soup be met with spices.

Portable soup was such a convenient discovery that it became popular with families and travelers, too. In 1690, "bouillons en tablettes" appeared in Antoine Furetière's *Dictionnaire universel*, referencing consommé in tablet form or a broth that could be carried by pocket. A recipe by Mrs. Ann Blencowe revealed *veal glew*, paper-wrapped slabs of veal jelly, in her *Receipt Book* only four years later. About half a century thereafter, a more elaborate recipe appeared in a subscription journal, adding a host of warm spices, a touch of anchovy, and a heel of bread.[14] A simpler version was offered by William Byrd II, a botanist from the South, who recommended his "Glue-Broth" as a wholesome solution for fatigued travelers.[15] By the late 1700s, newspaper advertisements were promoting canisters of portable soup as a pleasing sipper for gentlemen on long trips.

Despite the documented origins of portable soup, it was a female innkeeper who received credit for the invention by the Royal Navy in 1756. The widow of a French chef, Mrs. Dubois won a contract to produce portable soup for the fleet, enough to provide sailors with a daily ration. Filling and nutritious, portable soup was believed to prevent scurvy at sea. Successors honored her place in history, printing acknowledgment on advertising materials long after the contract was complete: "Successor to Messieurs Bennet and Dubois, The Original Portable Soup-Makers to His Majesty's Royal Navy."[16]

And so, portable soup became cargo on vessels set for long journeys. Aboard both of his South Seas voyages, Captain James Cook mandated consumption of the reconstituted broth by his sailors, flogging those who refused. Combined with hot water and *pease flour*, a meal made from yellow field peas, portable soup was an unappealing porridge. Punishment might've been easier to endure.

Alongside an extensive list of goods packed for transport—double sets of oars, matching pairs of stockings, arms and accoutrements, presents set aside for Indians—there was little in the way of comestibles among the stash on Meriwether Lewis's and William Clark's Corps of Discovery. Subsistence was to be achieved through self-sufficient means—hunting by land, fishing by sea, and trading with foreigners along the way. Yet portable soup was supplied in abundance. *National Geographic* reports:

> *Under Provisions and Means of Subsistence, Lewis lists assorted spices, three bushels of salt, and 193 pounds of "Portable Soup," which last—a reduced and dehydrated mix of beef broth, eggs, and vegetables—was the nineteenth century's version of space food. It was intended for periods of dire dietary emergency.* [17]

Seventeen months into the expedition, with fewer pheasants foraged than men to feed, portable soup was removed from storage and put on the menu. The taste was so revolting that the men decided to sacrifice a horse instead.

There is a certain emphasis on the convenience of pocket soup throughout history; rarely is it associated with pleasing the palate. When asked how long to simmer the mixture, one recipe advises until "the meat has lost its virtue." This is a sentiment shared by Hannah Glasse, author of *The Art of Cookery Made Plain and Easy*, an eighteenth-century cookbook that was written for household servants and the emerging middle class. In *The Far Side of the World*, the tenth historical novel of the Aubrey-Maturin series, Patrick O'Brian writes, "Dr. Maturin had flung his slabs of portable soup into the sea, on the grounds that they were nothing but common glue, an imposture and a vile job."

The invention of canned meats in the early 1800s quickly diminished the popularity of portable soup. An article about the comparative health of sailors appeared in 1815, debunking the nutritional benefits of portable soup. No longer would seamen have to endure drinking this sludge for sustenance.

Soldiers—forever the recipients of ready-to-eat meals—were not so lucky. French chef Alexis Soyer developed an improved version of portable soup for the malnourished troops of the Crimean War. More of a vegetal cake, his portable soup included carrots, turnips, parsnips, onions, cabbage, celery, leeks, and seasonings. When added to water, these large slabs, known as "coarse julienne," could feed one hundred men. The flavor was well received; presumably morale improved.[18]

Popular long before the release of Jell-O, these unctuous amber blocks were first the predecessor to industrial meat extract and bouillon cubes; portable soup

RECIPE FOR PORTABLE SOUP

The following is the complete recipe for Hannah Glasse's portable soup as it appears in *The Art of Cookery Made Plain and Easy*, first published in 1747 and still in circulation. Per the author's instructions, the dried glue can be dissolved in boiling water to make soup, gravy, or sauce, perhaps enhanced with truffles or morels, to your liking.

TO MAKE PORTABLE SOUP

Take two legs of beef, about fifty pounds weight, take off the skin and fat as well as you can, then take all the meat and sinews clean from the bones, which meat put into a large pot, and put to it eight or nine gallons of soft water; first make it boil, then put in twelve anchovies, an ounce of mace, a quarter of an ounce of cloves, an ounce of whole pepper black and white together, six large onions peeled and cut in two, a little bundle of thyme, sweet marjoram, and winter-savoury, the dry hard crust of a two penny loaf, stir it all together and cover it close, lay a weight on the cover to keep it close down, and let it boil softly for eight or nine hours, then uncover it, and stir it together; cover it close again, and let it boil till it is a very rich good jelly, which you will know by taking a little out now and then, and letting it cool. When you think it is a thick jelly, take it off, strain it through a coarse hair bag, and press it hard; then strain it through a hair sieve into a large earthen pan; when it is quite cold, take off the scum and fat, and take the fine jelly clear from the settlings at bottom, and then put the jelly into a large deep well tinned stew-pan. Set it over a stove with a slow fire, keep stirring it often, and take great care it neither flicks to the pan or burns. When you find the jelly very stiff and thick, as it will be in lumps about the pan, take it out, and put it into large deep china-cups, or well-glazed earthenware. Fill the pan two-thirds full of water, and when the water boils, set in your cups. Be sure no water gets into the cups, and keep the water boiling softly all the time till you find the jelly is like a stiff glue; take out the cups, and when they are cool, turn out the glue into a coarse new flannel. Let it lay eight or nine hours, keeping it in a dry warm place, and turn it on fresh flannel till it is quite dry, and the glue will be quite hard; put it into clean new stone pots, keep it close covered from dust and dirt, in a dry place, and where no damp can come to it.

and its derivatives were used as an expedient building block for cooking. To attest to the considerable shelf life of portable soup, one gentleman tasted a tablet in 1930 that was believed to be from Captain Cook's cargo. Well over a century old, the soup did not kill him. It is not surprising, then, that Jell-O, with its tacky texture and unlimited shelf life, was developed by the owner of a glue factory.[19]

As the years went on, palates progressed and portable soup lost its mobility. In the *Household Cyclopedia*, published in 1881, a variation on the standard recipe appeared that had a limited shelf life. Portable soup is also a precursor of Escoffier's glace de viande, which came many years later and remains a fundamental tool in French cookery to this day. Not much has changed: Processed bouillon is still convenient and bland; a homemade reduction, by contrast, requires patience in the kitchen and pleases the appetite. See Soup Cubes, page 335, for a modern-day version of portable soup.

The Science of Food Manipulation

One small box, one knife handle, or a dozen buttons made of bone: All of them correspond to a broth that has been robbed from the poor.

—ANTOINE CADET DE VAUX, chemist (1743–1828)

Throughout the late eighteenth century and well into the next, food scarcity was a hot topic in France, and in part, a catalyst for the French Revolution. When liberal economists effected a deregulation of the grain market, bread became less affordable; a frustration among consumers that led to revolt in times of poor harvests. Politicians—aware that food shortage was a threat to the stability of their power—turned to scientists for answers: How can we alter fresh food to extend supply and derive more nutrition?

It sounds like the same question asked by modern-day Monsanto and other industrial giants. Indeed, this was an era where manipulating fresh food or synthesizing new edibles was the government's solution to feeding more people. Historian E. C. Spary writes that "the authority of scientific and medical practitioners in France was not exercised at the individual level, but was derived from their membership of government-supported institutions."[20] This led to a common belief that refining and processing food through means of chemical extraction led to healthier products. It was perhaps the birth of industrial food: Regular flour, for instance, was enhanced into potato flour; meat and bones were reduced to extract.

With animal protein in limited supply, food chemists endeavored to prove gelatin from bones held as much nutritive value as meat. Some chemists theorized that gelatin was a worthwhile supplement for invalids in hospitals and an economical solution for the poor, and the government enjoyed this theory enough to encourage further development. One scientist, Antoine Cadet de Vaux, claimed that broth from one pound of bones was comparable to six pounds of meat. To him, bone was "a bouillon tablet formed by nature," and required recovery from industrial use—a time when buttons and dominoes were made from bone—and care in the kitchen as a means to assist the poor.

Inspired by de Vaux's work, Jean-Pierre-Joseph d'Arcet resolved to dedicate his life in pursuit of discovering a gelatin-based solution that could enhance nitrogen in food for impoverished communities. He developed an elaborate steam-extraction method that took five days to execute and produced a gel intended for hotels and hospitals to feed ill residents. Motivated by his initial results, d'Arcet opened a gelatin production plant and invented other mechanisms to extract gelatin, including a digester that dissolved bone with acid.

His broth, though certified as nutritious by medical faculty, was met with distaste by patients and criticism from peers. Many referred to his broth regimen as a starvation diet and some patients developed digestive problems. One hospital reported only a slight savings by using the gelatin over regular bouillon; it was not enough to justify the account. De Vaux's work was also accused of exaggerating results in an effort to advance his cause of feeding the poor.[21]

In 1831, the Academy of Sciences responded to industry criticism by forming a Gelatin Commission; its intentions were to conduct empirical research on the nutritional properties of gelatin. After nearly a decade of experimentation, the results belied the expectation: Their findings about gelatin were inconclusive; contradictory data introduced questions more about their methods than the subject itself.[22]

Some thirty years prior, the French military awarded Nicolas Appert 12,000 francs for validating a method of preserving food sealed in glass jars—a directive from Napoleon Bonaparte himself. Per the terms of his contract, Appert published *The Art of Preserving All Kinds of Animal and Vegetable Substances for Several Years*, which detailed his procedure for the public. He then opened the first canning factory in the world and proceeded to seek patents on foodstuffs in jars—from beef and poultry to milk and eggs. Appert's biggest claim to fame, however, was preserving an entire sheep in a crock.[23]

Appert also submitted a patent for dehydrated bouillon in the same year the Gelatin Commission formed and identified a method for extracting gelatin from bones without the use of acid. His bouillon patent was dismissed as being an unoriginal concept. And yet he succeeded in developing a heat-sealed technology without understanding the scientific relationship between microbes and food decay—a discovery attributed to Louis Pasteur over fifty years later.

At the same time Appert's research on dehydrated bouillon was under review, German chemist Justus von Liebig published a journal about organic chemistry that would establish him as the founder of the field. Liebig was known for his work in agricultural chemistry: He discovered the significance of nitrogen and other organic compounds in plant life and was responsible for the first nitrogen-based fertilizer. Perhaps shaped by his childhood experience with climate-induced famine—widely known as the "Year Without a Summer" (1816)—it was only a matter of time before Liebig would apply his theoretical findings to everyday needs, like subsistence.[24]

In the 1840s, Liebig shifted his attention from plants to animals for the same reason as his peers: He hoped to use scientific means to increase food supply for the poor. His research in plant and animal metabolism helped him develop theories about meat cookery. For instance, Liebig believed meat juices, in addition to meat fiber, were nutritionally significant, and he is responsible for the (now debunked) idea that meat retains its juices when seared.[25] Using this logic, he identified a method of reducing meat to what he thought was its most essential nutrients—a portable beef-based extract to be reconstituted in water. There was only one problem: The product was extraordinarily expensive to produce. His extract was of such substantial quality that it required thirty pounds of meat for every one pound of extract. It took fifteen years of small-batch production before a commercial plan came about—one that involved cheap land, plentiful with cattle, close to a port that could ship overseas.

With the first arrival of extract to Europe in 1865, Liebig and his partner finally launched a commercial enterprise: Liebig Extract of Meat Co., a concentrated meat base—thick as molasses—promoted for its medicinal properties. Advertisements were not shy to point out the virtues of tea made with the extract—those who imbibed it would soothe their digestion by day and experience "brain-excitement" by night. Liebig went so far as to promote meat tea as a treatment for typhus and pelvic inflammation. With an endorsement from the Royal Medical and Chirurgical Society of London, it wasn't long before hospitals began using the extract as part of patient regimen.

As momentum grew for the extract, so did skepticism about its nutritional significance. Analysis revealed that the product was low in protein and fat, and critics accused Liebig of misleading consumers. The company boasted that each batch was made from a large quantity of meat, and yet the quantity of nutrients in each jar was nowhere near comparable. The medical claims associated with the brand were unfounded and their customers were catching on.

Pressure from chemists, and perhaps even sabotage from competitors, forced the company to simplify their approach—from a medicinal application to a convenient way to make soup. Instead of marketing the product to hospitals for the infirm, the extract was advertised as indispensable to the home cook.

It was in this manner that concentrated meat base became a household staple, eventually adopted by soldiers in times of war. By the 1900s, Liebig Extract of Meat Co. was producing around 500 tons of extract each year.[26]

Over the next century, the company traded hands and transitioned into other products many times. But not before it left an advertising legacy: A year before Liebig's death, the company began producing print materials, such as calendars, stamps, children's games, and trading cards. Elaborate in design and varied in content, these cards were crafted by famous artists and were the first of their kind to be produced using lithography. The cards—arriving in series of a half dozen to a dozen and published in many languages—quickly became collector's items across Europe. The final printing was in 1975 (a full century of publication!), and cards can still be found in collections around the world.[27]

Soon after meat extract hit its commercial stride, and perhaps because its nutritional value had been discredited, chemists developed a cheaper version: a liquid bouillon that was quickly changed into a dehydrated format for ease of use and distribution. These are the little salty cubes that are common today. Three of the earliest bouillon companies remain in production: Maggi, Knorr, and Oxo, a companion company to Liebig Extract of Meat Co. The contemporary version of meat extract—sold as Oxoid Lab-Lemco Beef Extract Powder—is an industrial ingredient used for fermentation processes.[28]

Influence of the French

From eighteenth-century bouillon to nineteenth-century business, from miniature soup-cup to Rabelaisian excess, from sensibility to politics: these are the transitions that defined the term "restaurant."

—REBECCA L. SPANG, *The Invention of the Restaurant*

In sixteenth-century France, alongside the popularity of portable soup, street vendors were known to sell thick, cheap soup as a restorative elixir. These establishments were the first to use the word *restaurant*—from the French verb *restaurer*, to restore—and served a bouillon that would relax digestion and refresh the spirit.

Now refuted by some historians, the legend begins with a sign that advertised restorative soups in the shop window of a Parisian chef: *Venite ad me vos qui stomacho laboratis et ego restaurabo vos.* "Come to me, all who labor in the stomach, and I will restore you," read the sign. Remembered by his last name only, Chef Boulanger is reputedly the first restaurant owner to serve soup as an elixir. His endeavor was so popular that he added a sheep's feet stew to the menu for sustenance. Adding a second dish was an infringement on the strict regulations of the Caterers' Guild—the duality of his offerings proved disruptive to other establishments and led to a court settlement. The ruling favored Boulanger, an action that surprised many and gradually led to the popular use of the word *restaurant*. Here customers could find not only comfort in a warm cup of broth but also convenience in the selection of a variety of dishes.[29]

In *The Food of Paris*, Marie-Noel Rio explains the process of making a restaurant, or restorative meat broth:

> *The restaurant is made from beef, mutton, veal, capon; young pigeon, partridge, onions, root vegetables, and fine herbs. It is steamed, but without using any liquid, in a pot whose lid is sealed with pastry. The pot is put in a bain-marie for five to six hours, after which this decidedly succulent broth is sieved and the fat removed. Once this operation has been completed, then a loaf of bread is hollowed out and is filled with the minced and seasoned meat from capons and other fine cuts, before being poached in the bubbling broth. Before serving, it is garnished with cockscombs, calf sweetbread, and other delicacies browned in smoked bacon.* [30]

The restaurants of today—with their flexible à la carte menus, long hours of operation, and ability to accommodate parties of all sizes—did not fully materialize until after the French Revolution, when chefs of many fallen aristocrats were out of jobs and able to open their own establishments. It was around this time that the audience for cookbooks also shifted: Once designed only for professionals—chefs to noblemen, *traiteurs* of cookhouses, servants to the wealthy—recipes were also being written for a new middle class that emerged from significant political change. As advances in agriculture were creating an abundance of food, chefs were given license to expand their creativity and home cooks were invited to enhance their knowledge.

Tracing the lineage of pot au feu—the classic French "pot on a fire" of boiled beef and vegetables—helps elucidate these culinary advancements across the classes. Though the French did not document pot au feu until the Revolution, its origins can be found nearly two centuries prior during the reign of King Henry IV of France. A decree from the king acknowledged the efficiency of one-pot cooking: "I want no peasant in my kingdom to be so poor that he cannot have a *poule au pot* on Sundays." And yet his statement was one of wishful thinking, a politician's blind promise to infuse wealth across his land: While simmering a whole chicken with vegetables is an efficient way to feed a family, only the rich or the bold—those who endeavored to hunt illegally on royal land—could afford poultry at that time. The French soon adopted the term *pot-pourri*—a "rotten" pot—to describe combining a variety of food in one vessel and cooking it for a length of time. Together, the etymology of poule au pot and pot-pourri reveal the economy of the process more than the contents of the pot.

Carême published the earliest French recipes for pot au feu. Intended for a professional audience, his recipes were preceded by a description that spanned multiple pages and discussed finer merits of the dish—from its suitability for the infirm to its versatility across all classes. Of particular interest to Carême and his colleagues was the importance of the bouillon, the liquid in the pot—believed to be dense with nutrients—and the *bouilli*, the resulting meat, tender if simmered for an adequate length of time. Pot au feu was commonly served in courses—warm broth as starter, beef and vegetables as entrée—perhaps an indication of why Carême, who is credited with degustation dining in France, showed interest in the dish. Over time, pot au feu would appear in recipes as an ingredient, referring only to the leftover broth from the stew itself.[31]

Englishman Jules Gouffé documented the significance of bouilli in an economical pot au feu for the home cook, reserving an entire chapter to introduce its preparation.[32] With the rise of the middle class, home cooks were redesigning their kitchens—hearths transitioned from fireplace to stove, later fueled by gas and oil. Pot au feu was an ideal dish to be made at home, relying on residual heat to hold a steady simmer for hours after the stove was extinguished.

While Apicius appeals to some as the first celebrity chef due to his dramatic death, Carême more often receives the title, given his influence on global cuisine. In addition to his extensive documentation on French cookery, he is also responsible for designing a comprehensive list of sauces, categorized as four *mother sauces*. These original sauces are béchamel, Espagnole, velouté, and allemande—three of which begin with stock as a formative ingredient. About a century later, Escoffier revised Carême's structure in *Le Guide Culinaire* by grouping allemande within the velouté class and adding two additional mother sauces: hollandaise and tomate. These five mother sauces are still recognized today.

Escoffier is credited with the standardization of French cuisine in the early twentieth century. He refined Carême's approach to *haute cuisine*, streamlining the ornate and bringing order to the professional kitchen. Escoffier offered a streamlined approach to cooking while maintaining elegance. As the recognized architect of veal stock, it is no surprise that he used stock in everything, relying less on heavy cream-based sauces than his predecessors. Escoffier insisted stock was the workhorse of the kitchen, the backbone of good cooking—an essential building block that required time to produce and yet simplified the subsequent cooking experience.

Stock and Broth in Today's Kitchen

Unlike early French influence, when science was believed to unlock nutrition in plants and animals, many modern-day cooks have gone back to the source. On a happy farm, soil health determines agricultural methodology and quality of harvest, and ultimately what goes in the stockpot. Even fast food—impacted by a decline in sales and a consumer demand for transparency—is being reinvented. Some restaurateurs are showing an increased interest in quality sourcing and a decreased reliance on efficiency. Chefs are endeavoring to make food go further and lessen waste.

My education about stocks began with the influence of Thomas Keller and has evolved into an academic pursuit to better comprehend our agricultural construct. Fellow value-added producers, such as Jessica Prentice of Three Stone Hearth in Berkeley, CA, and conscientious chefs, like Marco Canora of Brodo in New York City, are helping shape a new broth category. Inherent to the success of this category is the significance of supporting a regional food system, making use of ingredients once destined for the incinerator. With it comes a promise that producers will select ingredients responsibly and treat them with integrity. Despite a suppressed economy, annual reports show that small-batch soup companies are gaining momentum while the Campbell Soup Company of old is in decline.[33] For the first time in the history of industrialized food, we have better options—from the supermarket and from our land—and this translates to a richer brew in the pot.

The first supermarket supposedly appeared on the American landscape in 1946. That is not very long ago. Until then, where was all the food? Dear folks, the food was in homes, gardens, local fields, and forests. It was near kitchens, near tables, near bedsides. It was in the pantry, the cellar, the backyard.

—JOEL SALATIN, *Folks, This Ain't Normal: A Farmer's Advice for Happier Hens, Healthier People, and a Better World*

CHAPTER FOUR

The Composition
of Stocks and Broths

In certain cultures, there is a dogmatic belief that the strength of an animal is absorbed by the person who consumes it—sometimes even a direct correlation from heart to heart, liver to liver, limb to limb. Tiger wine, for instance, is an elixir made from tiger bones and rice wine, available on the Chinese black market. It is believed to be a remedy for arthritis, improve circulation, and enhance overall *qi*, our circulating life force. Those who consume it trust they will gain the "strength of a tiger and the senses of a predator."[1]

The practice of drinking tiger wine is steeped in a rich history of Chinese medicine—every part of the tiger thought to remedy a long list of ailments. Following a recent ban on the domestic trade of tiger bone, some practitioners rejected the efficacy of tiger-based antidotes, and sales went underground.[2] Today, there are as few as 3,200 wild tigers around the world. As tiger populations continue to decline, their black-market value increases. All this even though there is little to no scientific evidence that validates the medical hypotheses believed by some practitioners.

Similarly, there is surprisingly little research in support of the popular notion that nutritive broths are a miracle cure.[3] Medical claims are many, ranging from the healing of a leaky gut to the strengthening of our bones; correlations made from the composition of various broths to unique parts of the body. And while most of the claims about bone broths do not have direct scientific evidence to back them up, the research that *does* exist shows a positive trend—for example, reduced inflammation and increased hydration. Yet there is much we don't know.

When customers ask if our animal products qualify as bone broths, I tell them they do. After all, we take high-quality bones and simmer them until properly rendered, extracting as much flavor and gelatin as possible without compromising culinary integrity of the product. We are as much a culinary stock company as we are a nutritive broth company; the secret is the quality of our source materials and the care with which our products are made. As an organization, we endeavor to support studies that prove our mothers right: We *want* chicken soup to cure what ails us!

The good news is that well-made stocks and broths are undoubtedly better for you than what you find in a box or a can. The bad news is that it might not be the cure-all we had hoped for. But what is a cure-all anyway? True health is more about our diet as a whole than any one part. Nevertheless, the known benefits validate the pursuit of additional research.

At the time of publication, Brooklyn Bouillon is designing studies to fill in the academic and industrial gaps that have occurred over the decades. We endeavor to explore how the body absorbs mineral and amino acid content when rendered in a stockpot. We hope to find evidence that well-sourced ingredients make as positive an impact on the body as they do on the land. For now, we'll review the research published to date while remaining content with the sublime knowledge that homemade stocks are good for the soul.

Assessing Bone Broths

There are many perspectives on how to make bone broth. Some recipes advocate soaking bones in vinegar to assist leaching minerals before heating; most suggest simmering bones upward of twenty-four hours in the same bath. In this text, I apply French culinary technique to their assembly: A remouillage separates the lengthy cook time, ensuring enough heat distribution to render bones without emulsifying the liquid. I insist on high-quality bones with healthy marrow content. I recommend skimming for clarity—I don't encourage cooking until the bones crumble. Soaking the bones in vinegar is optional. This modified approach takes existing studies and basic nutritional science into account and lands firmly in the belief that a nutritive broth should be as delicious as a culinary stock.

It appears that culinary arts and nutritional science were at a similar crossroads in the early part of the twentieth century. In 1934 a study was published in the *Archives of Disease in Childhood* to examine the nutritional components of bone and vegetable broths. The study was a response to the common practice of feeding bone broth to infants; its fortifying effects were widely believed to strengthen newborns despite a lack of empirical evidence. While the study is over eighty years old, the findings are still relevant.

Broths were prepared in the following manner:

The bones are chopped to expose marrow, covered with water containing a small amount of vinegar, and simmered for 4 to 9 hours. Chopped vegetables such as potatoes, carrots, greens, and onions are added, and the simmering is continued for a further hour. The bones and vegetables are then strained off, and the broth is set to a jelly. Most recipes advise that the final volume should be 1 pint per pound of bones. [4]

The study investigated the rate of protein and mineral extraction from bones and vegetables by three points: temperature, time, and acidity. A copper-reduction method that is still in use today was employed to identify sugars. Batches made in the kitchen were prepared in iron, enamel, and aluminum vessels; those constructed in a laboratory were made in glass. Commercial broths were also compared with those prepared for the study. As a final point of comparison, the research assessed the nutritional value of human and cow milk against the broth findings. Here is what they discovered:

TEMPERATURE

Mineral extraction from bones was compared between two batches of water: one kept at room temperature and another set at 212°F (100°C). To be expected, the loss of nitrogen was consistent over cook time and markedly less at room temperature, supporting the idea that soluble proteins diffuse during the conversion of collagen to gelatin in a heated environment. Of particular interest was the finding that greater amounts of iron, calcium, and magnesium were extracted from the bones set in room-temperature water.

For vegetables, the study confirmed that soluble nutrients of chopped produce were not lost in room-temperature water. This is because vegetables are alive and with their external membrane intact, as opposed to bones, which lose their semi-permeable membrane upon processing. When heated, however, vegetables quickly lost their nitrogen, calcium, iron, potassium, sugars, and starch.

TIME

When testing bones in water at 212°F (100°C) and at room temperature, the loss of potassium was rapid in the first hour for both temperatures and tapered off in subsequent hours. Calcium, iron, and magnesium were fully extracted within the first hour for both bodies of water. The only protein that was extracted from either was gelatin, and only from bones—extraction increased over the length of cook time. Fat was also extracted from the bones. All vegetables lost their soluble nutrients within one hour of being cooked in simmering water.

ACIDITY

The sample that included one tablespoon of acetic acid had the lowest pH as compared with a sample with no acid and another with twice the acid. The study concluded that the addition of vinegar had little impact on the rate of protein and mineral extraction. The expectation that acid would not affect the extraction of calcium was confirmed; this is because the acid is too weak to penetrate collagen, where calcium phosphate is embedded.

Other findings include the following:

- There was no difference in iron detected in broths made across all vessel types. The amount found in the broth was comparable to an amount typically found in cow's milk.
- All of the starch in the broth was extracted from vegetables; none came from bones.
- All fat in the broth was isolated from bones, as well as all phosphorous, copper, sodium, and chlorine.

This study concluded that milk is a better source of nutritional value for infants than bone broth. The supposition was based on earlier findings that protein in gelatin harnesses "limited biological value"—a claim that has been refuted since this study. While milk might contain more nutrients, bone broth is a good alternative for those who cannot tolerate lactose; it also contains less sugar than milk.

An interesting observation from the study is that minerals are extracted early in the cooking process. Trace minerals ebb off within an hour or two of simmering animal protein, and even less for vegetables. An extended period in the pot, then, is intended only to break down bones and extract gelatin into the liquid. This evidence supports my suggestion to measure cooking time based on the size of bones. For instance, chicken bones require less simmering time than beef bones.

I also recommend maintaining water temperature at 18 degrees lower than the 212°F (100°C) stated in the study—180°F (82°C). This measure helps prevent emulsification, and might lessen (but not prevent) the denaturation of nutrients in the pot. Brooklyn Bouillon has designed a study that intends to examine how various bone types respond to different points in time and temperature. Our theory is that the quantity of gelatin extracted is sufficient *before* bones crumble; that a law of diminishing returns might occur as the bones become spent—before they turn a satisfactory cooking stock into a muddy mess.

Consistent with the findings in the *Archives of Disease in Childhood* study, the USDA database reveals average mineral content found in homemade beef and chicken broth. In one cup of beef broth, calcium and magnesium account for 2 percent and 4 percent of the daily value, respectively, with less in chicken broth. Quantity of potassium is valuable but not significant, ranging from 7 to 12 percent of the daily value. Additional trace minerals include phosphate, glucosamine,

TABLE 4.1. Comparison of Commercial Stocks and Broths (per 100 g)

	Beef Stock (frozen)	Beef Broth (can)	Beef Broth, Lower Sodium (box)
Water	19.9 g	97.55 g	98 g
Energy	124 calories	7 calories	6 calories
Protein	9.5 g	1.14 g	1.2 g
Fat	5.1 g	0.22 g	0.08 g
Carbohydrate	10.1 g	0.04 g	0.21 g
Sugars	0.3 g	0.00 g	0.20 g
Calcium	55.4 mg	6 mg	2 mg
Iron	1.4 mg	0.17 mg	0.04 mg
Magnesium	7.7 mg	2 mg	1 mg
Phosphorous	46.9 mg	13 mg	10 mg
Potassium	124 mg	54 mg	23 mg
Sodium	103 mg	372 mg	180 mg
Zinc	0.4 mg	0.00 mg	0.32 mg
Thiamin	0.1 mg	0.002 mg	0.02 mg
Riboflavin	0.0 mg	0.021 mg	0.085 mg
Niacin	0.2 mg	0.78 mg	0.5 mg
Vitamin B_6	0.4 mg	0.01 mg	0.107 mg
Vitamin B_{12}	0.0 mg	0.07 mg	0 mg
Vitamin A	2.7 IU	0 mg	0 mg
Vitamin E	0.0 mg	0 mg	0 mg
Cholesterol	21.4 mg	0 mg	0 mg

chondroitin, glycine, phosphorous, hyaluronic acid, proline, sulfur, and sodium. Iron is also present in negligible quantities.[5] Not surprisingly, homemade broth contains significantly more protein—about 6 to 12 grams per cup—and considerably less sugar than commercial brands. A recent assessment of sugar in the American diet revealed that one 10.75-ounce container of Campbell's Classic Tomato Soup on the Go has the equivalent sugar content of two Krispy Kreme doughnuts.[6]

Most contemporary studies look at the impact of hydrolyzed supplements on our bodies (and sometimes only in rats) in research trials.[7] The challenge with this approach is twofold: Daily supplements are delivered in higher concentrations than found in a daily portion of bone broth, and supplements are processed in a manner that increases bioavailability. With all the approaches to making bone broth, and few actual studies using bone broth as the indicator, it is difficult to establish a baseline for bone broth's nutritional value. Nevertheless, a positive trend seen in these studies—from the strengthening of nails to a reduction in joint discomfort—justifies the need for more direct research.

Collagen in Bones, Gelatin in Broths

Collagen and gelatin have long been touted as versatile compounds across multiple industries—from pharmaceuticals to cosmetics. In the early 1800s, Napoleon employed gelatin to reinforce protein rations for his troops during the English blockade. Unlike the natural food movement of today, there was a scientific preoccupation with "purification, refinement, processing, and chemical extraction"[8] of unrefined foods—an attempt to manufacture edibles that were healthier than unprocessed options. Meat extract was one of the food developments from this era—a product that came from the belief that bone gelatin was as nutritious as meat.

One scientist, Jean-Pierre-Joseph d'Arcet, used acid to dissolve bone and extract gelatin; he went so far as to develop a gelatin production plant to house his digesters. By the early nineteenth century, gelatin gained popularity with chefs, evolving into the famed aspic of Carême's vision. The French held a continued fascination with gelatin, researching varied applications for decades before suspending the effort amidst global political conflict in the 1950s.

Elsewhere around the globe, gelatin has maintained a similar scientific allure for over a century. Gelatin has gone from sustaining soldiers during times of war to entertaining children with a colorful after-school snack. Over time, however, scientists arrived at the conclusion that gelatin has "limited biological value."[9] With all the attention given by the research community, what advanced the idea that these compounds are nutritionally deficient despite the popular perception that they are healthful?

The surface answer is in its basic composition. While gelatin is almost entirely composed of protein, its amino acid structure is incomplete. Gelatin is unusually high in glycine and proline—two amino acids that are considered nonessential because they are produced by the human body—and deficient in essential amino acids.

It was long believed that the body poorly manages food with incomplete proteins. The meat and dairy industries, for instance, have campaigned about the significance of complete proteins contained within their respective categories. Yet recent studies have shown that our bodies can combine complementary proteins over the course of a day, or even longer.[10] This means that gelatin might serve well as a *supplement* to a varied diet, especially one rich with plant matter.

This latter point is key: According to Dr. William H. Percy, an associate professor at the University of South Dakota, our digestive system breaks down collagen into amino acids, and our bodies apply them where they are needed. In other words, the consumption of collagen does not directly translate to the augmentation of collagen in or between bones. Instead, the body uses nutrients to support skeletal structure based on need, and passes unneeded amino acids from the body through urine. As with most balanced perspectives on nutrition, diet should not rely on only one source of protein; other nutrient-dense materials like leafy greens, legumes, and nuts should be consumed to round out a diet.[11]

In 1963 one study assessed the effects of orally administered gelatin on fingernails of healthy adults. Over the course of a month, the ingestion of two grams of gelatin per day resulted in significantly stronger fingernails and the improvement of small nail defects.[12] Another study identified a gelatin therapy in subjects with fungal infections of the nail, called *onychomycosis*. Additional research on the effect of gelatin in finger vascularity concluded "it is possible that the gelatin corrects a deficiency in one or more amino acids necessary for proper nail growth,"[13] adding that more proof was needed.

A recent medical examination of skin health saw increased firmness, decreased dryness, and a reduction in the appearance of wrinkles with the daily supplementation of hydrolyzed collagen over the course of three months.[14] (The supplement was further fortified with hyaluronic acid and additional vitamins and minerals.) Hydrolysis in collagen occurs when molecular bonds between individual strands are broken down into smaller peptides. This process increases the bioavailability of collagen in humans. The collagen found in bone broth, however, is *not* hydrolyzed, making it a less efficient source of this type of protein.

Another popular theory is that the collagen contained within bone broths might reduce joint pain. One powerful study illustrated a decrease in swollen and tender joints when patients with severe rheumatoid arthritis were treated with supplemental chicken collagen. The majority of the patients reported a reduction in joint discomfort, and four out of sixty patients showed complete remission—all within three months of treatment.[15] The theory for this study is that collagen is a significant protein in articular cartilage and might act as an autoantigen within inflamed joints. Additional proof of this theory comes from a more recent study: An extract made of hydrolyzed cartilage from chicken sternum, with the addition of chondroitin sulfate and hyaluronic acid, relieved joint discomfort in osteoarthritic patients.[16]

While the findings are meaningful, these studies make use of hydrolyzed collagen in a supplemental format. The collagen in bone broth is less concentrated, less accessible to the body, and an unreasonable quantity would need to be consumed to match the value found in supplements. Moreover, mixed results were seen in other clinical trials—one study showed improvements in a minority of subjects and another study found a worsening of conditions in patients. As a result, a response by the European Food Safety Authority Panel on Dietetic Products, Nutrition, and Allergies stated that no clear cause and effect has been proven between collagen hydrolysate and joint maintenance.[17] Researchers agree that there is a need for more controlled studies on the topic.

The Chicken Soup Theory

In defending my early professional decision to move from medical research to food systems, I remember telling my father: "Dad, I just don't want to devote my life to scientific trivialities. I mean, how long did it take for scientists to figure out why our pee smells funny after we eat asparagus?" The answer: A curiosity throughout the ages, the compound *still* intrigues scientific inquiry.[18] And the irony: Now more than ever, I want to support research that endeavors the little things, like how chicken soup might help cure the common cold.

As luck—or a keen collective intuition—would have it, a popular study that provides evidence in this direction was published in *CHEST Journal* at the beginning of this century. Affectionately called Grandma's Soup, samples from a traditional chicken soup recipe were gathered in vitro according to clarity and particulates, compared against commercially available soups, and assessed for their ability to mitigate inflammation associated with upper respiratory tract infection. The homemade soup showed strong indications of reducing inflammation in subjects, whereas the commercial soup showed inconsistent inhibitory effects. Of interest but without explanation, vegetables extracted from the broth had a mild toxic effect on cells, and yet no cytotoxicity was detected in the composite soup, notably made from well-sourced ingredients.

Admittedly limited in its scope, yet strict with its methodology, the results of this study provide one small point of control to substantiate that compounds in soup could be medically worthwhile. The researchers conclude by encouraging more evaluation of soup using "rigorous modern methods," but not before acknowledging in vivo studies that came before it, stating:

> *The social setting in which chicken soup is often taken is likely to contribute to a strong placebo effect . . . whole chicken soup may contain a mixture of active agents that synergize each other in order to achieve their beneficial effects. It is also consistent with the recommendation that the use of chickens of a certain age that are, perhaps, happy is more effective.*[19]

Rarely do you see research that includes subjective commentary about the social acceptance of placebo or the welfare of animals. For the popular assertions of the soothing nature of chicken soup, our grandmothers would not protest! We'll dig deeper into the nutritional merits of "happy" animals in the following section.

Another earlier study corroborates with their findings: Sipping heated chicken soup broke up nasal mucus for a sustained period of time—more than hot or cold water did—in healthy subjects. This research endeavored to compare the temperature of liquid on management of upper respiratory tract infections: Hot chicken soup, regardless of whether the results are attributed to aroma or taste, increased the velocity of nasal mucus significantly more than other liquids.[20]

Another deduction that nutritionists agree on is that both stocks and broths are excellent liquids for rehydration. The fluidity in broth returns water to the system, electrolytes restore sodium, and amino acids are transported to where your body needs them most. As a post-workout beverage, I recommend cooling down before drinking a hot broth, or simply sipping a tepid broth while your body temperature is elevated. This step ensures that your skin will perspire at a healthy rate and cool you down in the process.[21]

Upon reviewing research to date, perhaps it is best to consider bone broth as an important part of a rounded diet, and an integral component to health over the long haul. Instead of bingeing on bone broth lattes, learning how to incorporate them in our own home kitchens can be rewarded with long-term nourishment. This practice is merely a perpetuation of what traditional chefs (and grandmothers) have known for a very long time.

The Significance of Pastured Animals

Stepping onto fresh pasture, following the paths of cows and chickens, and taking in the rich smell of well-maintained land—this was my indoctrination to the merits of animals raised on pasture. Practitioners of ecological agriculture, including permaculture, say that grass-fed beef is better for every being involved: The land requires less energy to grow grass than grain, and soil health soars with rotational maintenance. The livestock breed, often heritage or rare, is selected for traits that are well suited for regenerative farming methods. It is raised in a natural environment, not squeezed into a feedlot and pumped full of hormones and antibiotics. These farmers are preserving significant genetic resources for future stock intended for pasture. And the consumer benefits from leaner meat with a beneficial fat profile. Overall, empirical research is illustrating how holistic land management helps restore biodiversity of plant and animal communities.[22]

As with bone broths, the scientific community has only recently begun to uncover the health benefits associated with raising animals on pasture. This is understandable when considering the state of the beef industry: Concentrated animal feeding operations, or CAFOs, appeared just over half a century ago, when antibiotics were introduced as a health management technology for confining large numbers of animals. The discovery of *tetracycline*—an antibiotic that suppresses harmful bacteria and encourages growth—accelerated the livestock industry into a post-war era, in response to a rising demand for meat.

Orville Schell, a cattle rancher and investigative journalist, was one of the first professionals to caution against the use of antibiotics and hormones in what he called the "pharmaceutical farm." He traced an exponential increase in the use of antibiotics over the course of two decades—from 1.2 million pounds in 1960 to over 19 million pounds in 2001. Within a decade of industrial-scale usage in Japan, microbiologists discovered resistant bacteria, a trend that continues to this day.[23] With each generation of bacteria that develops resistance, our global pool of effective antibiotics lessens for both animals and humans. Today, antimicrobial resistance is considered one of the greatest threats to human health worldwide.[24]

Before intensive animal farming, chickens, cows, lambs, and pigs were mainly raised on family farms. Chickens, for instance, were expensive, and prized more for eggs than meat. Poultry populations were small enough to fit and forage the land of each homestead; a limited supply of supplemental feed and the winter months helped regulate flock size. Management was dictated by the seasons, and the health of the land was an essential tool for success. Animals lived natural lives, and in turn, people consumed natural animals.

If we are to lean on the old adage "we are what we eat," a comparative review of an animal's diet becomes worthwhile:

> *A pig allowed to forage will find roots, grass, leaves, berries, fruit, grubs, insects, and if they're lucky, hazelnuts and acorns. Farmers commonly supplement with table scraps; sometimes whey makes it to the trough. Manure, in manageable amounts, becomes fertilizer. By comparison, hogs raised in a factory setting, are often confined within a gestation crate, commonly fed corn and soybean meal and given antibiotic and hormone supplements. Their diets are rich in calories and based entirely on grains; their waste is concentrated and difficult to manage in large quantities.* [25]

The diet of a well-raised animal should be evidence enough to encourage the careful selection of meat for your diet and bones for your stockpot. Despite the obvious benefits to land and animal, pastured meat can be a hard sell to the common consumer: Individual cuts are more expensive and often require a cooking approach that goes beyond searing in a hot pan. Labels can be confusing. To further complicate the marketing of pastured animals: Studies are tricky to design; a nutritive baseline is difficult to achieve when so many breeds exist and pastures vary.

Here is what research, albeit limited to date, has uncovered about beef, pork, and chicken raised on pasture:

BEEF

A university study that observed three decades of farming practices found consumption of grass-fed beef aligns with the goals of a nutrient-dense diet—one that is lower in saturated fat and higher in beneficial fats. Nutritional assessments show grass-fed beef to contain more omega-3 fatty acids, antioxidants, beta-carotene, and vitamins A and E while being lower in calories than CAFO-raised meat. [26]

Early critics within the meat industry stated that grass-fed beef contained a nominal increase in omega-3 fatty acids and consumption did little to change overall diet. Yet later studies illustrated significantly higher levels of omega-3 in the tissue of subjects who ate grass-fed beef when compared with those who consumed conventional meat. This points to how our bodies normalize omega-3:omega-6 intake: An internal competition for conversion enzymes found in these fatty acids achieves a better structural balance in grass-fed meat eaters.[27]

PORK

Similar to cows, pigs raised on pasture exhibit a significantly improved fat structure, yet their micronutrient profile isn't much different than that of their factory-farmed counterparts. A 2012 study by Compassion in World Farming discovered a nominally higher daily percentage of vitamin E and iron in pastured pork.[28]

The key here is diet and exercise: A roaming pig will enjoy a natural intake of leafy greens and acorns, both a significant source of omega-3s, unlike conventionally raised pigs, who are often confined in a barn. Many small farmers also supplement a pig's diet with whey—a nutritious by-product from yogurt and cheese production—and finish with barley and triticale, which contain half the quantity of omega-6 fats as corn. This type of regimen produces pork with less polyunsaturated fats, resulting in firmer meat and creamier fat.

Fat profiles are wildly different across breeds. Factory-farmed pigs are much leaner—more muscle than fat—than they were fifty years ago. Today, heritage breeds that are raised in a natural environment often have lard-type fat and well-marbled meat. The variance across breeds has resulted in different data sets, but the assessments in fat composition invariably favor pastured heritage-breed pigs.

CHICKEN

Research on chickens has resulted in similar findings: Pastured chicken offers an *improved* fat profile—a lower ratio of omega-3:omega-6 fatty acids—favoring dark meat over white meat. As with pigs, pastured chicken showed a high daily percentage of vitamin E and iron, but not in quantities that are considered significant to overall health.

The speed of development plays a key role in composition: Fast-growing hybrid breeds—those found in intensive farming environments—contain up to 50 percent more fat than slow-growing heritage breeds. This results in an unfavorable ratio of omega-6 to omega-3 fatty acids.

Studies show that selection of breed is directly related to beneficial fat composition: Heritage breeds tend to have long bodies, long legs, strong bones, and smaller breasts, all of which aid mobility.[29] The bird should come from a breed that is selected for climate, geography, and temperament—a measure that ensures health during the slower growing phase.

In all of the studies reviewed, bone health is either secondary to the composite animal, or an afterthought of the analysis. Brooklyn Bouillon is designing a comparative review of the composition of bones from animals raised in intensive settings versus pastured habitats. Nevertheless, it is safe to say that animals that roam natural environments are "happier" than those raised in factory farms, and we believe this translates to the quality of contents in a stockpot.

On the Criticisms of Bone Broth

"Another autumn, another slew of fawning stories about bone broth,"[30] begins one article about the bone broth phenomenon. The claims associated with bone broth have led to rigid criticism by some nutritionists. Chefs who have long been making stocks with good bones wonder what all the fuss is about. Let's review a few of these statements:

CRITICISM #1: VITAMINS AND ENZYMES IN BONE BROTH BECOME DENATURED FROM HEAT, MAKING THEM LESS AVAILABLE TO OUR BODIES.

As with most cooked foods, the nutritional composition of ingredients in bone broth is altered during the long simmering time. Each ingredient—whether animal or vegetable—responds differently to heat. Some nutrients are degraded while others are enhanced.[31] This is contrary to popular thinking about raw food diets: While heat *does* break down plant cell walls, the stored nutrients of some are released. For instance, processed tomatoes have higher lycopene content than uncooked tomatoes; boiled carrots have increased carotenoid levels and fewer polyphenols. A general rule: The cooking process protects fat-soluble vitamins and antioxidant compounds and degrades water-soluble nutrients and polyphenolics.[32]

One observer goes further to say:

All enzymes from food are denatured upon digestion in stomach acid, if they haven't been denatured first by cooking. Cooked foods may have marginally less vitamin content than uncooked foods, but humans have been successfully absorbing vitamins from cooked foods for a very long time. [33]

Time and temperature play a critical role here, too. Amino acids tend to be stable up to 248°F (120°C)—well above the recommended temperature for simmering stocks—with lysine being the least stable of all enzymes. A study that examined the stability of amino acids during the cooking of sweet potatoes found that baking the roots caused less degradation than canning or dehydration; lysine was the most affected in all cooking methods.[34]

Nevertheless, evidence shows that sustained temperatures below 248°F (120°C) exhibit limited alteration in enzymatic structure. For instance, one chicken broth study set liquids at two temperatures—185°F (85°C) and 210°F (99°C)—for four hours and measured no significant differences in amino acid content.[35] Another study set at a lower temperature showed a concentration of enzymes. The results, therefore, are inconclusive.

Since most of the existing research is on broth simmered at a higher temperature than suggested in this book (see "Guidelines for Making Stocks and Broths," page 88), Brooklyn Bouillon is interested in conducting an assessment of how the composition of bone broth is affected by time and temperature. The most logical conclusion, one that likely will not change, is to enjoy a diet with a variety of fruits and vegetables—both fresh and cooked—to ensure balance.

CRITICISM #2: IF BONE BROTH CONTAINS GOOD MINERALS, THEN IT MUST ALSO CONTAIN BAD ONES, LIKE LEAD.

Unlike vitamins and enzymes, minerals are less sensitive to sustained heat and tend to leach into boiling water. This applies to many minerals—the ones we want to consume and those we want to avoid. It's not surprising that a recent study went so far as to claim potential lead contamination in organic chicken broth.

Their findings showed the highest concentration of lead in a broth made with skin and cartilage (9.5 µg/L), a little less in broth made with bones (7.01 µg/L) and considerably less in broth made only with meat (2.3 µg/L). The quantity of lead found in simmered tap water (0.89 µg/L) was the least of all liquids tested.[36] As a point of reference, 15 µg/L is the recommended daily limit for lead in tap water, as set by the Environmental Protection Agency. The highest level of lead identified in the study is well below the defined limit.

Still, the risk of lead contamination is a serious matter, especially when young children are concerned. In our early developmental years, our bodies are susceptible to absorbing as much as 50 percent more lead through dietary intake. When you consider that the objective of the earliest bone broth study—from eighty years ago—was to determine if bone broth is good for infants, then you can understand the significance of this research.

Advocates of bone broth sought answers from the publishers of this study—asking after the type of cookware used, and going further to question the possible presence of fluoride in the tap water.[37] Their initial question resolved—the stainless cookware was not the culprit—there was still inadequate information about the chickens. They dug deeper into the quality of the poultry source, only to find the farm had been dissolved since the study was released. Was the water or soil available to the chickens contaminated? Were they exposed to pesticides on the farm? Without answers to these questions, many nutritionists dismissed this study as inconclusive, deferring again to the paramount importance of knowing your farmer.

Other research about possible lead contamination in broth discovered that most of the metal was found in unfiltered tap water. In a series of tests performed by The National Food Lab, there was no lead detected in pastured chicken broth or grass-fed beef broth as prepared by the reputable Three Stone Hearth Co-op in California. The water used underwent reverse osmosis and showed no presence of lead.[38] Regardless of your intentions to sip broth—whether for sustenance or restoration—these findings reiterate the significance of the quality of your source materials.

CRITICISM #3: EVEN THOUGH BONE BROTH IS MADE FROM BONES, IT IS NOT A SIGNIFICANT SOURCE OF CALCIUM.

It might come as a surprise—after all, the largest mineral deposit in bones is calcium phosphate—but this statement is true. Consistent with findings from the early 1934 study, milk remains a substantially better source of calcium than broth—both store-bought and homemade varieties. A recent review confirmed these findings: Broth made from a whole chicken, two chicken feet, and vegetables contained 2.31 mg of calcium per cup; whereas broth made with bones and vegetables contained 6.14 mg per cup. Similarly, only trace amounts of other minerals found in bone—such as sodium, magnesium, potassium, and sulfur—were present in the broth.[39]

Advocates of bone broth purport that the enzymes found in collagen, even after denaturation, are what humans use to manufacture our own collagen. We have reviewed the limitations associated with this assumption—namely that the body uses amino acids where they are needed, not necessarily where we want them to go. More research is required to test the hypothesis that consumption of bone broth has a direct influence on human bone development.

Of interest here is how lead and calcium interact in the body: Calcium competes with lead for a residence in the intestines. Studies have shown that dietary calcium—meaning, calcium concentrated in a supplemental form—can reduce gastrointestinal lead. Iron and B vitamins have also shown a reduction in lead toxicity.[40]

This all points to the complexity involved in how our bodies absorb minerals and counterbalance toxins. Whether broth contains good minerals, like calcium, or bad ones, like lead, the quantities detected are insignificant. There's no escaping the importance of well-sourced ingredients and the value of a balanced diet.

A Need for More Research

The scope of research—a curiosity that crosses cultures and spans decades— supports the simple idea that homemade stocks and broths serve as a healthy part of a balanced diet. But drawing parallels from the effect of concentrated supplements and hydrolyzed compounds to the health benefits of bone broth is messy science. Studies that compare the composition of meat (not bones) from animals raised in different conditions also tell us only part of the story.

The matter becomes even trickier when you consider that large food corporations are funding much of the research. These organizations endeavor to isolate methods that lead to improved efficiency—for instance, how to extract the most moisture to protein in iterative batches. Production time, here, is more important than quality of ingredients. And, as we have seen, there are few studies that go beyond the nutritional analysis as required for the label. History repeating itself!

There are other popular claims about the benefits of bone broths—for instance, a belief that daily consumption cures a leaky gut and detoxifies the body. Digging into scientific archives, however, shows little research on how glutamine affects the human intestinal tract or how glycine assists the liver in eliminating toxins. The research that does exist is performed on rats—an empirical step that often comes before trials on humans—and the nutrients are delivered in supplemental form. Even research that shows a positive healing correlation—such as injecting the hyaluronic acid found in racehorses' cartilage to treat osteoarthritis[41]—is limited in scope. To justify these claims, research that investigates how unprocessed forms of these nutrients are absorbed by the body could be useful to those who adopt an integrative approach to nutritional science.

There is also a popular modern belief that the cartilage in gelatin could help rebuild bone, connective tissue, and skin. This statement is built on evidence collected from studies that employ supplemental collagen; a mechanism that delivers a higher concentration of nutrients than, say, a cup of bone broth. The research is compelling, and yet the delivery method is telling.

All told, the large community of chefs and nutritionists who care about stocks and broths share a common interest in the quality of their source ingredients. Even critics agree that bone broth is delicious, hydrating, and packed with protein—when produced with intention. They simply suggest adopting a more moderate perspective on the extent to which these broths are beneficial.

Oftentimes, a balance is easy to find: For instance, if you want to enhance calcium content in broth, add fresh vegetables that are rich in calcium, such as carrots, parsnips, leeks, and fennel, near the end of the cooking time. (The calcium will denature in the broth if simmered for too long.) You can also boost calcium content by adding milk or cream to a finished broth.

The best way to achieve a baseline for examining content and effect of bone broths is to produce and compare consistent batches. Ingredients must have accurate weights and ratios; time in the pot and the maintenance of temperature must correspond across lots. Contrasts should be evaluated—for instance, how does the composition of a culinary stock—the bones passed through once—differ from that of a remouillage? What is the source of the ingredients? How do store-bought broths compare? With this foundation, we can design nutritional studies that help us decode its true impact on our biology.

In the meantime, there is no question that bone broths are better for you than packaged varieties. Just keep in mind that eighty years of limited research informs us of this simple conclusion: Stocks and broths start in the kitchen and are meant for cooking—the good, wholesome cooking that connects friends and brings family to the table. Bone broth is probably not a miracle elixir, but it is a healthy addition to a well-balanced diet. Placebo or no, bone broth is pleasurable to the palate and happy in the belly. I'm okay with these findings and curious about discovering more.

A Word on Vegetable Stocks and Seaweed

As with animal stocks and bone broths, the temperature at which you maintain a plant-based stock is important. While most minerals remain relatively stable in a heated stockpot, a rapid boil results in some vitamin loss, especially from a delicate plant structure. The goal is a steady simmer, almost a diffusion state, which extracts substance without destroying all nutrients. The temperature should hold steady on the stovetop at around 180°F (82°C).

Nevertheless, the heating process *will* minimize some vitamins while reinforcing others (see "On the Criticisms of Bone Broth," page 61). With all the hype about bone broth, vegetarians might find solace in knowing there is more calcium present in vegetable stock than bone broth, and both contain considerably less than milk.[42] To boost calcium in broth, add vegetables in the last ten minutes of simmering, or fold in milk or cream at the last minute. Making your own vegetable stock also allows you to control sodium content, unlike store-bought options, which boast more glutamates than essence. Homemade vegetable stocks are also low in fat and carbohydrates.

Regardless of nutrient content, vegetable stocks will never hold the viscosity of bone broths; this is because there is no collagen or fat rendered from vegetables into the pot. Add kelp if you desire a vegetable stock that maintains its structure; the alginate incorporates a gelatinous property to the liquid.

When carefully simmered, kelp exudes a slew of vitamins: An ounce of kelp holds about 15 percent of your recommended daily allowance of folate and about 25 percent of your daily allowance of vitamin K. A vitamin rarely found in vegetables, B_{12}, is also present in kelp. This type of seaweed absorbs minerals from seawater: It is rich in magnesium, iron, zinc, and calcium. Seawater also contains iodine, which, in reasonable quantities, is essential to a healthy thyroid. (Nevertheless, iodine is a trace mineral that should be consumed in moderation, and for those who have trouble assimilating it, with great caution.) Limited research shows that dietary kelp lowers estradiol levels, an important theory that could mediate the risk of breast cancer.[43]

The same criticism about mineral content in bone broths also applies to kelp in vegetable stocks: If seaweed gathers good compounds from its natural habitat, then it must also absorb bad ones, such as mercury, arsenic, and lead. Unlike bone broth, there is extensive research on seaweed. In many species, small quantities of toxic metals are detected, but most often as organic compounds that are not considered hazardous. Hijiki is the only type of seaweed that has been proven to possess harmful levels of heavy metals.

Stocks have always had a place in the kitchen. With the recent popularity of bone broths, more home cooks are replacing the convenience of boxed versions with the mindfulness of homemade ones. Even if stocks and broths are more energy drink than magic elixir, the nourishment they provide is undeniable. It is reassuring to learn there is an element of truth to the widespread belief that chicken soup is curative. For those of us who pay equal respect to vegetables, seaweed serves to thicken and fortify our plant-based foundations.

Nevertheless, the key to unlocking these nutritional benefits is in the careful sourcing of materials. The next chapter explains why knowing where your food comes from is crucial to the quality of long-simmering stocks and broths. With this information, you will be able to acquire the ingredients that develop a flavorful and nutritious foundation. Here, too, we can work toward a reality where good food acts as preventive medicine, where the kitchen is as much an apothecary as a hearth to the home.

CHAPTER FIVE

The Significance of Quality Sourcing

T he most important decisions you will make before simmering a day away have to do with the sources of your ingredients. The underlying context of this book is the significance of responsible agricultural practices: How caretakers treat the environment upon which they farm and the animals whose lives they harvest for our strength—every decision they make is reflected in the pot. A kitchen full of well-sourced ingredients extends the life of an animal or vegetable and produces the most flavorful and nutritious foundation. From here, your cooking will flourish, enriched by choices that help replenish the land.

Food as Medicine

"You are what you eat *eats*," says Michael Pollan. When you know your farmer, you begin to learn the story of how caretakers interact with their environment— by land and by sea. Meat, fish, and vegetables become more than how they are packaged for consumption. The humanity with which we treat animals carries through to how well they nourish the soil and water, how well they adjust to climate change, how well they feed us on the plate.

The sourcing suggestions in this book follow the premise that paying more for quality goods means you will pay less for health care over time. A focus on the humane treatment of animals and the health of soil and water translates to more density of nutrients and flavor. With quality meat—and its higher fatty acid profile—you can eat less. Your body requires less to sustain itself. Bones,

What we refer to as the beginning and end of the *food chain*—a field on a farm at one end, a plate of food at the other—isn't really a chain at all. The food chain is actually more like a set of Olympic rings. They all hang together. This is how I came to understand that the right kind of cooking and the right kind of farming are one and the same. Our belief that we can create a sustainable diet for ourselves by cherry-picking great ingredients is wrong. Because it's too narrow-minded. We can't think about changing parts of our system. We need to think about redesigning the system.

—DAN BARBER, *The Third Plate: Field Notes on the Future of Food*

when turned into stocks, and then compost, continue to feed us and enrich the soil long after the meat has been consumed.

It is important to know what you will and won't accept in the food you purchase. Some buyers require a farmer to hold certifications—Animal Welfare Approved, USDA Organic Seal, so on and so forth—while others find it sufficient to know when a farmer practices humane and sustainable methods without certification. Knowledge of where your food comes from teaches you about the land around you and ultimately what you are putting in your body. Every individual will have a different set of parameters for what is acceptable.

In this chapter there are lists of questions that will help you get to know livestock farmers, vegetable growers, and fishermen. These lines of inquiry are intended to encourage dialogue between you and the people who grow and harvest your food. A conversation with your farmer or fishmonger can lead to purchasing decisions that ensure you are consuming the healthiest food and supporting the most responsible producers. With these answers, you will also be able to determine your personal comfort level with varying farming practices. Let the discussion guide you in developing your own standards for consumption. The inquiry provided about livestock and vegetable farmers are based on suggested questions for consumers that were created by GRACE Communications Foundation, a not-for-profit that advocates for a sustainable food system. Consult appendix A for additional sourcing guidelines.

Pastured Animals, Healthy Bones

On cold market days, among frozen meat and poultry, I would often find the farmers of Grazin' Angus Acres sipping homemade chicken broth from a thermos to stay nourished and warm. It's a good sign of quality when a farmer is smiling over his own goods despite below-zero weather, at the ready to boast about the welfare of their animals and the quality of their soil.

Farmers Dan and Chip have been supporters of the bouillon business since the beginning, and it is using their ethics that we select source materials for our broths. The standards of permaculture practices are mirrored between the land and the pot: Slow-growing heritage chickens follow Angus cows on pasture, scratching and feeding at manure, managing parasites, and enhancing overall soil conditions. When harvested in a reduced-stress environment, these animals produce bones rich in flavor and dense with nutrients. The resulting stock is packed with gelatin and holds a healthy ratio of fatty acids—a reflection of the *terroir* and welfare of the animals. And what of the land! Stepping onto pasture, the nose is met with the vitality of protein-heavy grass and nitrogen-rich clover mixed with an undeniable tang of plush manure. Trust me: It's intoxicating. This is the best land a farmer can offer and the finest cuts a butcher can convey.

The significance of small livestock farms and responsible butchers goes beyond health and nutrition. When you buy from the source, you know your food hasn't traveled far, and that your dollars support the local economy. Farmers and butchers are part of a small network—with the processor as the bridge between them—and they can answer questions about how the animal was raised and harvested. Buying local offers better assurance that your bones come from one traceable source, often from the same animal. Your choice also helps producers make use of their entire animals, reducing waste from the agricultural level to your plate.

With the rise in popularity of bone broth, you might find that quality bones are more difficult to locate. In the early years of Brooklyn Bouillon, I would often vie for attention from farmers who already had buying commitments from conscientious chefs. Over time, as our little outfit became a known buyer, farmers and butchers would save bones for us, even seek partnerships. This is another reason to get to know your farmer: The promise of quality goods in exchange for your loyalty—a reciprocal transaction.

The bones highlighted in appendix B are recommended for concentration of flavor and density of collagen; however, if you happen upon bone types other than those listed, you can still make a stock or broth. Keep

We work to preserve the land through our actions for future generation of farmers. We work to preserve rare breeds to save these great breeds from extinction and improve our bio-security through biodiversity. We work to promote other family farms to help preserve farmland in our region so more people can enjoy their world-class products. It is through cooperation, trust, personal responsibility that we all do better.[1]

—**MIKE YEZZI**, Flying Pigs Farm, Shushan, NY

QUESTIONS TO ASK YOUR CATTLE FARMER

Does the animal receive hormones?

Does the animal receive antibiotics? If so, when? Why?

Are the animals confined? If so, when?

Are the animals on pasture? If so, when?

Are the animals fed hay during their growth? If so, when? For how long?

Are the animals finished on hay? If so, for how long?

Is the pasture mix made of regional or native grasses? If not, is it coastal hay?

When is the animal finished?[2]

in mind that the result might not be as flavorful, nor will the liquid gel without sufficient collagen. If this type of stock is less appealing to you, I recommend keeping it on hand as a secondary stock, and then making other products from the bones, such as dog food or bone meal.

Changing Tides, Responsible Catch

Years ago, I worked as a pastry chef in Pike Place Market—a bustling public market located in the heart of Seattle, Washington. I would often arrive as early as the fishmongers, passing by their assembly of glistening fish displays on my way to the kitchen, well before the sun would rise. It was groggy-eyed conversations with these fishermen that influenced me to add wild salmon to my diet, a decision that would end a decade-long commitment to vegetarianism. Wild salmon from the Pacific Ocean, they taught me, are a regional catch, abundant in supply and managed by responsible fisheries. They insisted it would make my skin glow. And almost overnight, it did.

Consuming wild salmon became a bi-monthly indulgence, a treat that would deliver essential fatty acids and fuel me for hours, yet it also introduced me to a difficult conversation. It seemed whenever I would research the active seafood populations or fishing methods associated with various fish species, there would be a controversy brewing between business interests and conservation alliances. One side would oppose evidence of environmental impact, such as global warming, on the health of water and fish populations; while the other would insist that safeguarding mechanisms were a necessity for the sustainability of environment and industry. As a curious consumer, it was challenging to gain a clear perspective on the state of fishing, even when considering a regional catch.

My education on wild salmon opened a Pandora's box of inquiry and ultimately a realization that the status of fish and their populations shifts as swiftly as the tide. To this day, I consult private interest groups such as Monterey Bay

AN ETHICAL DILEMMA

This anecdote is about a homesteader and his pet cow. Together they tilled the land and managed the soil, until the grazer met an untimely end. For me, this was a lesson about animal welfare and the ultimate cost of meat, and not an easy one to tell.

A couple of years ago, I received word from an upstate New York acquaintance that his pet cow—intended as a summer grazer—had been mauled by a neighborhood dog. His recovery options were limited: Find a winter home for the unfortunate cow and nurse it back to health; or harvest it before winter, eliminating the possibility of infection. Neither of us were farmers: We were met with an ethical dilemma.

The challenge in locating a proper winter home for the cow was inherent to its breed: Jersey cows are best used for dairy production—the girls, anyway—and land management. The cow would need to survive the winter to be useful to the landowner. Known more for being robust than for the quality of its meat, this cow had been fed supplemental feed of poor quality; there had been no intention of raising him for consumption. The idea of harvesting him as a means to prevent waste was not ideal.

We consulted with farmers, landowners, even butchers and chefs; limits on time and resources prevented anyone from assuming responsibility. Sadly, no one wanted a cow that held an uncertain return. Failing to locate a good home, we ended up taking his life, swiftly and with the assistance of an expert hunter. This act left me with the first-time task of butchering a whole bovine. It felt like I was breaking all my rules—harvesting an animal under questionable conditions, encouraging consumption of an animal raised on GMO feed—and yet what seemed paramount was making a commitment to use every part of the animal.

It was then that I felt some distant empathy: Imagine the loss a farmer might feel when an animal he invests in, and cares for, is met with a premature demise or a rejection during inspection. I wanted to know that we were making the right decision. A phone call to Chip from Grazin' Angus Acres granted the permission I was seeking. He confided, "Our cows hardly ever get sick. Which is sort of the point of raising them on grass. We administer antibiotics in acute cases of, say, pink eye and a few other minor infections, but the percentage is wildly low. We're more likely to lose a cow to a broken leg or a chicken to a predator than to illness."

What I didn't realize at the time was this lesson was about more than animal husbandry: It was a hands-on education about the significance of quality sourcing. We shared the primal cuts and made a plan for how to make use of all remaining portions. It was to our great surprise that the beef was tender despite being lean. Portioned and frozen, the meat from this one animal alone fed us for over a year.

Yet when I endeavored to make a classic stock from the bones, all we could taste was his hardy constitution. The result was entirely barnyard in flavor, and the odor—all leather and sweat—had no redeeming culinary quality. It was perhaps a signature left from the poor quality of the feed, and it was destined for dog food.

The adage "we are what we eat" never rang truer. Animals, too, are the composite of their consumption. And bones reflect terroir. A realization, for me, that lessens the divide between a cow grazing on pasture and meat wrapped and sealed for purchase.

Aquarium Seafood Watch and Marine Stewardship Council, to determine best practices when purchasing and consuming seafood. Groups like these stay on top of geographic nuances found across species—from how populations are managed to types of fishing methods used by area fisheries. Luckily, a simple search can now inform responsible consumer choice.

The decision to add Sustainable Fish Fumet to our product line came about with the introduction of Community Supported Fisheries (CSF) in the city. These organizations are largely funded by the consumer. They enable the buying of fish direct from the docks, often paying fishermen in advance for their potential catch. The type of fish is rarely guaranteed, dictated by seasonality and environmental conditions, with only an annual benchmark to guide probability. Sometimes the same fish is delivered week after week; other times the weekly catch is varied. And yet the unique offering is fully transparent: When one type of fish disappears, there is always an explanation—one grounded in responsible decisions made by the fisherman. Acquiring bones from CSFs means we sometimes shift ingredients for the fumet. As if transferring my education about salmon, it was now my turn to explain to customers why each batch might exhibit subtle differences.

This buying philosophy also explains why shrimp is omitted from this text. While some good options exist for locating sustainably caught shrimp, over 90 percent of shrimp sold in the United States is imported from questionable sources around the world.[3] The farther away from the source, the more difficult it is to buy with integrity. With our production in the Hudson Valley, nowhere near the wild Alaskan seafood supply or other areas where closed-tank productions are managed, shrimp is simply not on our menu. Alternatively, you'll find an enthusiastic endorsement for other shellfish: When managed responsibly, mussels, clams, and oysters are beneficial to their habitat. We also indulge on an occasional lobster—those seasonally caught from responsible fisherman.

When setting out to make fish fumet, focus your search on the bones from a white fish. Our choice cold-weather formula at Brooklyn Bouillon includes a

QUESTIONS TO ASK YOUR FISHMONGER

What fish is in season?
When was your fish caught?
Is your fish wild-caught or farmed?
What method was used to catch your fish?
Are any preservatives used to enhance the
    appearance of your fish?
Is your fish certified or rated by marine-
    friendly organizations?

majority of bones from mild white fish, such as grouper, with small amounts of monkfish tail for a mild oyster flavor and skate wing for texture. Shellfish is more straightforward, both in procurement and stock production. The key to a good shellfish stock is to start with the live animal and to cook it close to when you want to eat. That way, you can capture the liquor from the shells in the liquid and consume the meat separately, or as in our kitchen, as the stock simmers to fruition.

Rich Soil, Wholesome Vegetables

About an hour from Manhattan there is a special stretch of land—a relatively flat patch of jet-black soil that extends for twenty-two square miles. Appropriately named the Black Dirt region, this part of Orange County, NY, is known for producing some of the country's best onions. The locals call the land "muck soil," an affectionate reference to glacial pockets that possess considerable amounts of organic matter, a sulfur-rich landscape ideal for growing spicy alliums. These are the hard, yellow onions that last forever in your cupboard, the sugary toiler that rewards patience with a perfect caramel in the pan. When cut, these are the onions that make you cry. This is the onion you want for stock.

Lucky for us, this region is only a short drive from our kitchen. A hardy vegetable, perfect for storage, its regional abundance means we have year-round access to an essential ingredient. Onions, like bones, are heavy. So at times of pick up, I am thankful for remaining committed to our local economy, a scale fit to my physical size, if only for the preservation of my back.

When suspended in liquid, the brassiness of onions combines with the sweetness of leeks and carrots to balance flavor. These vegetables, simply cleaned and chopped, form the vegetal foundation of most stocks. Together they blend into the background, allowing flavors of animal or other vegetables to come forward; or roasted, they become the purpose. As with bones, the key to an intensely flavored vegetable stock lies in the richness of the soil from where the vegetables are plucked. The health of the land enriches vegetables and encourages the growth of vibrant grass that feed animals.

In this book, I have fun with vegetables, highlighting individual types in place of bones, an homage to those days when plants replace animal protein in your diet. I acknowledge the basic idea that charring an onion adds color to any stock and go further to illustrate how an onion releases different flavors and textures throughout unique phases of its agricultural development. Garlic, as another example, arises with scapes, the stalk that grows from the bulb, and advances through aged—marked by a rich, amber sweetness that evolves as the plant develops in,

QUESTIONS TO ASK YOUR
VEGETABLE FARMER[4]

How do you control pests on your farm?
How do you fertilize your soil?
What types of crops do you grow?
Do you rotate crops?
Do you grow heirloom varieties?
Is your farm certified organic, biodynamic
    or naturally grown?

and then out, of the soil. In stock form, an essence emerges that follows the growth of a vegetable; an approach that expands their application in the kitchen.

Look for firm onions, yellow or white, reserving red onions for other culinary endeavors (they discolor a stock). Leeks should also be firm and preferably tall, ensuring a healthy ratio of white bulb to light green stalk. Reserve the tops of leeks for assembling *bouquet garni*, a tidy package of herbs for the pot. In most cases, the top of one or two leeks is acceptable for a stock, but too many will also discolor the liquid. Carrots should be bright orange for most stocks, though lighter varieties can be used for those recipes that have no need for an infusion of beta-carotene. They can be small and tender or large and bulbous; size doesn't matter much here. You will see other vegetables—tomato for depth of flavor, or parsnips, which impart more earth than sugar—yet onions, leeks, and carrots form the backbone of most stock recipes.

Should you happen upon a farm stand full of seconds produce, don't hesitate to load up and head straight to the hearth. Seconds, sometimes referred to as "ugly vegetables," are often just as fresh as their primary counterparts; separated if oddly shaped or blemished, and labeled according to what the market demands. What matters to common retailers does not matter to a stockpot, making seconds an ideal pursuit for a savvy cook. Keep in mind that seconds are sometimes discounted for ripeness and need to be used soon after acquired. While freshness ensures a greater density of nutrients in the pot, you can also make use of a crisper full of neglected vegetables. Your stockpot shouldn't be used like a kitchen sink, yet these measures will help eliminate food waste from the farm to your fridge.

Kelp: The Missing Ingredient

When a colleague told me about a kelp farmer in Maine, I jumped at the opportunity for an introduction. A type of seaweed, kelp is packed with essential vitamins and nutrients (see "A Word on Vegetable Stocks and Seaweed," page

65), offering a gelatinous boost to plant-based stocks where collagen from animal bones is absent. A white powder binds to the exterior surface of dried kelp; this is a naturally occurring source of glutamic acid, which adds intense umami when dissolved in water. Bound by a commitment to source locally, kelp was a key ingredient our vegetable stocks were missing.

For years we struggled with wanting to add a healthy ingredient that would infuse body to our plant-based stocks. Most seaweed options come from overseas, and starch thickeners were out of the question. Instead, we relied on the integrity of the formative ingredients, and we preserved flavors through freezing within two hours of batch completion. Luckily, kelp is a reasonable substitute for *kombu*, a type of sea plant that comes from East Asia and forms the foundation for most seaweed-based broths. With the addition of kelp harvested within our region, our vegetable stocks now have a nutrient-dense viscosity that rivals our bone stocks. Vegetarians, rejoice!

The trouble with home-cooked vegetable stock is that it lacks body and loses flavor quickly—often limp from the ladle with few structural compounds to shape the liquid. The extraction of flavor from vegetables happens quickly in a warm stockpot. Muscle proteins in vegetables tighten when heated, creating tension that breaches plant cells and forcefully releases contents into the liquid. This makes for a quick-cooking stock, one that also loses flavor in a refrigerator within a day or two. The alginate in kelp augments body that holds everything together and acts like a natural preservative.

In these stock recipes, kelp is listed as an optional ingredient. You don't need kelp to make a quality stock; however, it is an ingredient that introduces an undeniable mouthfeel to a dish. Should you live near Maine, I encourage you to seek a local or regional source. Otherwise, seek kelp that has not been overly processed: Sometimes sodium alginate is added *after* seaweed has been blanched and dehydrated, an unnecessary redundancy. Much seaweed on the market also contains sweeteners, food coloring, and preservatives.

The kelp you want is aged for less than three years and yields a characteristic clear, delicate broth, such as *rishiri*. If graded, look for a green or red (as opposed to purple or brown) band on the top of the package; this indicates an inspection result of the highest ranking, based on factors such as color, weight, thickness, and presence of white powder on the surface.[5] Should you live near clean, open waters, you can also forage kelp, simply rinsing it in water to remove sand and setting on a clothesline until dry.

As consumers, our buying decisions can support the land, animals, and caretakers that provide our nourishment. The benefit to us is that food tastes delicious while also being wholesome. This is the secret to what makes stocks and broths meaningful—in the kitchen and in our bodies. You don't need a fancy kitchen to make a good foundation; you only need well-sourced ingredients and quality time at the stove. The next chapter reviews the tools and equipment, as well as a few additional staple ingredients that will assist in the making of well-developed stocks and broths in your kitchen.

CHAPTER SIX

Setting Up Your Kitchen for Making Stocks and Broths

If you cook at home often, your kitchen is likely supplied with the equipment you need to make a good stock. At a minimum, a stockpot, a strainer, and a reliable heat source will produce worthwhile results; for the serious cook, the addition of a scale and thermometer will help attain precision. The tools outlined in this chapter will guide you in maintaining the right temperature; achieving the right color, clarity, and consistency; and ensuring a safe environment to produce and preserve your stocks and broths. A review of staple ingredients, such as water and salt, is also included.

Tools and Equipment for the Home Cook

There's no real magic to making a good stock or broth at home, only a commitment to tend the pot and an ability to be patient, sometimes very patient. Correct tools will help you achieve the best results—proper color, concentration, and clarity—as will measures that ensure food safety. There's a good chance your home kitchen is already equipped, ready to enrich your household with warmth that emanates from the pot. If you are limited on space, time, and equipment, or are a stickler for energy efficiency, consider cooking stocks and broths in a slow cooker or pressure cooker (see "Simplified Methods," page 363).

SCALE

A scale allows you to measure the weight of ingredients to achieve precise concentration and consistent results. A scale for this purpose can be digital or analog; it is optional for small batches and recommended for large batches. If you require consistency across batches, then you'll want to weigh the bones and vegetables. The recipes in this book list primary ingredients, such as bones, meat, fish, and vegetables, by weight; all recipes include metric conversions for accuracy of measurement.

OVEN

An oven is used to roast and defat bones and vegetables for brown stocks. The process of roasting creates a golden-brown crust on the bones and vegetables; it also develops a fond, the caramelized drippings that stick to the bottom of the pan, which is responsible for the darkened color and depth of flavor in a stock. When marrow bones are roasted, much of the fat is rendered, which helps clarify the stock before adding water.

You can use a conventional oven or a convection oven to roast your ingredients. A conventional oven—the standard for most home kitchens—works by radiating heat up and pushing cold air down. This mechanism can cause uneven baking; simply turn the bones or stir the vegetables throughout cooking to ensure even distribution. Alternatively, a convection oven is outfitted with a fan that circulates air around the inside, and results in more evenly cooked food. This type of oven typically requires less cooking time because it heats the contents faster. Regardless of oven type, it's always a good idea to keep an oven light on to observe the cooking process.

STOCKPOT

Selecting the correct pot is an important step in building a quality foundation. Appropriately, the stockpot—a wide pot with a flat bottom, straight sides, and an opening that extends the full diameter of the pot—is intended for making large quantities of stock or broth. Two handles should reside on the sides, and though not all stockpots come with a lid, one with a top handle can be useful.

Stockpots circulate liquids through convection and are wide enough to accommodate frequent skimming from the top. The height of a stockpot determines rate of evaporation. For a stock or broth, you want a tall, narrow pot, which limits evaporation during a long simmer.

The most common materials for stockpots are stainless steel or aluminum. Stainless steel has many advantages over aluminum, except the price. Stainless steel is heavier and therefore manages heat better; unlike aluminum, it has a nonreactive surface, which means you can cook acidic or salty foods. Stainless steel can be used on a gas or electric range, as well as an induction surface (provided it is magnetic stainless steel and contains some iron); aluminum cannot be used on an induction surface, unless it is constructed with a magnetic layer on the bottom surface. Anodized aluminum exists to solve the challenges that aluminum presents and offers a solution that is less expensive than stainless steel. You can find more expensive options in copper, vitreous enamel (most often as enamel-coated cast iron), and layered metals that are all designed to improve heat conductivity.

If you plan on making stocks on a consistent basis, go one step further and consider the gauge—or the thickness—of the pot. A heavy-gauge stockpot ensures even heat distribution and durability during lengthy simmering times. Remember that the numbering system for gauge structure is in reverse: The smaller the number, the thicker the gauge. If no number is listed, look for a description that mentions "heavy-gauge" and examine the base of the stockpot for multiple-ply construction. Even the smallest heavy-gauge stockpot will possess heft.

You can select the correct capacity based on the size of your kitchen and the quantity of stock you plan to use or store at a time. I recommend an 8- to 12-quart (8- to 12-liter) pot for home kitchens, a 20-quart (20-liter) pot for restaurants, and upward of a 60- to 80-quart (60- to 80-liter) pot for commercial productions. Jacketed steam kettles are also wonderful for commercial use, though they require a specialized ventilation system and certified installation procedures.

You can use other pots—such as a saucepan or even a slow cooker. Make sure you have enough room in the pot to cover all solid ingredients with water.

KITCHEN STOVE

An obvious heat source, the kitchen stove is mentioned here because of its significance to the process. The stovetop allows you to control the rate of heat as it transfers to the pot, which dictates the temperature of your liquid and therefore the amount of simmering time. Whether gas, electric, or induction, it is important that your stovetop can maintain a steady temperature for a long period. If it cannot, refer to methods using a slow cooker or pressure cooker (see "Simplified Methods," pages 363) to achieve similar results.

BURNER PLATE

If your gas stove runs hot or you are using an induction range, a burner plate will help diffuse the heat and assist with even cooking. Look for a plate made of cast iron or stainless steel; skip those made of aluminum. The plate should be thick and heavy and fit over the burner to lock in heat.

THERMOMETER

The best thermometer to use when making stock is one that clips to the pot. Select a deep-fry or candy thermometer, which are typically outfitted with a built-in clip. For those thermometers that aren't, such as instant-read thermometers, you can improvise with a binder clip: Clip it on the edge of a pot with one arm arranged over the liquid and the other lifted toward the outside of the pot; insert the probe into the former and rest the digital reader on the latter—the probe will securely settle into the liquid. The temperature range of your thermometer should reach 100°F (37°C) on the low end.

SKIMMER

A skimmer is an easy and effective tool for removing fat and impurities from stock or broth. Choose a fine-mesh skimmer with a long handle and a flat bottom. I keep my skimmer handy—set in a bowl next to the stockpot and close to the sink for periodic cleaning. You can attribute the clarity of a stock in part to the skimming process; it helps eliminate impurities as they rise to the surface, making this tool an essential part of the mise en place of stock making.

STRAINERS

There are three types of strainers that are ideal for finishing a stock: A conical strainer, called a *China cap*, and a reinforced bowl-shaped strainer, simply known as a *double-mesh strainer*, are used most frequently. Use the China cap for passing large objects, such as bones, and the double-mesh strainer to catch smaller particles. If you can't locate a double-mesh strainer, simply lay cheesecloth in a single-mesh strainer to catch finer bits. At Brooklyn Bouillon, we first ladle our stocks from the pot through a China cap, and twice more through a double-mesh strainer. To further refine the texture of a sauce, you can add a *tamis*, also known as a drum sieve, to your strainer collection.

COOLING ICE PADDLE

An important food safety measure when making stock is the rapid cooling period that comes after removing a pot of stock from the stovetop. This step helps prevent harmful bacterial growth that can occur when hot liquids are suspended in the danger zone—from 135°F (57°C) to 41°F (5°C)—during their transition from stove to refrigerator. If you are in the business of producing stock, or find yourself making multiple batches at home, consider acquiring an ice paddle, typically found at restaurant supply stores. Ice paddles are simple to use: Simply fill with water and freeze until needed. When added to hot liquid, the frozen paddle cools liquid from the inside out in a quick and even manner. Alternatively, you can make an ice bath in your kitchen sink or in stainless steel hotel pans (found at restaurant supply stores) to achieve the same effect.

STORAGE CONTAINERS

Always have clean containers on hand for your finished stocks. You can store liquids in plastic containers with tight-fitting lids in the refrigerator or freezer. Stocks will also hold well in sealed plastic bags. Lay the securely sealed packs flat in the freezer with kitchen towels between each layer to prevent sticking.

Alternatively, if you dislike plastic, transfer and store the liquid in glass jars. If you plan to freeze the stocks in glass, make sure to chill the liquid in an open jar until frozen; this allows the liquid to expand during the freezing process and prevents the glass from breaking under pressure. When the liquid is frozen, seal the jar with a lid.

My preferred container sizes are pint and quart containers. Depending on the recipe, a pint is a sufficient amount of stock for one meal; a quart will provide enough base to feed a small family. A clever tip for freezing in small portions: Pour the liquid into ice cube containers, freeze until solid, and transfer the cubes to a container that is easily accessible in the freezer. Keep in mind that the cubes will be exposed to more surface area, which encourages freezer burn; plan to use the cubes more quickly than stocks stored in larger containers. In all instances, label your stocks with a name and date.

COLD STORAGE

Another obvious yet essential asset to the stock making process is cold storage. After the initial cooling stage, you can store a batch in the refrigerator for a few days or in the freezer for much longer. For large batches made in a professional kitchen, a blast chiller is recommended. This commercial appliance rapidly cools hot liquids to a safe temperature, typically within ninety minutes. Any fat in the stock will solidify on the top when chilled, allowing for easy removal. If preserving in the freezer, you can store and stack sealed bags or pour into ice cube trays for single portions.

DEHYDRATOR

Invest in an electric dehydrator if the idea of making dried bouillon cubes and gelatin powder appeals to you, or if you are limited on freezer space. Dehydrating is a healthy method for preserving nutrients in food while extending shelf life. Look for a dehydrator that heats through convection and is outfitted with

MY "SEASONAL" KITCHEN

For those of us who adore good food, the word *seasonal* evokes memories that match ingredients to time and place—cider apples in fall, root vegetables in winter, lamb in spring, and endless nightshades in summer. The appearance of our kitchens might reflect the seasonality of what we pick from the land or find at market—perhaps a big, heavy enamel pot takes residence on the stove throughout the cold months, and a canning operation moves in at the end of the warm ones. Indeed, this movement from season to season is how I perceive the functional use of a kitchen, and yet, in my world, the kitchen itself is not a constant, knowable thing.

In the tough real estate market of New York, the life of a conscientious broth maker is a mobile one—yes, there are days spent skimming pots and producing stocks in bulk, but much of the work includes meeting with farmers, courting investors,

and assessing infrastructure. The truth of our trade is that slaughterhouses have fallen out of commercial favor over the past generation, and professional kitchens are rarely outfitted to meet the needs of small producers. Living between urban industry and rural farmland means my personal cooking spaces are also in flux—from the compact commonplace kitchen of a Brooklyn apartment to the rickety kitchen expressions of an old farmhouse.

As a commercial broth maker, my ideal industrial kitchen includes steam-jacketed tilt kettles and perhaps deep braising pans; other less ideal spaces offer multiple well-ventilated heat elements that can accommodate huge stockpots. I sometimes deliver filtered water to the pot from a food-grade hose; in rare, less-than-satisfactory instances, a spigot assists with transferring finished product from pot to sieve-lined container. The setup of the kitchen dictates ease of production:

stackable trays. You will also need non-stick drying sheets that fit on your dehydrator trays. The manufacturer often sells them as an accessory.

TERRINE MOLD

Though a terrine mold is not a tool for making stocks, it is a great piece of equipment to have around if you are regularly cooking with them. Terrines are typically packed with forcemeat or vegetables that are held together by a chilled gelatinous stock, or aspic; they are commonly served as an appetizer. A terrine mold can be rectangular or oval in shape, has vertical sides and is fitted with a lid. Traditionally crafted from glazed earthenware, modern terrine molds tend to be made with enameled cast iron. If you do not have a formal mold, you can use a regular loaf pan; simply line it with parchment and weight the contents with full cans in lieu of a fitted lid.

Heat in a jacketed kettle, for instance, is managed through steam, which stabilizes temperature better than the heating element on a stove. This feature requires less monitoring once the stock is settling in for a long simmer. The tilt mechanism on both kettle and braiser eliminates the need for heavy lifting; enormous stockpots, the cumbersome alternative, require more than two hands to manage. Admittedly exhausted by the end of a production day, I sometimes invite friends or colleagues to assist with hand-labeling units. For these instances, the kitchen is almost always equipped with a stock of wine.

Over the years, my home kitchens have garnered an enviable collection of beautiful, functional pots and pans. These vessels rarely travel with me, but knowing they exist is comforting: Each pot has a unique feature—say, a conductive property that improves the structure of a sauce or a visual vibrancy that invites guests to gather in the kitchen. I have a similar adoration for my collection of shiny sieves and strainers, knowing they hold the secret to proper viscosity and silken texture of foodstuffs. Still, the mobility of my business has forced me to become agile in the kitchen. One day of producing stocks will build a frozen arsenal for future cooking experiences—whether a quick, late-night meal for one, or a multicourse production for friends. These days, my personal kitchens are as utilitarian as my commercial production space; the romance is less about fancy equipment and more about lasting nourishment.

This confession isn't intended to discourage you from building a well-stocked kitchen. There are few greater pleasures in life than owning a warm, developed kitchen, one that encourages friends and family to join in the cooking experience. Instead this view into my mobile culinary life is an invitation to cook without interference from limited resources. Regardless of how well a kitchen is outfitted, it is almost always possible to make stock. And with a good stock, nourishment is within reach.

A Note on Staple Ingredients

In addition to basic equipment, there are a few ingredients that, when sourced with consideration, will produce a better-tasting stock or broth. The quality of your water, for instance, plays a significant role in the quality of a foundation; water, after all, is what carries the flavor and holds the texture of the infusion. The choices you make when selecting other staple ingredients, such as salt, oil, and tomato paste, also make a difference in the pot.

QUALITY WATER

It is easy to overlook a basic ingredient like water, which is provided to our kitchens as a natural municipal resource. Water makes up the largest-volume ingredient in a stock or broth, however, and treated well water will always produce a healthier result. Toxins, such as chlorine, reside in our water supply and can counteract the benefits of a good bone broth. I recommend learning about the quality of your water so you have better control over the end product.

The Environmental Protection Agency sets standards and regulations for which contaminants are allowable in the public water supply.[1] Ask your community water supplier for an annual Consumer Confidence Report to learn more about the quality of your local drinking water. You can acquire a low-cost test kit from your local hardware store to determine what is coming out of your tap.

Based on the contaminants in your water supply, select a filtration system that is qualified to remove those toxins. A reverse osmosis filter, which purifies by pushing tap water through a semi-permeable membrane, is highly recommended. If you are making only a small quantity of stock, store-bought filtered water or countertop filtration carafes are sufficient. If neither home filtration nor store-bought water is an option, proceed with the water on hand, but be aware that the purity of the stock might be compromised.

SALT

Salt is a naturally occurring mineral found in abundance on earth—mostly in seas and oceans, but also from dried surfaces and underground deposits. Most commercial salt, such as table salt and kosher salt, is produced through a process called solution mining. This method injects fresh well water into salt beds to dissolve the salt, after which the brine is pumped out and delivered to plants for evaporation. Alternatively, sea salt is gathered through solar evaporation, where the wind and sun assist salt collection from shallow pools.

Though the chemical composition of commonly used salt is the same, there are some considerable differences in texture and density across type and brand. These nuances, once known, might make a difference in the way you approach cooking. Table salt, which is denser than other salt and often contains stabilizers and conditioning chemicals, as well as an off-putting metallic taste, has no place in my kitchen. Kosher salt, which is less processed than table salt, is employed for curing and blanching; sea salt, itself with endless variations, is often reserved for finishing dishes, a final enhancement before the meal reaches the table.

The recipes in this book rely on a singular brand of kosher salt and specific types of sea salt, depending on the application. Kosher salt offers coarse grains that coat ingredients well without dissolving, making it an ideal salt for seasoning meat and vegetables before cooking. Its affordability also makes it a good choice for blanching and brining. The size and density of kosher salt flakes depend on the evaporation process. This means that each brand of kosher salt has a different weight. For consistency, the recipes in this book use Diamond Crystal Kosher Salt, which weighs 135 grams per cup.

All stocks and broths in this book call for sea salt, preferably unrefined, the most natural type of salt available for cooking. Sea salt is collected around the globe from evaporated seawater, and its color variations are indicative of trace minerals that are specific to its origin. Gray sea salt (also known as Celtic sea salt) from France, for instance, gets its color from the clay bottom pans of salt marshes where it is harvested by hand. Other types of unrefined sea salt include Real Salt, which is mined from salt deposits in Utah, and Himalayan sea salt, a rose-colored flake from Pakistan. For finishing dishes, I prefer Maldon Sea Salt, a soft, pyramidal flake that exhibits a clean flavor and an almost effervescent texture. These salts contain trace minerals, which are imparted into the dish when cooking and add to the overall nutritional value of stocks and broths. If you cannot locate unrefined sea salt, you can substitute refined sea salt, which might be processed for flake consistency and could contain an anti-caking agent.

This book does not make use of table salt. It is commonly fortified with iodine—a global health initiative that introduces iodine in societies where it is deficient, an effort that unfortunately lends an unpleasant metallic taste to the salt.

GRAPESEED OIL

The roasted stocks in this book use grapeseed oil to coat and cook bones and vegetables before simmering in water. Grapeseed oil is recommended for this purpose because it has a higher smoke point and a more neutral flavor than olive oil. This means it does not turn rancid during the roasting step, and the oil does not interfere with the flavor of ingredients.

Grapeseed oil is extracted from the seeds of wine grapes after the juice is pressed from the fruit. As you might imagine, the seeds of grapes do not contain much oil and therefore require a method that coaxes oil from seeds. Unfortunately, cold pressing, the healthiest method, is not effective with grapeseeds, and solvent extraction, the most harmful method, should be avoided. Instead, look for expeller-pressed grapeseed oil, a process that uses a mechanical press to release the oil. Keep in mind that grapeseed oil is high in omega-6 fatty acids and should be used sparingly. Lastly, do not confuse grapeseed oil with rapeseed oil, which is made from the flowering plant of the Brassicaceae family and is otherwise known as canola oil.

TOMATO PASTE

Some classic brown stocks, such as veal, lamb, and duck, benefit from a boost of flavor and color; the char from bones can sometimes darken liquid to an unpalatable tint. For these roasted stocks, tomato paste is the ingredient that provides necessary enhancement. A roasted duck stock, for instance, goes from a dull brown to a deep mahogany when the tomato paste is folded in. This step also mellows gaminess from the bird by adding the natural umami found in concentrated tomatoes.

As with most of the ingredients reviewed, the type of tomato paste you use makes a difference in your cooking. Most commercial tomato paste is made from flavorless tomatoes—those hard fruits that are picked from the vine too early. It is also sometimes fortified with citric acid to improve shelf stability and/or sugar to balance overall acidity. The canned version often tastes metallic—the acidity of the tomatoes competes with the packaging material. Even though tomato paste is used sparingly, the combination of these factors is detectable on the palate.

Time permitting, I recommend stocking up on many pounds of late-summer tomatoes and making your own tomato paste. One day of preserving will produce enough *conserva* for your winter pantry. The freshness of the fruit combined with the slow touch of a home kitchen promises a tomato paste that is silky in texture and caramelized in flavor. The recipe for tomato paste (page 273) includes honey as a natural component to further mellow the concentration. If you are unable to make your own, look for tomato paste in a jar, tube, or can, that lists only one ingredient: tomatoes.

———————

Whether making a small batch for your home or a large batch for a crowd, the tools and equipment required to make stocks and broths are straightforward—a vessel, a heat source, and cold storage. It might be tempting to throw all your ingredients in the pot and leave them to simmer, but there are nuanced details that go into producing an excellent foundation. The next chapter explores each step of the process—from tending the pot to cooling for safety—and the science involved therein. Combined with great ingredients, this culinary knowledge offers a sincere approach to cooking—slow and steady, thoughtful, and meditative.

CHAPTER SEVEN

The Basic Science of a Good Foundation

When I first got into the business of making stocks, my friends called me "The Queen of Flavored Water." It was a joke that both endeared and endured—after all, what are stocks but a long-winded infusion?

As it turns out, there's a lot of science that goes into the making of a good stock. Water temperature, heat distribution, surface area, simmering time, fat and protein ratios—these are just a few of the factors to consider when mastering a stock. But don't let the details intimidate you: If you have good bones, basic vegetables, clean water, a vessel to hold them in, and a heat source, you can make stock at home.

At its highest level, time in the pot affects how much gelatin is extracted from bones and how many nutrients are preserved in vegetables. It varies by type. For instance, it takes less time to break down chicken bones than it does beef bones. Carrots, when processed, develop an increase in carotenoid levels and a decrease in polyphenols. Knowing how a specific animal or vegetable reacts in liquid will help guide you in creating superb stocks and broths at home. What comes before and after the simmer—the where, what, how, and why of sourcing and handling ingredients—is where technical mastery of a stock resides.

People often tell me that they simmer the carcass of a store-bought roasted chicken to make a quick stock at home. This is a perfectly acceptable way to extend the life of a bird, and by following a few tips, you can end up with a quality stock with less effort, one that is far healthier than most commercial options.

Guidelines for Making Stocks and Broths

This section will guide you through the technical process of making stocks and broths. Each step is intended to develop structure, define appearance, and refine flavor, such that the finished product will serve as a proud staple in your kitchen. Technique defaults to a classic French approach and aims for a foundation with visual clarity; however, other methodologies, such as those used in Asian cultures, are also referenced throughout the guidelines.

SOURCE GREAT INGREDIENTS

As I've already said—the quality of a dish is as good as its ingredients—and this is also true of a homemade stock and broth. The way your farmer treats his animals and manages his land will have a lot to do with the quality of raw materials.

Not all bone types are equal in nutrients. You want the parts of the animal that are richest in collagen and minerals—knuckles and marrow bones from grass-fed beef; necks, backs, and especially feet from pastured chickens. I use a small portion of skate wing (when available from certified sustainable seafood sources) in fish fumet, which adds a gelatinous texture as seen in its meaty counterparts.

When making a culinary stock, you can use bones from other parts of the animal, though the end product might not be as flavorful or concentrated. For bone broths, always use the suggested bone types to ensure a result dense with gelatin.

The size of the bones dictates length of simmering time, especially when making bone broths. A slow, steady simmer allows the collagen in bones to be extracted as gelatin. Large beef bones will take longer to render than small chicken bones. Whenever possible, ask your butcher to split the calf's foot—this allows the foot to render at the same speed as the other bones.

For vegetables and aromatics, locate a mixed vegetable farmer who practices responsible growing methods. Vegetables in a stock are basic—onions, leeks, carrots, sometimes fennel, and tomatoes—and always in a quantity less than your bones. Ask your farmer about seconds—those funky-looking vegetables that might not fit the supermarket model—and you may save a few dollars.

A farmer doesn't have to be certified organic to have healthy land, happy livestock, and vigorous vegetables. Many small farmers prefer to spend time farming and do not have the resources to qualify for the certification. There's no better way to know the quality of your ingredients than by building a direct relationship with your farmer.

TREAT BONES WITH CARE

Store bones according to when you plan to cook with them. Place in the freezer if you do not intend to use them within a couple of days. If received frozen, and you are planning to cook within two or three days, you can slowly defrost them in the refrigerator—they can take up to a full day to thaw. Alternatively, you can defrost bones in cold water (40°F [4°C] or lower), which reduces the thawing time to less than thirty minutes, or quick-thaw in a hot-water bath (around 100°F [37°C]), which requires less than fifteen minutes. The former two methods are approved by the Department of Agriculture to minimize bacterial growth; the hot-water bath method was successfully tested for safety in an USDA laboratory and published in *Journal of Food Science and Food Control*.[1] Be sure to weigh the defrosted bones before proceeding, or simply note the weight before removing any packaging.

When you are ready to make a batch, thoroughly wash your bones in cold water, removing all traces of blood and any other impurities. Remove any organs that might remain attached, and continue to wash the bones.

For a white stock, simply wash or blanch the bones before placing in the final water bath. If a thorough rinse does not remove the impurities, then blanch the bones in barely simmering water. A proper blanch is achieved by covering rinsed bones with cold water in a stockpot and slowly heating the contents; as the water temperature increases, scum will release from the bones and rise to the surface, where it is easily captured. The bones are blanched once the water arrives at a ripple and before it breaks into a boil; rinse again before placing in the final water bath. Some chefs insist on blanching, though a thorough rinse will often suffice for the home cook.

For a brown stock, you will roast the bones until they are deep brown, a method that adds flavor and color to the stock. Both blanching and roasting bones serve the same purpose: to remove surface impurities and coagulate exterior proteins before the bones are introduced to the final water bath.

If you aren't using the bones immediately, store them in the refrigerator before proceeding. For bone broths, should you want to soak the bones in vinegar first, make sure to start with cold bones, which is said to open pores for easier penetration. See the section "Soak in Vinegar" (page 91) to learn more about the optional vinegar soak.

USE THE CORRECT STOCKPOT

A stockpot—with its height greater than its diameter—is designed to prevent rapid evaporation, making it the ideal vessel for a long-simmering stock. The pot should have tall, straight sides, a flat bottom, and a wide opening with handles on either side. This structure circulates liquids by convection and provides easy access to the top—a requirement for all the skimming you'll be doing!

Consider outfitting your kitchen with a stainless steel or anodized aluminum pot—both have a nonreactive surface that manages heat well. On the higher end, copper and enamel-coated cast iron are excellent stockpot materials, should your budget allow. Aluminum is the least expensive type and can be used in a pinch on conventional or gas stoves. Regardless of material, a heavy-gauge stockpot, or a pot with heft, is recommended; the thickness provides additional protection against long exposure to heat.

Select the pot's capacity based on how much stock you intend to make—an 8- to 12-quart (8- to 12-liter) stockpot is usually sufficient for a home kitchen. The capacity of the pot should also reflect the type of stock you are making: A small quantity of chopped vegetables can be managed in a smaller pot than, say, a portion of beef bones. The size of the pot should also match the size of the burner to ensure even cooking and prevent heat loss. Most stockpots come with a lid, unnecessary while simmering a stock, but helpful for storing a full vessel in the refrigerator.

Start with Cold Filtered Water

As I mention in the previous chapter, working with quality water is very important when making a good stock or broth. After all, majority of the end product is liquid—it makes sense that a quality water source is significant to the process. Check your municipality to assess toxins that might appear in your local drinking water, and always filter water—whether through a sophisticated system, such as reverse osmosis, or a countertop carafe—before placing it in the pot.

Also important is beginning with cold water: Place your prepared bones in the stockpot and add cold, filtered water to just above where the bones rest. A slow, gentle heating allows the soluble proteins to release into the liquid and rise to the surface, where they can be captured by skimming before they have a chance to cook and cloud the liquid.

If you are making a vegetable stock, sauté the vegetables in neutral oil, preferably expeller-pressed grapeseed oil, at this point. (While canola oil also has a neutral profile, it is partially hydrogenated oil that is likely to be genetically modified. I recommend avoiding it.) Read the section about preparing the vegetables ("Clean and Chop the Vegetables," page 94), and then proceed with heating the liquid slowly.

Soak in Vinegar (Optional)

For bone broths, some nutritionists recommend soaking cold bones in vinegar to help draw nutrients into the liquid. However, as I mentioned in chapter 4, an early study on bone broth determined that the introduction of vinegar did little to extract protein and minerals from bones. It went further to state that vinegar is too weak to extract calcium that is embedded within collagen.[2] For these reasons, I consider the vinegar soak to be optional when making bone broths.

If you decide to incorporate this step, use cold bones during the soaking process—the pores of bones close when heat is applied and will prevent the absorption of vinegar. For bone broth made with chicken or other poultry, use 2 tablespoons vinegar to 1 gallon water. For those made with beef or other large animals, use ½ cup vinegar to 1 gallon water. Use a vinegar type that has a pleasing flavor, such as raw apple cider vinegar. Recommended soaking time is one hour before heat is applied. Do not rinse the soaked bones; simply soak in the stockpot and start heating from there.

Note that culinary stocks do not employ a vinegar soak because it changes the fundamental flavor and acidity level of the final liquid. To achieve a similar extraction, chefs simply use collagen-rich bones and simmer the stock for the period of time appropriate for each animal, skimming often, and monitor the end result for a clear, gelatinous state, reducing further if necessary. Most chefs care more about clarity of stock than nutrient density of the final liquid.

Slowly Heat the Liquid

One of the most important steps in creating a clean stock is heating your liquid slowly in an uncovered stockpot. When water comes to a boil too quickly, impurities that rise to the top have an easy chance to cook, and these cooked proteins will add an off flavor to the stock. A rapid boil will also suck impurities to the bottom of the pot, which emulsifies and clouds the liquid.

Heating the liquid slowly allows the protein and scum to coagulate at the surface where they can easily be skimmed off. An uncovered pot ensures cooling of the liquid during evaporation, which helps maintain a steady simmer, and also dehydrates the scum that rises to the top, aiding in more streamlined removal.

If you step away from a slowly heating pot only to return to boiling water, not to worry, simply lower the temperature of the stove and bring the liquid back to a sustained simmer. You will have a chance to clarify the stock at the end of the process, if desired. The liquid should hold steady at around 180°F (82°C).

Start Skimming (and Don't Stop)

Impurities will start to rise to the top as soon as there is enough heat to lift them from the solids in the liquid. Begin skimming the moment you see scum at the surface; continue to skim for as long as impurities continue to rise to the top, even after you add the aromatics. If you skim appropriately, you will see less scum by the time you reach the aromatics stage. This is by design, as it is easier to remove impurities before you add vegetables, which float amidst the scum at top. Don't forget to rinse your skimming utensil after each removal, or else you'll reintroduce extracted impurities by dipping a dirty tool into your clarifying liquid.

You might be tempted to avoid the skimming process and settle for a cloudy stock. After all, this step is where most of the active work is required, and it is simpler to set ingredients to a simmer and walk away. A chef will argue that the clarity of stock is essential to building clean flavors, and nutritionists confirm that surfacing scum is a colloid devoid of nutritional value. While I encourage you to skim with diligence, don't fret if you end up with a cloudy stock. You can clarify your stock with a protein raft or ice filtration (this method removes gelatin content) after it simmers. It will still taste wonderful and be healthier than most stocks or broths available at your supermarket.

Simmer the Liquid

Once the liquid begins to tremble, immediately lower the temperature, so that the liquid calms. A happy stock while simmering is one that gently bubbles, or smiles, a French term that refers to a liquid in a state of diffusion. You should maintain a smile once proper heat distribution is achieved and for only as long as the bones and aromatics require to break down. The ideal holding temperature of a slow-simmering stock is 180°F or 82°C—hot enough to infuse contents in the pot but cool enough to exhibit few bubbles on the surface.

Keep in mind that some types of cuisine encourage a rolling boil when making stocks. This technique applies to many Asian dishes, including Korean Ox Bone Soup (page 130) and Japanese Tonkotsu Ramen (page 318). I apply this method sparingly throughout this book, relying more often on French technique to produce clarified stocks.

Remove Fat and Impurities

A liquid that smiles allows you to continue to skim off impurities with ease. Follow the skimming tips above to remove most impurities from the bones in liquid, before you add aromatics to the pot. This step is repeated here because it is important to be diligent about skimming your liquid throughout the simmering process. It might seem like an endless course of action, but you will see fewer impurities rise to the surface as time goes on.

For fat removal while simmering, especially with white stocks such as chicken or those not blanched after washing, you can add ice when the liquid comes to a simmer. This measure will chill the liquid and thicken the fat, assisting in removal by skimming before adding the remaining ingredients. This step is suggested but not required.

Consider the Simmering Time

For animal stocks and broths, you will have only bones and water in your stockpot at this point, and you should be skimming with frequency to remove impurities. This is a good time to consider your simmering time, a parameter dependent on the type of animal or vegetable in use, as well as the purpose of the final liquid state.

For culinary stocks, simmer only as long as the bones require to extract flavor while maintaining clarity in the liquid. As a general rule, the size of the bones will dictate length of time cooking. For example, a white chicken stock will take less time than a brown beef stock because chicken bones are smaller than beef bones; they require less time to break down in the liquid. Similarly, fish fumet takes minimal time as compared with, say, lamb stock, for the same reason.

Another culinary explanation for time in the pot is that a white chicken stock—one that is light in body and flavor—is intended to carry the flavor of more prominent ingredients in the final dish, while a roasted beef stock is intended to guide the flavor of a final dish. The longer the simmering time, the more concentrated the flavor. If you are new to making stocks, you can follow the guidelines for each stock type in part 2 of this book. With experience, however, you will gain an intuition, observing the stock as it simmers to determine viscosity and tasting it near the end to satisfy proper salinity.

For vegetable stocks, the flavor from the vegetables is imparted to the liquid much faster than from bones. If the vegetables in an animal or vegetable stock are simmered too long, then they begin to disintegrate into and absorb the liquid. A coarsely chopped vegetable in an animal stock requires only ninety minutes of simmering time; a finely chopped vegetable for a vegetable stock will be fully extracted in forty-five minutes. If you are pressed for time, you can start a vegetable stock at the beginning of your cooking process and extract a liquid that is more flavorful than water in about fifteen minutes.

For a bone broth, some cooks simmer the liquid for multiple days—twenty-four to seventy-two hours, depending on the type of animal—to ensure maximum extraction of gelatin. To some, a sign of readiness is that the bones crumble in the final stages. This state is alarming to chefs who are concerned with the clarity of their stocks, as a brittle bone will emulsify and cloud the liquid. It will also make the broth taste bitter. Instead, I recommend simmering the bones across two batches of water and marrying both strained stocks at the end. This technique, called a remouillage, allows you to simmer for a length of time that ensures a healthy extraction without clouding the stock. Refer to the guidelines in appendix B for further information on recommended cooking times.

Clean and Chop the Vegetables

Just as clean bones are important to a quality stock, so are clean vegetables. I peel onions and brush carrots. Some chefs suggest that you include vegetable skins. This is an acceptable step, but keep in mind that skin and peels might discolor your stock. (Given my dislike for food waste, I can't blame a home cook for including them.)

The color of the vegetable matters: Beta-carotene from carrots will brighten a stock; chlorophyll from dark greens will darken a stock. You will see parsnips in some recipes, which impart sweetness without adding color. Parsley—which is hardy enough to prevent discoloration—is the only green we add to stock. Remove the tops from carrots, the dark green tips from leeks, and the fronds from fennel, as the green pigment will discolor the stock. Never use red onions, only white and yellow onions.

You might notice that celery does not appear in any stock or broth recipe in this book. This is because celery tends to add bitterness to the liquid. Instead, fennel is used when a watery vegetable is required to balance the sweetness of carrots and the pungency of onions. Fennel puts forth a subtle anise flavor that blends well in a stock. Alternatively, celery root (also known as celeriac) does find its way into some stocks—unlike the stalk, celery root is sweet and earthy, a nice root vegetable to add to the mix.

When carefully handled, however, celery can be delicious. In this book you'll find celery is reserved only as a vegetal addition to finished dishes, as seen in the sofrito broth that accompanies Skillet Eggs with Garlicky White Beans (page 277). Here, the celery in the final broth is simmered for fifteen minutes, enough to extract flavor without introducing bitterness. Two recipes that feature cardoon, a bitter Italian celery that is closely related to the artichoke, are also included—the key here is that hearty stalks are soaked in vinegar and blanched to strip bitterness, before roasting or braising to encourage sweetness. Unlike celery, cardoon is strong enough to withstand the twice-cooking mechanism that eliminates bitterness.

The size of mirepoix, a combination of chopped aromatic vegetables, is determined by type of stock and intended simmering time. A fine or medium cut allows for a quicker simmering time; coarse vegetables can stay in the pot longer. For animal stocks, vegetables should be coarse to hold up to the longer simmering time; for fish and vegetable stocks, vegetables can be chopped fine in order to expedite the extraction. Raw vegetables break down faster than sautéed or roasted vegetables.

In most cases, it is best to chop your vegetables by hand, since a food processor will yield an uneven chop, often liquefied if taken too far. A hand-chopped pile of vegetables will illustrate control over your cuts and allow a more straightforward cooking time. For some fish and vegetable stocks, however, a food processor is suggested to yield a fine chop for a bulk quantity. You should pulse the vegetables in small batches to prevent liquefaction. This increases the surface area in the pot (meaning, how much vegetable matter is in contact with water) and decreases cooking time, a measure that quickly extracts flavor without clouding the stock.

Add Vegetables and Aromatics

Aromatics refer to any ingredient—vegetable, herb or spice—that is used to enhance flavor in food or drinks. A classic French combination of chopped onions, carrots, and celery, called mirepoix, serves as the vegetal base for many dishes. Stocks in this book, however, split the onion component with leeks, and substitute fennel for celery. I still refer to the combination as a mirepoix, since my foundation is a commonly adopted variation of the traditional form. Standard herbs and spices in stocks are thyme, marjoram, bay leaf, and peppercorns. Sea salt should always be added at the end of the simmering time (more on adding salt at the appropriate time in a moment).

Once the bones have simmered according to their appropriate cooking time and the liquid has been skimmed of most impurities, add the prepared vegetables and aromatics to the pot. They will rise to the top and rest there while simmering, which is why it is important to remove as many impurities as possible before adding them.

At a steady simmer, uncooked vegetables will extract their flavor and nutrients in as little as forty-five minutes, or until fork-tender, depending on vegetable size and water temperature. Too much time in the liquid will break down vegetables into a mushy state where particles float in the liquid and cloud the stock. Vegetables that are sautéed or roasted before being added to the stock become concentrated during the heating process and can remain in the pot longer without clouding the stock.

You can add herbs and spices directly to the pot to be strained alongside other solids, or you can create a bouquet garni or herb sachet for an elegant delivery of herbs to the pot. A bouquet garni is made by tucking loose herbs, such as

BOUQUET GARNI

Translated from the French, *bouquet garni* simply means "garnished bouquet," an herb package used to flavor stocks, soups, stews, and sauces. You can substitute other herbs, such as marjoram, depending on what flavors work best in a recipe. If using whole spices, like black peppercorns, wrap the aromatics in cheesecloth instead of the leek tops.

ACTIVE TIME: 5 minutes | **TOTAL TIME:** 5 minutes | **YIELD:** 1 bundle

1 leek, green tops only
4 sprigs flat-leaf parsley

4 sprigs thyme
2 bay leaves

Separate two green leek top leaves and trim them to the same length, about 6 inches (15 cm) each. Nestle the parsley, thyme, and bay leaves into the leek tops. Arrange the leeks facing each other to form a neat package; the herbs should be concealed within the leeks. Tie butcher's twine around the bouquet, secure enough to contain the herbs while cooking. Place the bouquet garni in the pot alongside other ingredients, and cook according to the recipe instructions. When the cook time is complete, remove the bouquet with a fork and discard.

thyme and bay leaves, into a dark green leek top, and securing it with butcher's twine. An herb sachet is made by wrapping herbs and spices in a piece of cheesecloth and binding it with twine. These packages can be thrown in the pot, left to float alongside vegetables, conveniently removed before straining. They are particularly useful when you intend to repurpose bones or vegetables after the simmering time. You simply locate and toss the package instead of handpicking each spent sprig.

Add Salt

The correct amount of salt—just enough to balance flavor—is important to the quality of a stock or broth. I recommend unrefined sea salt due to its clean flavor and higher mineral content. You can use refined sea salt if unrefined is unavailable, or kosher salt in a pinch. See "A Note on Staple Ingredients," page 83, for more about selecting salt.

You should add salt to a stock or broth only at the end of the simmering process. This is because the meat and vegetables release their own salt into the liquid and this concentrated flavor is exhibited in the reduction. A homemade stock requires only 1 teaspoon of salt for every gallon of water to both equalize flavor and add minerals. If your stock requires additional concentration, wait until after you reduce the liquid before adding salt.

Adding salt to your stock also helps minimize the need for excess seasoning while cooking. When preparing a final dish, it is standard practice to adjust seasonings at the end of the cooking process. If you start with an unbalanced stock, however, then the final dish requires many adjustments to achieve the correct equilibrium.

Keep in mind that you will need to add more salt when making a dish if you add a thickener to your stock or broth. Thickeners, such as flour or cornstarch, reduce the intensity of flavor, simply because thickening agents rarely have flavor of their own. A gradual reduction through evaporation maintains—often intensifies—flavor because the molecules have already been bound during the early simmering process.

Rest the Stock

When your stock or broth is complete, it is important to let it rest so any remaining particles can settle to the bottom of the pot. Turn off the heat and leave the pot on the stove for about ten minutes; moving the pot will agitate the liquid.

Ladle from Pot to Strainer

Instead of pouring the final stock or broth from pot to container, it is better to gradually ladle it into a strainer set over a container. This method prevents any remaining impurities from being forced through the strainer. Use a China cap for the first pass—the conical structure holds solids while passing liquid on all sides—followed by a second pass through a fine-mesh strainer. Never press on solids as they fall into the strainer. Some recipes recommend lining the strainer with cheesecloth before straining. Separate bones, vegetables, and other aromatics as you go, reserving the bones for a double or triple stock or to grind for dog food. See the dog food recipe (page 356), which makes use of partially spent bones. In some rare cases, simmered vegetables have an extended purpose, but more often than not, they are discarded at this point.

Discard Sludge on the Bottom

At the bottom of the pot, the base layer might be cloudier than the top majority of the liquid. This is where impurities settle during the resting process—a mixture that should not be reintroduced to the final stock. I recommend reserving it for compost or dog food.

Strain More than Once

No matter how much skimming you perform while simmering a stock or broth, some particles will always remain in the liquid when complete. Straining the stock multiple times helps eliminate many of these lasting particles; or straining through gelatin filtration will produce a crystal clarity (see "Clarify if Cloudy," page 100). (This latter method also strips the stock of gelatin and should be reserved for times when a certain type of consommé is required.) I recommend straining at least one additional time after ladling from the pot. Line the strainer with fresh cheesecloth if particles appear fine. Never force solids through a strainer, as this will push impurities through and cloud the resting liquid.

Cool in an Ice Bath

An important safety measure when making a stock or broth is to rapidly cool the liquid in an ice bath. The temperature danger zone is 135°F (57°C) to 41°F (5°C)—the range where bacteria can multiply quickly. According to the FDA Food Code,[3] rapid cooling should occur within the first two hours with a total of six hours for full cooling. An ice bath will help you cool the stock to 70°F (21°C) in less than an hour, at which time you can slowly finish cooling in a refrigerated environment.

If you are making stock or broth at home, you can build an ice bath in your sink, and then place the container into the ice water. Stir often, until there are no traces of steam. For commercial quantities, I recommend a cooling ice paddle or a commercial blast chiller to assist with rapid cooling. Cooling in stainless steel hotel pans will also facilitate heat transfer.

Start a Second Extraction (Optional)

If bones from the initial simmer are still strong, you can simmer them again to make a remouillage, or a second stock. The purpose of a secondary extraction is to maximize the conversion of collagen into gelatin from the bones without clouding the stock. Veal bones are used to make a classic remouillage, as illustrated in Two-Day Veal Stock (page 111), but bones from other large land animals, such as cow and lamb, can be applied here. This method is employed for many of the bone broths in this book.

To determine if the bones are strong enough for a second extraction, pick them up with tongs and look for any remaining marrow in the pockets. The bones should be strong enough to stay within the clasp of the tongs with some residual marrow left for rendering. If the bones are weak or brittle, do not use them for a second stock; instead, reserve to grind for compost or dog food. If they remain sturdy, place them in a clean stockpot, cover with cold, filtered water, and slowly heat as you would an initial simmer. Repeat the resting, straining, and cooling steps before proceeding to the next step. In some cases, the remouillage will be married with the initial extraction and reduced together to create a balanced stock. This step is reviewed below, after both extractions rest in the refrigerator overnight.

Chill Overnight

Some stocks are fattier than others—chicken with its schmaltz, beef with its tallow, pork with its lard—and resting the liquid in the refrigerator overnight encourages excess fat to suspend on the top. The fat from beef, pork, and lamb stock will harden into a cap and can easily be removed before using the final stock or broth. The fat from chicken stock is more viscous, requiring a gentle skim once chilled.

If you do not have time to chill the stock, you can blot the surface with a clean cloth, kitchen towels, or plastic blotters that are designed for this purpose.

If you like some fat in your final stock, such as the flavorful, nutritious variety found in the marrow of beef or veal bones, you can scrape it from the fat cap and reintroduce it to your stock while heating. Keep in mind that despite adding a wonderful flavor and texture to the liquid, this step might also cloud your stock. Do so sparingly and be mindful of when and why you add fat back into your stock, especially since you spent so much time skimming at the front.

You can also reserve certain fats for use as a medium for cooking. Simply remove the solid fat from the stock, pat it dry with kitchen towels, and store in the refrigerator in a sealed container. Another use for the fat from meat stocks is to make salve and soap. See "Using Animal Fats for the Body," page 347, for instructions.

Adjust Concentration

Once strained, rested, and chilled, examine your stock or broth for signs of preferred concentration, consistency, and flavor. If your liquid seems too thin, return it to a clean pot and gently simmer until reduced. If your liquid seems too thick, simply heat the liquid and add filtered water to achieve the desired consistency. If your liquid is the correct concentration and consistency but lacks depth of flavor, try adding sea salt to achieve balance.

If you are making a remouillage, this is when you marry the first and second extractions. In separate stockpots, gently heat both extractions before combining them. You can reduce the combined stocks if the mixture is too thin—this will produce a silky, sophisticated stock that makes the most of your ingredients.

Keep in mind that heat level, length of cooking, and quality of ingredients all play a role in the consistency of your stock. Gelatin can break down if heat is too high or if the broth is simmered for too long. You will also find a variance in bones made from conventionally raised animals: Since most live in lots that limit their range, these animals never get the chance to use muscles and ligaments that enrich bones with high levels of collagen. I can't state it enough—always buy from known farmers who are raising their animals in the most humane conditions. Finally, the use of collagen-rich bone types, such as beef knuckles and chicken feet, will help ensure a proper gel.

Clarify if Cloudy

If your resulting stock or broth is cloudy, or if you are making consommé, you can clarify the liquid in a variety of ways. The classic method, called a raft, applies solid protein to extract emulsified particles; an updated technique, called ice filtration or gelatin filtration, clarifies by slowly thawing and straining frozen stock.[4] The former method is useful when you need to quickly clarify stock, but it has the disadvantage of removing flavor. Filtering a frozen stock requires additional time and removes gelatin content, yet preserves flavor and yields a crystal-clear liquid.

A raft clarification can be performed by stirring whisked egg whites and egg-shells into the cold stock, followed by slowly heating the mixture and holding at a simmer for about an hour. The egg whites form a network that captures large proteins in the liquid, and these proteins rise to the top, where they can be collected. After the raft is skimmed and the liquid is strained, your stock or broth will be clearer.

The introduction and removal of egg proteins reduces flavor and gelatin content from the liquid. To counter this loss of flavor, add a small amount of finely chopped meat and vegetables to the stock alongside the egg whites and eggshells. Alternatively, you can follow the Chinese culinary method of clarifying with meat proteins only. To do this, simmer finely chopped meat in the cloudy stock until particles collect around the solids; strain and repeat until the liquid becomes clarified.

If you have adequate time and sufficient space, ice filtration will produce a clear stock without loss of flavor. Devised by Harold McGee, this method is also known as gelatin-filtered consommé. It requires a stock that has been concentrated to achieve a gelled state when refrigerated. Since this process removes gelatin from the stock, it is only recommended for culinary stocks that need to be light in body and intense with flavor.

To clarify a stock through ice filtration: If the stock does not gel when chilled, temper the liquid with gelatin, preferably grass-fed, or agar-agar. (See table 7.1, page 102, for measurements.) After the stock is concentrated and before it is chilled, pour it into containers that fit in your freezer. You can divide the stock into ice cube trays for single-portion use or quart containers for stackable units. Keep in mind that the size of the container will dictate the amount of time the stock takes to thaw. A day or two before you need clear stock, line a strainer with a coffee filter or cheesecloth and set it over a container large enough to hold the liquid. Remove the stock from the freezer, place it in the filter, and put the setup in the refrigerator. When the stock is fully defrosted, the liquid in the container will be clear and flavorful. The gelatin and fat remaining in the filter can be used for dog food.

Thicken as Needed

Thickening agents, often called a *liaison*, will add viscosity to a stock or broth and come in many forms—a variety of gelatin, seaweed, or starch. In traditional French cookery, *liaison* refers to a mixture of egg yolks and heavy cream used to

TABLE 7.1. Thickening Agents for Stocks, Broths, and Finished Dishes

Type	Quantity (per cup of liquid)	Instructions	Notes
GELATIN			
Gelatin, Powder	1 tablespoon	Sprinkle gelatin over half of cold liquid; rest for 1 minute to hydrate. Stir into remaining warm liquid.	Grass-fed is available.
Gelatin, Sheets	3 sheets	Place gelatin sheets in cold water; bloom for 3 minutes. Remove from cold water, and add to remaining warm liquid, stirring until fully dissolved.	Grass-fed is not available.
Gelatin, Granulated	1 envelope (1 tablespoon)	Sprinkle gelatin over half of cold liquid; rest for 1 minute to hydrate. Stir into remaining warm liquid.	Grass-fed is not available.
SEAWEED			
Agar-Agar	½ teaspoon	Add agar-agar to water; stir to dissolve. Bring to a boil to activate gelling property.	Agar-agar achieves a thicker gel than kelp.
Kelp (or kombu)	1 to 2 strips	Add strips to boiling liquid; simmer for 10 to 20 minutes. Remove kelp and reserve for another use.	Kelp adds a subtle viscosity to liquid.
STARCH			
Arrowroot	1 tablespoon	Whisk arrowroot with 2 tablespoons cold water until blended. Whisk slurry into remaining hot liquid until combined.	Organic is available. Contains no gluten. Contains no corn.
All-Purpose Flour	1 tablespoon	Whisk flour with 2 tablespoons cold water until blended. Whisk slurry into remaining hot liquid until combined.	Organic is available.
Cornstarch	1 tablespoon	Whisk cornstarch with 2 tablespoons cold water until blended. Whisk slurry into remaining hot liquid until combined.	Organic is available. Cornstarch should not contain gluten; however, some brands do. Review the label.
Potato Starch	1 tablespoon	Whisk potato starch with 2 tablespoons cold water until blended. Whisk slurry into remaining hot liquid until combined.	Organic is available. Contains no gluten.
Potato Water	2 tablespoons, or more as needed	Whisk potato water into simmering liquid. To thicken more, add 1 tablespoon potato water at a time until desired viscosity is achieved.	Use organic potatoes. Contains no gluten.

thicken sauce; however, the term has evolved to refer to any binding agent. You might need to employ a liaison if a stock does not gel through volume reduction or when further reduction compromises necessary yield. You might also need to add a liaison if the dish requires a gradual release of flavor, an effect that comes from thickened liquids.

If a concentrated stock or broth requires additional viscosity, you can simply add gelatin powder or gelatin sheets to achieve the effect. It is easier to locate grass-fed gelatin in powder than sheet form. Seaweed can also lend additional viscosity to a liquid and is a good alternative to animal-based or starch thickeners. Agar-agar is a fibrous powder obtained from red algae; but be careful, it can have a laxative effect if consumed in large quantities. Similar to gelatin, agar-agar will create a thick gelatin; it is often used as a substitute for pectin in jam. If you need a small increase in viscosity, adding kelp to the liquid is sufficient. A good example of how to enhance the body of a vegetable base using kelp is found in the recipe for Velvety Vegetable Stock (page 247).

Though I rarely use starch-based thickening agents in cooking, the historical telling of stocks and sauces is not complete without acknowledging them. The sauces of Escoffier, for instance, rely on flour to bind compounds within a liquid and cornstarch to add a finishing gloss. These additions are also important in understanding how commercial manufacturers have evolved to create products that rely on processed additives, many of which derive from starchy roots and vegetables that are chemically synthesized to stabilize packaged ingredients.

I recommend using starch only when thickening a dish (rarely for stock), following the recipe to determine expected viscosity. The addition of starch to a stock will cloud and discolor the liquid. Use sparingly. Make a slurry by whisking a small amount of arrowroot, flour, cornstarch, or potato starch into a portion of liquid, and then temper into the remaining stock over moderate heat. Arrowroot is the most expensive starch listed but produces the clearest result. If none of these options are on hand, you can use the starchy water left over from simmering potatoes to thicken soups, stews, and sauces.

It is important to use starches in moderation in order to impart a neutral taste and to minimize the dilution of flavor. For all starch-based thickeners, you will need to add salt to restore any taste and aroma that were absorbed by the starch. If using cornstarch, look for an organic brand, especially if your other ingredients are sourced from local farmers.

Store in Refrigerator or Freezer

Stocks and broths keep well in the refrigerator for immediate use or in the freezer for long-term use. Vegetable stocks have a shorter shelf life and lose their flavor more quickly than bone stocks due to a lack of protein structure. As a rule, you can store your stocks in a sealed container in the refrigerator up to two days for vegetable stocks, a little longer for stocks made with bones, or in the freezer for up to six months. Vacuum-seal packs are ideal for bulk freezing, or freeze in ice cube containers and store in freezer bags for easy access to smaller portions.

If you need to keep a refrigerated stock in short-term storage for a bit longer, you can bring the liquid to a simmer, strain, cool, and chill the stock to extend its shelf life by a couple of days. If your stock ever smells off, err on the side of caution and toss it.

Use Your Stock or Broth

At this point, your stock or broth is ready to be used for cooking or sipping. You can use your stock as a fundamental soup or stew base, or to add a savory component to vegetable dishes. A quick dash of gelled liquid will glaze meats and vegetables in the pan.

You can further enhance your stock into a double or triple stock. This is done by using your stock as the base liquid for a fresh extraction from meat, bones, and vegetables. Alternatively, you can reduce your stock to a clear, solid jelly, called glace de viande or "meat glass," if reduced by ten times its original volume; or demi-glace when combined with a classic brown sauce and reduced by half its original volume. Both of these techniques concentrate amino acids yet flatten aroma, making the glaze ideal for building rich, voluptuous sauces.

You can heat your bone broth and sip it, as is, for a restorative beverage. Turn it into a tonic by adding ingredients such as ginger, turmeric, cayenne pepper, or even ghee, to enrich the flavor and to add nourishment. See chapter 13 for tonic recipes.

Finally, save any leftover braising liquid by straining out the solids and freezing the remaining liquid. Instead of using unseasoned stock or broth, you can use the reserved braising liquid as a base. This repetitive measure concentrates natural glutamic acid, which enhances the umami flavor and silky texture of your foundation.

When assessed at this level of detail, the process of making stocks and broths might seem overwhelming; however, once you have all the materials and equipment in place, the practice shows its inherent fluidity. The act of making stocks blends into the background of your kitchen, providing a constant source of warmth and a gentle encouragement to explore the joys of slow cookery.

PART TWO

Stocks and Broths in the Kitchen

With materials found and foraged, and sharp knives at the ready, you are ready to explore the fundamentals of developing a rich foundation—this is where excellence in the kitchen begins. This section provides detailed instructions on how to make a full range of culinary stocks and broths—built from land animals, fish and seafood, and a variety of vegetables—and use them to build flavor and enhance texture in finished dishes. These complete meals highlight the value chain associated with each ingredient—from farmer to butcher to chef. A farmer will endeavor to cook with, say, a tough rooster; a good butcher will make use of lesser-known parts, like lamb breast; a chef will see value in not just the carrots but also the carrot tops. The recipes begin with well-developed foundational stocks and progress to a deeper exploration of culinary methods, both simple and complex, for omnivores and vegetarians.

Before setting out to make stock or broth with these recipes, read the detailed guidelines in chapter 7. These step-by-step instructions explain the nuance of the process—for instance, how the structure of a stockpot minimizes evaporation, and why you won't see celery or red onions in the base recipes. Keep in mind that my favored methodology follows classic French technique: A long, slow simmer at a steady temperature produces the clearest stock, intended as a versatile foundation. Any deviation from this process—whether due to type of cuisine or ingredient—is described within the guidelines or preceding the recipe.

BEFORE YOU BEGIN

Here are a few tips to remember when reviewing this section:

Sourcing. Each recipe holds the fundamental tenet of careful sourcing and waste management. For the best results, purchase your ingredients from the most responsible farms and markets in your area.

Intention. Stock and broth recipes are separated by purpose: A stock is built to act as the foundation, a broth is further developed in a finished dish, and a bone broth is simmered at length to extract significant amounts of gelatin.

Butchery. For meat and poultry stocks, the size of the animal and the way the bones are cut will determine length of simmering time. Lamb bones, for example, will take longer to render than rabbit bones.

Approach. There is little crossover in each section—lamb stock is used for lamb-based recipes, mushroom stock is used for mushroom-based dishes—as a way to emphasize the unique characteristics of each animal and vegetable. In some instances, however, recipes will include a mixture of stocks to develop a rich composite.

Variations. Take note about subtle variations in ingredients, especially when you arrive at the vegetable stocks. A parsnip, for instance, might be listed where a carrot is typically found—a distinction that imparts earthiness without adding color. Refer to appendix B for a high-level overview of how stocks and broths vary by ingredient and cook time.

Yield. The stock and broth recipes made from animal and fish bones yield between 2 and 4 quarts (1.9 to 3.75 liters), and those made with vegetables produce between 1 and 3 quarts (.9 to 2.8 liters). The yield on shellfish stocks is lower—around 1 quart (960 ml) or less—because the flavor comes from the small amount of liquor that is released from shellfish when they are cooked. These yields are intended as guidelines only; always taste your stock at the end of the cooking process to determine if it needs to be diluted or concentrated. Recipes for basic bulk stocks are provided at the end of the book (chapter 15).

Range. On average, the finished dishes in this book are designed to feed a small family and can easily scale up as necessary. One to 4 quarts of stock or broth (.9 to 3.8 liters) is enough to prepare multiple dishes, depending on the focus. Soup, of course, will require more broth; whereas a sauce will start with less liquid and be further reduced to a glaze.

Efficiency. Think twice before throwing away spent bones and animal fat. There's an entire chapter, as well as tips throughout, devoted to making use of these ingredients—such as dog food and fertilizer from dehydrated bones, an aromatic spread and hand cream from excess animal fat (see chapter 14). If you don't have time to work with spent bones or washed fat, you can label and freeze them for later use.

CHAPTER EIGHT

Meat Stocks, Broths, and Dishes

This section is devoted to large land animals, both ruminant and swine—calf, cow, lamb, and pig. The bones of each animal develop a distinctive stock or broth, each intended for different culinary purposes. Where veal stock is neutral and blends within a dish, beef stock is bold and acts as a guiding flavor. Lamb stock lends a subtle gaminess to dishes, and pork stock adds an undeniable mouthfeel that leaves your taste buds wanting more: All are fundamental to good cooking.

As with all recipes in this book, the quality of your source ingredients is critical, especially when it comes to bone broths. Look for farmers who practice rotational grazing—this is nature's way of helping both the animals and the soil get what they need to be healthy. Pay attention to the bone types listed in each recipe: Specific types of bones, such as marrow bones or knuckles, will help you achieve the intended viscosity for the intended purpose. Some stocks are lighter in body; others jiggle like Jell-O when chilled.

Ask your butcher to split calves' feet, as they tend to take longer to break down than other bones. Remember that the process for making bone broths is typically less fussy about clarity than culinary stocks. To balance this approach, a remouillage—the re-wetting of bones to produce a second extraction—is employed to yield a technically accurate broth, both clear and gelatinous.

VEAL

In *Le Guide Culinaire*, Escoffier begins his seminal text with a recipe for *fond brun de veau*, or brown veal stock, identifying it as the foundation of good cooking. While Escoffier's veal stock is a simplified version of Carême's approach, it still requires a full day of preparation—the length of time required for the bones to impart quality to the liquid.

The goal of veal stock is to achieve umami while avoiding dominant flavors—no forward saltiness, sweetness, bitterness, or sourness should be present on the palate. For this reason, a properly made veal stock offers a neutral quality that takes on the essence of a dish while laying a solid foundation. Umami is both elusive and addictive: A dish made with veal stock should encourage an eater to take another bite. For most chefs, there is no substitute for the craving stimulated by a well-made veal stock.

In its simplest form, a white veal stock can be used as you would a chicken stock. For more complex presentations, reduce it to a glaze, known as glace de viande, and use it like a sauce; or marry it with a second extraction to develop a sophisticated remouillage. Veal stock is useful for braising meats—not only beef, but also lamb and duck, even rabbit—and delicious with mushrooms and roasted vegetables.

When sourcing veal bones, it is especially important to know your farmer. A farmer with humane practices will provide calves with access to their mothers' milk on pastured grass. Younger animals have more collagen in their bones—not just in knuckles and marrow bones—and this is what gives veal stock a sublime mouthfeel. The best bones to use for veal stock include knuckle, neck, back, and a small amount of marrow bone. You can also ask your butcher for veal breast, preferably cut into smaller pieces.

Basic Veal Stock

This white veal stock begins by blanching veal bones to remove initial impurities, resulting in a neutral base. Use it to enhance the flavor of an ingredient or to intensify the base of a dish—the natural concentration of glutamates from the bones will add favorable umami to your food. This stock is a versatile foundation that is worthwhile to keep on hand in any kitchen.

MEAT STOCKS, BROTHS, AND DISHES

ACTIVE TIME: 2 hours | TOTAL TIME: 7 hours (including heating, blanching, simmering, and initial cooling) | YIELD: Makes about 3 quarts (2.8 liters)

8 pounds (3.6 kg) veal bones (necks, breast, and backs), preferably rose veal

1 calf's foot, preferably grass-fed or pastured (optional)

8 quarts (7.5 L) filtered water, cold, plus water for rinsing and blanching

½ pound (225 g) white onions, cut into large dice

1 pound (455 g) leeks, dark green parts removed, cut into large dice

¾ pound (340 g) carrots, cut into large dice

6 sprigs thyme

6 sprigs flat-leaf parsley

2 bay leaves

Sea salt to taste

Rinse the veal bones under cold water until the water runs clear. Place the veal bones and calf's foot, if using, in a large stockpot, and add enough cold water to cover the bones by a few inches. Turn the heat to medium-high and slowly heat the liquid. Using a fine-mesh strainer, skim any scum that rises to the surface. When the liquid starts to ripple, but before it breaks into a boil, remove the pot from the heat. Do not boil the liquid; boiling extracts flavor that should be preserved for the long simmer.

Drain the bones in a large colander, and rinse under cold water. Thoroughly clean the same pot. Return the bones to the pot and add the filtered water. Heat the pot over medium-high, and slowly bring the liquid to a tremble, skimming as soon as scum appears. When the liquid ripples, reduce the heat to medium-low and maintain a simmer, or smile. Never let the liquid boil, as impurities will be sucked to the bottom of the pot and emulsify into the liquid.

Simmer the bones and water for 4 hours, skimming frequently. Add the onions, leeks, carrots, thyme, parsley, and bay leaves, and continue to simmer, another 90 minutes, carefully skimming around the vegetables as necessary. Do not add the sea salt at this time; it will be added later.

Turn off the heat and rest the stock on the stove, about 15 minutes. Set a fine-mesh strainer over a container large enough to hold the liquid contents of the pot. Line the strainer with cheesecloth. Carefully ladle the stock from the pot into the strainer, leaving any cloudy liquid at the bottom of the pot. Skim any fat that appears at the surface.

Taste the stock to determine desired concentration. If the stock tastes too watery, return it to a clean stockpot and simmer until reduced to a desirable consistency. Taste and season with sea salt.

Place the container in an ice bath to rapidly cool the stock. When the stock no longer steams, transfer to the refrigerator. Once chilled, remove the fat cap and reserve as tallow for cooking or making cosmetics (see chapter 14). Refrigerate the stock for up to 2 days or freeze in smaller containers for longer storage.

Roasted Veal Stock

This brown veal stock requires roasting the veal bones and deglazing with red wine to add color and depth of flavor to the liquid. The calf's foot reinforces gelatin in the stock that might be lost during the roasting process.

ACTIVE TIME: 2 hours | **TOTAL TIME:** 10 hours (including roasting, heating, simmering, and initial cooling) | **YIELD:** Makes about 3 quarts (2.8 liters)

---

8 pounds (3.6 kg) meaty veal bones (necks, breast, and backs), preferably pastured rose veal

1 calf's foot, preferably grass-fed or pastured

¼ cup (60 ml) grapeseed oil, divided

2 cups (480 ml) dry red wine, such as Bordeaux

8 quarts (7.5 L) filtered water, cold, plus water for rinsing

½ pound (225 g) white onions, cut into large dice

1 pound (455 g) leeks, dark green parts removed, cut into large dice

¾ pound (340 g) carrots, cut into large dice

¾ pound (340 g) tomatoes, coarsely chopped

6 sprigs thyme

6 sprigs flat-leaf parsley

2 bay leaves

1 tablespoon black peppercorns

Sea salt to taste

Preheat the oven to 425°F (220°C).

Rinse the veal bones and calf's foot under cold water until the water runs clear. Make sure that all visible blood is removed from the bones. The rinsing of blood will help eliminate proteins that could cloud your stock. Pat the bones dry with kitchen towels. Place the calf's foot in the stockpot and all remaining bones in a single layer on a large roasting pan. Coat the bones in the pan with half of the grapeseed oil and roast for 20 minutes. With tongs, turn the bones over and continue to roast until golden brown, another 20 minutes. Remove and transfer the excess rendered fat from the pan; reserve for another use (see chapter 14). Lower the oven temperature to 400°F (200°C).

Transfer the roasted bones to the stockpot with the calf's foot. Add the red wine to the hot pan, place over medium heat, and scrape to loosen the browned bits and glazed juices. Pour into the stockpot. Cover the roasted bones with the filtered water and turn on the heat to medium-high. Slowly heat the liquid, skimming as soon as scum appears at the top, until the surface starts to ripple. Lower the heat to medium and maintain a simmer, about 6 hours, adding water if any content evaporates during the lengthy cook time. Continue to skim, especially during the first hour of simmering.

While the stock is simmering, spread the onions, leeks, and carrots onto a sheet pan and coat with the remaining grapeseed oil. Roast in the oven until golden brown, about 25 minutes. Remove the vegetables from the oven and hold, covered, until needed.

When the bones have completed their initial simmering time, add the roasted vegetables, tomatoes, thyme, parsley, bay leaves, and peppercorns to the stockpot. Do not add the sea salt yet; you will adjust the seasoning at the end. Continue to simmer, another 2 hours.

Turn off the heat and rest the stock on the stove, about 15 minutes. Set a fine-mesh strainer over a container large enough to hold the liquid contents of the pot. Carefully ladle the stock from the pot into the strainer, leaving any cloudy liquid at the bottom of the pot. Skim any fat that appears at the surface.

Taste the stock to determine desired concentration. If the stock tastes too watery, return it to a clean stockpot and simmer until reduced to a desirable consistency. Taste and season with sea salt.

Place the container in an ice bath to rapidly cool the stock. Skim any fat that congeals at the surface. When the stock no longer steams, transfer to the refrigerator. Once chilled, remove the fat cap and reserve as tallow for cooking or making cosmetics (see chapter 14). Refrigerate for up to 2 days or freeze in smaller containers for longer storage.

Two-Day Veal Stock

This stock is for the devoted, but don't let it daunt you. Your efforts will be rewarded with excellence: While the process yields less than a batch of basic or roasted stock, the final reduction is undeniably sophisticated. A remouillage is a marriage between two extractions from one set of bones, ensuring that the gelatin from within is fully released. To achieve clarity, maintain a low, steady heat and skim often.

ACTIVE TIME: 3 hours | **TOTAL TIME:** 2 days (including heating, blanching, simmering, and chilling) | **YIELD:** Makes about 2 quarts (1.9 liters)

8 pounds (3.6 kg) meaty veal bones (necks, breast, and backs), preferably pastured rose veal
1 calf's foot, preferably grass-fed or pastured
16 quarts (15 L) filtered water, cold, divided, plus water for rinsing and blanching
½ cup (130 g) tomato paste (page 273)
½ pound (225 g) white onions, cut into large dice
1 pound (455 g) leeks, dark green parts removed, cut into large dice

¾ pound (455 g) carrots, cut into large dice
¾ pound (340 g) tomatoes, coarsely chopped
1 head garlic, halved
6 sprigs thyme
6 sprigs flat-leaf parsley
2 bay leaves
1 tablespoon black peppercorns
Sea salt to taste

Follow the initial cooking instructions for Basic Veal Stock to carefully rinse and blanch the bones. Thoroughly clean the same pot. Return the bones to the pot and add half of the filtered water. Heat the pot over medium-high, and slowly bring the liquid to a tremble, skimming as soon as scum appears. When the liquid ripples, reduce the heat to medium-low and maintain a simmer, or smile. Never let the liquid boil, as impurities will be sucked to the bottom of the pot and emulsify into the liquid.

When the liquid comes to a simmer, stir in the tomato paste. Slowly return to a simmer, skimming as necessary, and cook about 2 hours. Stir in the onions, leeks, carrots, fresh tomatoes, garlic, thyme, parsley, bay leaves, and peppercorns. Continue to simmer, another 2 hours.

Turn off the heat and rest the stock on the stove, about 15 minutes. Set a fine-mesh strainer over a container large enough to hold the liquid contents of the pot. Line the strainer with cheesecloth. Carefully ladle the stock from the pot into the strainer, leaving any cloudy liquid at the bottom of the pot. Reserve the bones and aromatics for the second extraction. Place the container in an ice bath to rapidly cool the stock. When the stock no longer steams, transfer to the refrigerator.

Thoroughly clean the same pot. Return the bones and aromatics to the pot and add the remaining 8 quarts (7 L) filtered water. Heat the pot over medium-high, and slowly bring the liquid to a tremble, skimming when scum appears. Maintain a simmer, skimming as necessary, another 4 hours. Repeat the resting, straining, and cooling with the second extraction, transferring the contents to a clean container. Place in the refrigerator and rest both extractions overnight.

Once chilled, remove the fat cap from both extractions and reserve as tallow for cooking or making cosmetics (see chapter 14). Transfer both extractions into a clean stockpot. Place over medium-high heat and slowly bring the liquid to a simmer. Reduce the heat and simmer until reduced by half, or until your desired consistency is achieved. Taste and season with sea salt. Repeat the resting process and strain the stock twice. Strain again if any particles remain in the liquid. The stock should be silky and viscous. Cool in an ice bath. Refrigerate the stock for up to 2 days or freeze in smaller containers for longer storage.

Classic Demi-Glace

A classic demi-glace is a transformative tool to have in the kitchen: The smallest addition melts into a pan sauce and lifts ingredients without overwhelming a dish. A foundation that is both neutral and decadent—this is the achievement of demi-glace in French cookery.

Demi-glace is made by reducing a combination of brown stock and Espagnole sauce, a basic brown sauce that is one of Escoffier's classic mother sauces.

Reduced by half, a demi-glace will coat the back of a spoon and serve as a savory icing—from the French word *glace*—to be built up with butter and poured over meat or to sauce a plate.

Though a demi-glace is traditionally made with veal, you can substitute beef or poultry as the base. You can also use a white stock as the foundation to be matched with brown sauce for the reduction. Do not confuse demi-glace with glace de viande, which is simply a meat stock reduced to a glaze; however, it is acceptable to use these interchangeably, if applied in small quantities. Due to concentration of amino acids, no salt is added at the end of the reduction.

ACTIVE TIME: ½ hour | **TOTAL TIME:** 2 hours (including heating and simmering) | **YIELD:** Makes about 2 cups (480 ml)

ESPAGNOLE SAUCE

2 tablespoons unsalted butter
½ cup (80 g) white onions cut into medium dice
¼ cup (38 g) carrots cut into medium dice
¼ cup (30 g) fennel cut into medium dice
2 tablespoons all-purpose flour

3 cups (720 ml) Roasted Veal Stock
2 tablespoons tomato paste (page 273)
4 sprigs flat-leaf parsley
1 bay leaf
1 tablespoon black peppercorns

In a medium saucepan, melt the butter over medium-high heat. Add the onions, carrots, and fennel, and stir until coated. Sauté the vegetables until they begin to caramelize, stirring often, about 5 minutes; take care not to burn the mirepoix.

Sprinkle the flour over the mixture, and stir with a wooden spoon until it thickens into a roux. Lower the heat to medium and continue stirring until the roux begins to brown. Using a whisk, slowly beat in the veal stock and tomato paste until both are well incorporated. Continue to whisk until smooth.

Return the mixture to a boil, and then lower to maintain a simmer. Stir in the herbs and spices. Simmer while stirring often until the mixture reduces by one-third, about 45 minutes. Skim the surface of impurities if scum appears.

Set a fine-mesh strainer over a container large enough to hold the liquid contents of the pot. Carefully pour the reduced sauce into the strainer and let it filter into the container. If you plan to complete the demi-glace immediately, keep the sauce warm. Alternatively, you can put a lid on the container and store it in the refrigerator until ready to use.

DEMI-GLACE

2 cups (480 ml) Roasted Veal Stock,
    warmed

2 cups (480 ml) Espagnole Sauce, warmed
Bouquet garni, or a bundle of herbs

In a clean medium saucepan, combine the veal stock and Espagnole sauce. Add the bouquet garni. Turn the heat to medium-high, and slowly bring the mixture to a boil. Reduce the heat to medium-low, and maintain a gentle simmer until the liquid is reduced by half, about 45 minutes.

Set a fine-mesh strainer over a container large enough to hold the liquid contents of the pot. Carefully pour the reduced sauce into the strainer and let it filter into the container. Use immediately or cool in an ice bath. Refrigerate the demi-glace for up to 1 week or freeze in a small container for longer storage.

Smoked Sweetbread Pâté

Confusing to the ear, sweetbreads contain neither sugar nor bread. Instead, *sweetbreads* refers to two glands—the thymus and pancreas—found in a calf or lamb. When properly handled, they have a mild flavor and a tender and creamy texture, ideal for gentle smoking or frying.

According to the *Oxford Companion to Food*, sweetbreads were first mentioned in the sixteenth century. Specific to the period, *sweet* could stand as contrast with the savory flavor of prime cuts, and *bread* might have its origins in the *brede*, or roasted meat, of Chaucer's time.

As an animal matures, specifically after it has been weaned, these glands will disappear, so it is important to find a source of healthy young calves. For this recipe, ask a farmer or butcher of rose veal for the sweetbreads, perhaps even before the animal goes to harvest. This will ensure not only humane treatment of the animal but also availability of this ingredient.

ACTIVE TIME: 2 hours | TOTAL TIME: 9 hours (including soaking, smoking, cooking, and chilling) | YIELD: Makes 12 to 14 servings

SMOKED SWEETBREADS

1 pound (455 g) milk-fed veal sweetbreads
2 cups (480 ml) whole milk

1 tablespoon kosher salt
Wood chips, such as cherry or apple wood

Rinse the sweetbreads, then place in a bowl filled with cold water. Soak for at least 6 hours or overnight, changing the water once or twice. This draws impurities out of the sweetbreads. Using a sharp knife, carefully remove sinew from membranes. Mix the milk with the kosher salt, stirring until combined, and submerge the soaked sweetbreads in the liquid. Soak for another 2 hours.

In a stovetop smoker, heat the wood chips, covered, over medium heat, until they start to smoke—about 10 minutes. Turn the heat off. Remove the sweetbreads from the milk and pat dry with a paper towel. Place the sweetbreads in the smoker, and replace the cover. Smoke with the heat off for 12 to 15 minutes. Remove the sweetbreads and chill in the refrigerator.

VEAL PÂTÉ

2 tablespoons olive oil
5 small shallots, minced
1 clove garlic, minced
½ pound (225 g) veal liver, cubed
2 tablespoons Two-Day Veal Stock
¾ pound (340 g) veal shoulder, cubed
1 pound (455 g) lean pork loin, cubed
¼ pound (115 g) pork fatback, cubed
¼ cup (60 ml) heavy cream

2 tablespoons Armagnac
1½ tablespoons finely chopped
   flat-leaf parsley
2 tablespoons green peppercorns
Pinch allspice
Pinch ground cloves
Pinch cayenne pepper
Salt and pepper
Smoked Sweetbreads (above)

Heat the oven to 325°F (165°C). Brush oil on a terrine or loaf pan; line with plastic wrap. Place a dish towel in a roasting pan large enough to fit the terrine. Reserve.

In a small sauté pan, heat the olive oil until hot but not smoking. Add the minced shallots and garlic; cook until the onions sweat. Stir in the liver and sear on all sides, about 2 minutes. Don't overcook. Deglaze the pan

with veal stock. Remove from the heat and set aside to cool.

In the bowl of a food processor, combine the veal, pork, and fat and pulse until the mixture is somewhat coarse. Transfer to a bowl and stir in the liver mixture. Stir in the cream, Armagnac, parsley, green peppercorns, and spices. Mix well.

Tightly pack one-third of the mixture into the prepared pan. Place the reserved sweetbreads in the middle of the terrine. Carefully pack the remaining mixture around and on top of the sweetbreads. Tap the pan on the counter to release air bubbles. Cover with the terrine lid or aluminum foil. Place in the roasting pan and pour in hot water until it reaches halfway up the sides of the mold. Bake until an instant-read thermometer inserted into the center of the terrine reads 140°F (60°C), about 1½ hours.

When cooked, remove the terrine, uncover, and place in an ice-water bath to cool. Remove the cooled terrine from the water bath, and seal it well with plastic wrap. Rest the terrine lid or a weight on top and refrigerate overnight. To serve, unmold the terrine and slice into ½-inch (1.25 cm) portions. Serve with toast points, grainy mustard, and pickled vegetables.

Rose Veal Marrow Dumpling Soup

In addition to making a delicious stock, the marrow from rose veal is excellent on its own. Here the marrow is blended with spiced meat, stuffed into semolina dumplings, and poached before settling into a rich, yet simple, broth. This soup is an ideal starter for pasta or meat courses.

ACTIVE TIME: 2½ hours | **TOTAL TIME:** 3½ hours (including chilling) | **YIELD:** Makes 4 to 6 servings

DUMPLINGS

1¼ cups (150 g) all-purpose flour
½ cup (85 g) semolina flour
¾ teaspoon sea salt
6 eggs, divided
1 teaspoon olive oil
¼ pound (115 g) ground veal
¼ pound (115 g) ground pork
2 ounces (58 g) veal marrow (page 118)

1 small onion, minced
¼ cup (55 g) steamed and chopped
   Swiss chard
1½ tablespoons finely chopped flat-leaf parsley
2 tablespoons heavy cream
Pinch cayenne pepper
Freshly grated nutmeg
Salt and pepper

FOR THE DOUGH: In a deep bowl, mix together both flours with the sea salt until

thoroughly combined. Make a well in the flour mixture, and crack 4 eggs into the center. Add the olive oil. Slowly stir the mixture until it comes together to form the dough. Transfer to a lightly floured work surface, and knead until smooth, about 10 minutes. Wrap in plastic and refrigerate for at least 1 hour.

FOR THE FILLING: In a large bowl, mix the veal, pork, marrow, onion, Swiss chard, parsley, heavy cream, cayenne pepper, nutmeg, and salt and pepper to taste. Add 1 egg and mix until well combined. Set aside.

FOR THE DUMPLINGS: Divide the dough into four pieces. Working with one piece at a time, pass the dough through a pasta roller, following the settings from thick to thin, until the sheet is translucent. Alternatively, if you don't have a pasta roller, use a rolling pin: Lightly dust a surface with flour and roll each dough piece into a long, thin rectangle. It should appear translucent when picked up. Lay

the pasta sheet on a work surface, and spoon or pipe the filling in a straight line across the lower edge, leaving about ¼ inch (.6 cm) at the bottom. Gently lift the length of the filled dough away from you and back onto itself to form a long tube.

In a small bowl, whisk the remaining egg and brush the dough just above the filled portion. Gently roll the tube forward to form a tight seal. Trim any excess by running a paring knife or pasta roller down the length of the dough. At consistent 1½-inch (3.8 cm) intervals, use your finger to firmly press the dough into individual dumplings. Separate the dumplings with a paring knife or pasta roller. Place cheesecloth or a damp kitchen linen over the dumplings so they don't dry out.

Bring a pot of salted water to a rolling boil, add the dumplings, lower the heat to a rapid simmer, and continue to cook until they float, about 10 minutes.

BROTH

1 tablespoon olive oil
2 medium leeks, thinly sliced
3 cups (720 ml) Basic Chicken Stock
1 cup (240 ml) Basic Veal Stock

½ cup (125 g) vegetables (such as carrot, parsnip, and tomato) cut into brunoise (a fine dice of vegetables)
Snipped chives, for garnish

FOR THE BROTH: Heat the olive oil in a medium stockpot, and add the leeks, stirring often, until lightly caramelized, about 5 minutes. Add both stocks and bring to a simmer. Stir in the brunoise and cook until al dente, about 3 minutes longer. Season with salt and pepper.

TO FINISH: Place three to four dumplings in a shallow bowl and ladle hot broth over the dumplings. Garnish with chives. Serve immediately.

ON SAVING ROASTED MARROW FAT

When preparing veal and beef bones for a brown stock, you should roast them first to deepen color and enhance flavor. While roasting, the solid marrow will caramelize and protrude from the bone, and some of the marrow will render onto the roasting pan. While the fat does not belong in the stock, rendered marrow should not be wasted.

If you're like me, you can't help but scoop out some of the marrow from roasted bones destined for the pot. I whip it with butter for a delicious spread, detailed below, or set it aside to be used as an ingredient, as with the veal marrow called for in Rose Veal Marrow Dumpling Soup. Don't be greedy: Keep most of the solid marrow in the bone cavity for the stock making process; it will strengthen the flavor of the stock. Any remaining fat will separate once the stock is strained and chilled, provided the stock was skimmed properly while simmering.

Here's how to make whipped marrow butter: Pour the rendered fat through a fine-mesh strainer and into a small saucepan. Add a healthy pinch of sea salt and other spices, such as peppercorns, cloves, star anise, whatever you fancy, and infuse over low heat. Strain again into a mixing bowl. Leave it at room temperature to congeal, and then add equal parts softened unsalted butter. Using a hand beater or a standing mixer, whip until soft peaks form. Pack into ramekins and store in the refrigerator, covered. Slather on crusty bread and serve alongside soups and stews as a stand-in for pure butter. See also Pink Marrow Butter, page 136, for a version with red wine.

Osso Buco with Salsify and Pearl Onions

Osso Buco is a classic Milanese dish that translates to "bone with a hole," referring to how the marrow bone is revealed within a cross section of the shank. As the meat cooks, the bone becomes more prominent and the marrow serves as a succulent part of the dish; scoop it out with a teaspoon and combine it with the sauce for a perfect bite. Use hind shanks if you desire a meatier portion, which is better for sharing, or foreshanks for a more delicate presentation. For a perfect winter meal, serve the shanks atop risotto, a common accompaniment to this dish.

ACTIVE TIME: 1½ hours | **TOTAL TIME:** 4 hours (including braising) |
YIELD: Makes 6 servings

VEAL SHANKS

6 veal shanks (about 5 pounds [2.3 kg] total),
    each about 1½ inches (3.8 cm) thick
¼ cup (32 g) all-purpose flour
1 tablespoon semolina flour (optional)
1 teaspoon smoked paprika
Salt and pepper
3 tablespoons olive oil
3 tablespoons unsalted butter
2 medium onions, finely diced
1 small fennel bulb, finely diced, fronds reserved

2 medium carrots, finely diced
2 cloves garlic, minced
1 cup (240 ml) dry white wine, such as
    Pinot Grigio
1 cup (240 ml) Roasted Veal Stock
5 medium tomatoes (about 700 g), blanched,
    peeled, and chopped
2 sprigs thyme
1 bay leaf
1 orange, zested and juiced

FOR THE VEAL: Heat the oven to 350°F (175°C). If the veal shanks seem delicate at the edges, tie butcher's twine around the perimeter. Mix the flours, smoked paprika, and a generous amount of salt and pepper in a bowl. Lightly dredge the veal shanks in the flour mixture, shaking to remove the excess.

In a large sauté pan, heat two-thirds of the olive oil and butter over medium-high heat. Add enough veal shanks to cover the bottom of the pan without crowding it, and sear, about 3 minutes per side. Remove and hold in a roasting pan while you repeat with the remaining shanks.

Pour off the used oil without removing the browned bits on the pan. Lower the heat to medium, and add the final third of the olive oil and butter. Add the onion and fennel to the pan, and cook, stirring often, until slightly caramelized, about 10 minutes. Stir in the carrots and garlic; continue to cook until the carrots are al dente, about 5 minutes.

Pour the wine into the hot pan, and simmer to reduce by one-half, stirring to dissolve the pan juices. Add the veal stock, tomatoes, thyme, bay leaf, and orange juice and zest. Season with salt and pepper. Bring the mixture to a boil, and pour over the shanks in the roasting pan. Add stock or water if necessary to bring the liquid to halfway up the sides of the shanks. Cover with a lid or aluminum foil.

Transfer the shanks to the oven, and braise until fork-tender, 1½ to 2 hours. Check the liquid occasionally, adding stock or water if the liquid has cooked down. When the shanks are tender, remove from the roasting pan and reserve to rest the meat. Remove string if used. Strain the sauce and reserve in a separate bowl.

VEGETABLES

2 tablespoons unsalted butter, divided
2 tablespoons olive oil
6 salsify roots or parsnips, peeled and
  diagonally sliced
24 pearl onions, trimmed, blanched and peeled

2 tablespoons Two-Day Veal Stock
2 tablespoons vegetables (such as carrot,
  parsnip, and tomato) cut into brunoise
  (a fine dice of vegetables)

While the veal is braising, make the vegetables. In a small sauté pan, heat 1 tablespoon butter and olive oil over medium-high heat. Add the salsify and pearl onions and cook, stirring often, until the salsify is al dente and the onions start to brown. Deglaze the pan with veal stock, mounting with the remaining butter, and stir in the brunoise. Set aside.

GREMOLATA

1 cup (60 g) chopped
  flat-leaf parsley

3 cloves garlic, minced
2 lemons, zested

Mix the parsley, garlic, and lemon zest in a bowl. Stir to combine, and reserve for plating.

TO SERVE: Spoon the braising liquid on the center of a plate, portion the vegetables on the sauce, and top with a veal shank. Sprinkle gremolata on the meat. If you are feeling decadent, serve with risotto.

Vitello Tonnato

In medieval times, fatty fish such as sturgeon and salmon—dense with calories and yet difficult to preserve—were a royal commodity and subject to priestly rationing. As such, mock recipes that created surrogates for meat and fish were a popular method of the time. One of particular interest—*Mock Sturgeon Made from Veal*—is perhaps a precursor to the marriage of veal and tuna in this classic Italian dish.

The Food of Paris, by Marie-Noël Rio, provides a recipe for *Esturgeon Contrefait de Veau* (circa 1393), whereby one calf head per person was scalded and boiled in wine until the meat fell from the bone. Cooled, sewn, weighted, and left to rest overnight, the end result—thinly sliced gelatinous veal—was paired with parsley and vinegar and delivered to the table as mock sturgeon.

Here roasted veal is chilled, sliced, and covered in a sauce of tuna, anchovies, capers, and parsley. When buying canned tuna, look for pole-caught skipjack, also known as light tuna. This species doesn't qualify as sushi grade, mostly due to its color, and is therefore not overfished.

ACTIVE TIME: 2 hours | **TOTAL TIME:** 6 to 10 hours (including chilling) | **YIELD:** Makes 8 servings

VEAL

1 top round veal (about 2½ to 3 pounds [1.1 to 1.4 kg])
Salt and pepper
2 tablespoons grapeseed oil
2 cups (480 ml) Basic Veal Stock

1 cup (240 ml) dry white wine, such as Pinot Grigio
3 sprigs marjoram
2 bay leaves
3 medium carrots, peeled and sliced into 3-inch (7.5 cm) cylinders

Tie the veal with butcher's twine as you would a roast; this helps the meat stay firm and cook evenly. Season with salt and pepper. In a large Dutch oven, heat the oil until hot but not smoking; add the veal and sear until golden brown on all sides, about 10 minutes. Carefully transfer the veal to a plate. Add the veal stock and wine to the pot; reduce by half, about 5 minutes. Stir in the marjoram and bay leaves. Return the veal to the pot, cover, and simmer until an instant-read thermometer reads 135°F (57°C), about half an hour. Add the carrots about 15 minutes before the roast is done.

When the veal reaches the correct temperature, transfer it to a plate to cool. With a slotted spoon, remove the carrots and hold with the veal. Strain the broth and return it to a clean pan. Over medium heat, reduce the broth to 3 tablespoons and set aside. Cover the veal and sauce and transfer to the refrigerator, at least 4 hours or overnight.

SAUCE

⅓ cup (46 g) capers, divided
⅓ cup (18 g) flat-leaf parsley, divided
1 can (5 ounces) oil-packed tuna, drained
3 tablespoons champagne vinegar

4 egg yolks
4 anchovy fillets, drained
2 lemons, divided
1 cup (240 ml) olive oil

In the bowl of a food processor, add half the capers and parsley with the tuna, vinegar, egg yolks, and anchovies. Top with the zest of one lemon. Pulse until combined, then slowly add the olive oil until emulsified. Thinly slice the remaining lemon; reserve for garnish.

TO SERVE: Remove the veal and reduced stock from the refrigerator half an hour before you plan to eat. In a small saucepan, gently warm the stock until it melts and immediately remove from the heat. Thinly slice the veal and moisten with the reduced stock. Arrange on a platter and spoon the sauce over the sliced veal. Place the carrots and lemon slices around the veal; garnish with the remaining capers and parsley.

BEEF

Many chefs value the velvetiness and versatility of veal stock over the heartiness of beef stock, and some cookbooks even omit the recipe for beef stock altogether. In my opinion, however, a well-made beef stock is the key to enriching a warm winter stew. It is a fine match for deeply caramelized onions, a counter to the earthiness of root vegetables, and a requirement for many noodle bowls throughout the world. Even though they come from the same animal, beef stock is very different than veal stock. It is rich and bold, and should guide a dish and form the base of a meal.

With proper attention and well-sourced ingredients, beef stock can also achieve a rich, silky consistency. Locate a farmer who either raises cattle entirely on grass or finishes animals with healthy grain during the last few months leading to harvest. The best bones to use for beef stock are knuckle, neck, and marrow. Ask your butcher to split the knuckle, which will lessen your simmering time, or if not split, plan for a secondary extraction, or remouillage. If using marrow bones, make sure the ratio to other bone types is balanced: Two or three medium marrow bones to each knuckle will yield a rich stock without too much fat. No tendons are called for in these recipes, as they tend to muddy the liquid.

Basic Beef Stock

This white beef stock adds blanched bones to a mirepoix—in this case, a coarse chop of onions, leeks, carrots, and parsnips—softened in white wine. Garlic is included to enrich the foundation.

ACTIVE TIME: 2 hours | **TOTAL TIME:** 9 hours (including heating, blanching, simmering, and initial cooling) | **YIELD:** Makes about 3 quarts (2.8 liters)

6 pounds (2.7 kg) meaty beef bones (from the neck or leg), preferably grass-fed or pastured
1 calf's foot, preferably grass-fed or pastured (optional)
8 quarts (7.5 L) filtered water, cold, plus water for rinsing and blanching
3 tablespoons grapeseed oil
1 pound (455 g) leeks, dark green parts removed, cut into large dice
½ pound (225 g) white onions, cut into large dice
2 cups (480 ml) dry white wine, such as Sauvignon Blanc
½ pound (225 g) carrots, cut into large dice
½ pound (225 g) parsnips, cut into large dice
1 head garlic, split in half, broken into pieces
3 sprigs thyme
3 sprigs flat-leaf parsley
2 bay leaves
1 tablespoon black peppercorns
Sea salt to taste

Rinse the beef bones under cold water until the water runs clear. Place the beef bones and calf's foot in a large stockpot, and add enough cold water to cover the bones by a few inches. Turn the heat to medium-high, and slowly heat the liquid. Using a fine-mesh strainer, skim any scum that rises to the surface. When the liquid starts to ripple, before it breaks into a boil, remove the pot from the heat. Do not boil the liquid; boiling extracts flavor that should be preserved for the long simmer.

Drain the bones in a large colander, and rinse under cold water. Thoroughly clean the same pot. Return the bones to the pot and add the filtered water. Heat the pot over medium-high, and slowly bring the liquid to a tremble, skimming as soon as scum appears. When the liquid ripples, reduce the heat to medium-low and maintain a simmer, or smile. Never let the liquid boil; if it does impurities will be sucked to the bottom of the pot and emulsify into the liquid. Simmer the bones and water for 5 hours, skimming frequently.

In a large sauté pan, heat half the grapeseed oil over medium-high heat. Add the leeks and onions and cook, stirring, until they sweat, about 7 minutes. Stir in half the wine and simmer until reduced by half, about 3 minutes. Transfer the alliums to a bowl and reserve until needed. Using the same sauté pan, heat the remaining oil and repeat with the carrots, parsnips, and remaining wine. Add the finished vegetables to the onions and leeks in the bowl.

When the bones have completed their initial simmering time, add the sautéed vegetables, garlic, thyme, parsley, bay leaves, and peppercorns to the stockpot. Continue to simmer, another 90 minutes, carefully skimming around the vegetables as necessary.

Turn off the heat and rest the stock on the stove, about 15 minutes. Set a fine-mesh strainer over a container large enough to hold the liquid contents of the pot. Carefully ladle the stock from the pot into the strainer, leaving any cloudy liquid at the bottom of the pot. Taste and season with sea salt.

Place the container in an ice bath to rapidly cool the stock. When the stock no longer steams, transfer to the refrigerator. Once chilled, remove the fat cap and reserve as tallow for cooking or making cosmetics (see chapter 14). Refrigerate for up to 2 days or freeze in smaller containers for longer storage.

Roasted Beef Stock

This brown beef stock employs roasted bones and caramelized vegetables to achieve a deep mahogany liquid. The charred onion adds color and flavor to the pot, a recommendation acquired from Thomas Keller. Though optional, a calf's foot reinforces gelatin in the stock that might be lost during the roasting process.

ACTIVE TIME: 2 hours | **TOTAL TIME:** 10 hours (including roasting, heating, simmering, and initial cooling) | **YIELD:** Makes about 3 quarts (2.8 liters)

---

6 pounds (2.7 kg) meaty beef bones (from the neck or leg), preferably grass-fed or pastured

1 calf's foot, preferably grass-fed or pastured (optional)

3 tablespoons grapeseed oil, divided

8 quarts (7.5 L) filtered water, cold, plus water for rinsing

1 pound (455 g) white onions, 1 onion halved, the rest cut into large dice

1 pound (455 g) leeks, dark green parts removed, cut into large dice

¾ pound (340 g) carrots, cut into large dice

1 head garlic, split in half, broken into pieces

3 sprigs thyme

3 sprigs flat-leaf parsley

2 bay leaves

1 tablespoon black peppercorns

Sea salt to taste

Preheat the oven to 425°F (220°C).

Rinse the beef bones and calf's foot under cold water until the water runs clear. Make sure that all visible blood is removed from the bones. The rinsing of blood will help eliminate proteins that could cloud your stock. Pat the bones dry with kitchen towels.

Place the calf's foot in the stockpot and all remaining bones in a single layer on a large roasting pan. Coat the bones in the pan with half of the grapeseed oil and roast for 20 minutes. With tongs, turn the bones over and continue to roast until golden brown, another 20 minutes. Remove and transfer the excess rendered fat from the pan; reserve for another use (see chapter 14). Lower the oven temperature to 400°F (200°C).

Transfer the roasted bones to the stockpot with the calf's foot. Add water to the hot pan, place over medium heat, and scrape to loosen the browned bits and glazed juices. Pour into the stockpot. Cover the roasted bones with filtered water and turn on the heat to medium-high. Slowly heat the liquid, skimming as soon as scum appears at the top, until the surface starts to ripple. Lower the heat to medium and maintain a simmer, about 6 hours, adding water if any content evaporates during the lengthy cook time. Continue to skim, especially during the first hour of simmering.

While the stock is simmering, heat a cast-iron skillet over medium-high heat. Place the split onion halved-side down on the dry skillet and cook until charred, about 20 minutes. Set aside. Spread the remaining onions with the chopped leek and carrot on a sheet pan and coat with the remaining oil. Roast in the oven until golden brown, about 25 minutes. Remove the vegetables from the oven and hold, covered, until needed.

When the bones have completed their initial simmering time, add the charred onion, roasted vegetables, garlic, thyme, parsley, bay leaves, and peppercorns to the stockpot. Continue to simmer, another 2 hours.

Turn off the heat and rest the stock on the stove, about 15 minutes. Set a fine-mesh strainer over a container large enough to hold the liquid contents of the pot. Carefully ladle the stock from the pot into the strainer, leaving any cloudy liquid at the bottom of the pot. Skim any fat that appears at the surface.

Taste the stock to determine your desired concentration. If the stock tastes too watery, return it to a clean stockpot and simmer until reduced to a desirable consistency. Taste and season with sea salt.

Place the container in an ice bath to rapidly cool the stock. Skim any fat that congeals at the surface. When the stock no longer steams, transfer to the refrigerator. Once chilled, remove the fat cap and reserve as tallow for cooking or making cosmetics. Refrigerate for up to 2 days or freeze in smaller containers for longer storage.

Beef Bone Broth

This bone broth incorporates a proper ratio of marrow bones to render healthy fat and gelatinous protein into the liquid. The calf's foot is necessary for achieving a proper gel, and soaking the bones in vinegar is optional. A remouillage is employed to achieve a full extraction of collagen without muddying the stock.

ACTIVE TIME: 3 hours | **TOTAL TIME:** 2 days (including roasting, heating, simmering, and chilling) | **YIELD:** Makes about 2 quarts (1.9 liters)

5 pounds (2.3 kg) meaty beef bones (from the neck or leg), preferably grass-fed or pastured
1 pound (455 g) beef marrow bones, preferably grass-fed or pastured

1 calf's foot, preferably grass-fed or pastured
¼ cup (60 ml) apple cider vinegar (optional)
3 tablespoons grapeseed oil, divided

16 quarts (15 L) filtered water, cold,
   plus water for rinsing
1 pound (455 g) white onions, 1 onion halved,
   the rest cut into large dice
1 pound (455 g) leeks, dark green parts
   removed, cut into large dice
¾ pound (455 g) carrots, cut into large dice

1 head garlic, split in half, broken
   into pieces
3 sprigs thyme
3 sprigs flat-leaf parsley
2 bay leaves
1 tablespoon black peppercorns
Sea salt to taste

Preheat the oven to 425°F (220°C).

Rinse the beef bones, marrow bones, and calf's foot under cold water until the water runs clear. Make sure that all visible blood is removed from the bones. The rinsing of blood will help eliminate proteins that could cloud your stock. Pat the bones dry with kitchen towels. Place the calf's foot in the stockpot with the apple cider vinegar, if using.

Arrange all remaining bones in a single layer on a large roasting pan. Coat the bones in the pan with half of the grapeseed oil and roast for 15 minutes. With tongs, turn the bones over and continue to roast until golden brown, another 15 minutes. Remove and transfer the excess rendered fat from the pan; cover and chill for later use. Lower the oven temperature to 400°F (200°C).

Transfer the roasted bones to the stockpot with the calf's foot. Follow the instructions for the Roasted Beef Stock to complete the first extraction. After straining, reserve the simmered bones and aromatics for a second run. Place the cooled stock in the refrigerator.

Thoroughly clean the same pot. Return the simmered bones and aromatics to the pot and add the remaining 8 quarts (7.5 L) filtered water. Heat the pot over medium-high, and slowly bring the liquid to a tremble, skimming when scum appears. Maintain a simmer, skimming as necessary, another 4 to 6 hours. Repeat resting, straining, and cooling process with the second extraction, transferring the contents to a clean container. Place in the refrigerator to chill both extractions overnight.

Once chilled, remove the fat cap from both extractions and add to the reserved fat from roasting the bones. Use tallow for cooking or making cosmetics (see chapter 14). Transfer both extractions into a clean stockpot. Place over medium-high heat and slowly bring the liquid to a simmer. Reduce the heat and simmer until reduced by half, or until your desired consistency is achieved. Repeat the resting process and strain the stock twice. Strain again if any particles remain in the liquid. Taste and season with sea salt. Cool in an ice bath.

When reheating the broth for sipping, mount with a small spoonful of the reserved fat to add essential fatty acids and exceptional flavor. Refrigerate for up to 2 days or freeze in smaller containers for longer storage.

Beef Heart Confit with
Caponata Stuffing and Sorrel Vinaigrette

A cow's heart is a muscular organ, and when cooked properly, it boasts the texture of steak. Many recipes for beef heart start with thin slices and rely on quick cooking techniques, such as searing or grilling. Here the entire heart is first stuffed with caponata and formed into a *roulade*—a French term for filled, rolled meat—before entering the oven where a confit is used. The heart is slowly roasted in a blend of tallow and duck fat, both reserved from their respective stocks—this keeps the heart moist during cooking. The accompanying vinaigrette is very acidic and makes a nice foil to the richness of the meat.

Note that the age of the animal will dictate the size of the heart; look for a heart of average size, about 3 to 4 pounds (1.3 to 1.8 kg). If your butcher provides a whole heart that has already been sliced open, it likely means the heart was inspected after harvest—a sign of a well-monitored processor. Soak the heart in salt water for half an hour before cooking with it; this step brings blood from the tissue to the surface, where it can then be washed away.

ACTIVE TIME: 2 hours | **TOTAL TIME:** 10 hours (including baking) |
YIELD: Makes 6 to 8 servings

CAPONATA

¼ cup (60 ml) olive oil
1 small red onion, chopped
½ serrano pepper, minced
3 cloves garlic, minced
1 medium red bell pepper,
   coarsely chopped
1 small eggplant, coarsely chopped
1 medium zucchini, coarsely chopped
2 tablespoons Beef Bone Broth

1 small tomato, chopped
1 anchovy fillet, chopped
1 tablespoon aged sherry vinegar
2 tablespoons capers
2 tablespoons chopped mint
¼ cup (15 g) chopped flat-leaf parsley
1 lemon, zested and juiced
½ cup (20 g) fresh bread crumbs, toasted
Salt and pepper

In a large sauté pan, heat the olive oil over medium heat. Add the red onion, and cook until it sweats, about 3 to 5 minutes. Toss in the serrano pepper and garlic, and continue to cook, stirring, about 3 minutes. Stir in the red bell pepper, eggplant, and zucchini, and cook until caramelized, another 5 to 7 minutes. Deglaze with the beef broth. Add the tomato, anchovy, and sherry vinegar; cook, stirring often, until the mixture comes together. Remove from the heat and transfer to a large bowl. Stir in the capers, mint, parsley, lemon zest, lemon juice, and bread crumbs. Taste and adjust the seasoning. Set aside to allow the flavors to develop.

BEEF HEART

1 beef heart (about 3 to 4 pounds [1.3 to 1.8 kg]), soaked in salt water for 30 minutes
Caponata (above)

Salt and pepper
½ cup (100 g) beef tallow
1 cup (205 g) duck fat
Olive oil, as needed

Heat the oven to 190°F (85°C).

Rinse the heart under cold water, and pat it dry with a dishcloth or kitchen towel. If the heart has not been cut open, slice into one side, starting from the hole on top, without cutting all the way through. Trim off the excess fat. Remove any visible stringy bits, arteries, or blood vessels.

On a work surface, lay the heart fat-side down, and stuff it with the caponata. (You should have some remaining, which can be served alongside the finished dish.) Roll the heart into a tight roulade, and secure it with butcher's twine. Season with salt and pepper.

Place the tallow and all but 2 tablespoons of the duck fat in a Dutch oven. Set the heart in the fat, making sure the heart is submerged. Add olive oil if you need more fat to cover the heart. Place in the oven and slow-cook for 8 hours. (This is a great way to use the oven overnight.) When the heart is tender, remove from the oven and cool slightly. Using tongs, carefully remove the heart from the fat and rest on a plate or cutting board.

In a large sauté pan, melt the remaining duck fat over medium-high heat. When the pan is very hot, sear the beef heart until golden brown, about 2 minutes per side. Remove the heart from the pan, and set aside to rest, about 15 minutes.

SORREL VINAIGRETTE

½ cup (30 g) sorrel leaves
2 tablespoons flat-leaf parsley
2 tablespoons apple cider vinegar
2 tablespoons lemon juice

1 tablespoon maple syrup
1 teaspoon grainy mustard
¼ teaspoon cayenne pepper
Salt and pepper

While the heart is resting, make the vinaigrette. Place all the dressing ingredients in a blender and process until well combined. Adjust the seasoning. The vinaigrette will be very acidic.

TO FINISH: Carefully slice the beef heart on the bias, and serve with the vinaigrette. Serve the remaining caponata on the side.

Ox Bone Soup with Tatsoi Kimchi

Years ago I had a chance meeting with Korean food writer Maangchi at a picnic in Prospect Park. After learning about my passion for stocks, she insisted we visit Gahm Mi Oak, a popular Koreatown destination, for seolleongtang, or "snowy thick soup," made from rendered oxtail bones and served with rice, scallions, sea salt, and plenty of kimchi. This restaurant sadly retired from service after two and a half decades, but the dish remains one of my favorite ways to highlight a good stock.

This is one recipe where maintaining the liquid at a boil is encouraged; the final goal is a milky white stock, which requires a hard simmer to achieve emulsification. Salt is not traditionally used when building this broth; instead, it is served in an unbalanced state, made rich from the rendering only. Salt and scallions are offered as an accompaniment so guests can season to their desire. Kimchi is also served tableside to enhance the umami of the dish. Here, the kimchi is made with tatsoi—a type of Chinese cabbage that is softer than other types of cabbage, which results in a faster fermentation. Feel free to substitute napa cabbage or green cabbage for the tatsoi, and make sure to start the process at least one day before making the soup.

The origins of this dish are found within a royal decree to increase the food supply in Korea. Here the bones are extended in liquid as a way to feed more people. You can go a step further by saving the bones and tallow for other uses, such as bone meal and homemade soap (see chapter 14).

MEAT STOCKS, BROTHS, AND DISHES

ACTIVE TIME: 4 hours | **TOTAL TIME:** 2+ days
(including fermentation, simmering, and cooling) | **YIELD:** Makes 6 servings

KIMCHI

1 pound (455 g) tatsoi

2 tablespoons sea salt, plus a dash to soften
the tatsoi

2 tablespoons sugar

2 teaspoons minced fresh ginger

1 teaspoon minced garlic

2 tablespoons Korean red pepper flakes
(*gochugaru*)

1 tablespoon high-quality fish sauce or
white miso

2 teaspoons toasted sesame oil

1 tablespoon white sesame seeds

One to two days before you make the soup, trim the tatsoi: Remove the root ends, and separate into leaves with stems intact. Place in a bowl and toss with a dash of sea salt. Set aside to soften, about 30 minutes. In a small bowl, combine the 2 tablespoons sea salt with the rest of the ingredients. Gently rinse the tatsoi and toss with the dressing. Cover and marinate in the refrigerator. The flavor of this kimchi intensifies as it ages.

SOUP

1 whole oxtail (about 4 pounds [1.8 kg]),
cut into 2-inch (5 cm) pieces

2 small beef marrow bones (about
½ pound [225 g])

15 quarts (14 L) filtered water, cold,
divided

2 quarts (1.9 L) Basic Beef Stock

2 small daikon radishes, chopped (about 3 cups)

1 medium white onion, chopped

4 cups (800 g) cooked jasmine rice

1 bunch scallions, thinly sliced on the bias

Toasted sesame oil

Salt and pepper

Kimchi (above)

Rinse the oxtail and marrow bones in cold water to remove surface blood and impurities. Fill a large stockpot with 3 quarts (2.8 L) of filtered water, and add the bones. Soak for 30 minutes. Remove the bones and thoroughly rinse in cold water. Discard the water in the stockpot; clean and reserve the pot for blanching the bones.

Bring 3 quarts (2.8 L) of filtered water to a boil over high heat. Place the bones in the pot, reduce the heat to medium-high, and maintain a hard simmer for about 8 minutes. Carefully remove the bones with tongs, and rinse under cold water. Discard the water in the stockpot; clean and reserve the pot for the soup.

Return the bones to the clean stockpot, and fill with beef stock and 3 quarts (2.8 L) filtered water. Add the daikon radish and onion to the pot. Over medium heat, slowly return the water to a boil, and then reduce the heat to maintain a hard simmer, about 3 hours.

Remove the pot from the heat, and carefully pour the broth into a holding container, leaving the bones in the pot. Store the broth in the refrigerator while you continue building the broth. Add 3 quarts (2.8 L) filtered water to the bones in the pot and return to medium heat. Slowly bring the water to a boil, reduce the heat, and simmer for another 3 hours. Repeat this step one

more time, with the last 3 quarts (2.8 liters) of filtered water, adding each batch of broth to the holding container and reserving in cold storage. Chill the final broth overnight. After the final simmer, transfer the bones to a bowl until cool enough to handle. Carefully shred the meat from the bones, and reserve in the refrigerator. Save the spent bones for another use.

The next day, remove the chilled broth from the refrigerator and scrape off the congealed fat from the top. Save the tallow for another use. Warm the broth over medium-high heat. Add the oxtail meat to the broth to heat through.

Place a scoop of rice in the bottom of a deep bowl, add some oxtail meat, and top with a generous portion of broth. Serve with scallions, sesame oil, sea salt, black pepper, and kimchi on the side.

Coconut-Braised Short Rib Pie with Maple-Ginger Broth

This recipe is an adaptation of the ultimate comfort food—chicken potpie—instead featuring beef short rib in a rich coconut sauce and encased in a leaf lard pastry. The filling begins by making a roux, a mixture of fat and flour that thickens the sauce and holds the meat and vegetables together. The maple-ginger broth can also stand on its own as a sipping beverage.

ACTIVE TIME: 3 hours | **TOTAL TIME:** 16 hours
(including resting, marinating, braising, and baking) | **YIELD:** Makes 8 servings

PASTRY

2 cups (240 g) pastry flour, plus additional for dusting

¾ teaspoon sea salt
¼ teaspoon baking powder

¼ cup (58 g) leaf lard, cut into small pieces, kept frozen, or lard reserved from Basic Pork Stock

½ cup (115 g) unsalted butter, cut into small pieces, kept frozen
6 to 7 tablespoons ice water

Place the flour, salt, and baking powder in the bowl of a food processor. Pulse to combine. Distribute the frozen lard over the flour mixture and pulse to a coarse meal. Repeat with the frozen butter. Add the ice water and pulse until the mixture loosely comes together. Turn the contents onto a clean work surface. Using the heel of your hand, knead the mixture with firm forward strokes to incorporate the fat into the flour. Shape the dough into a rectangular block. Wrap in plastic and refrigerate for 30 minutes.

Unwrap the dough and place on a lightly floured work surface. Roll the dough into a long rectangle. Fold the bottom third up onto itself and the top third down; turn the folded dough a quarter turn, so the folds are facing you. Flour the work surface and repeat the process twice. Wrap the dough again and refrigerate it for another 30 minutes. Repeat this rolling and folding process two more times—for a total of six turns. Refrigerate the dough for at least 1 hour and up to 2 days. This pastry also freezes well.

SHORT RIBS

3 small Thai chili peppers, sliced
¼ cup (28 g) peeled and sliced fresh ginger
2 stalks lemongrass, peeled and sliced
3 small shallots, sliced
3 cloves garlic, sliced
2 tablespoons brown sugar
½ teaspoon sea salt

½ teaspoon black pepper
3 pounds (1.4 kg) boneless beef short rib, cut into 2-inch (5 cm) cubes
2 tablespoons all-purpose flour
2 tablespoons grapeseed oil
1 can (13.5 ounces [400 ml]) coconut milk
2 cups (480 ml) Maple-Ginger Beef Brew

Place the chilies, ginger, lemongrass, shallots, garlic, brown sugar, salt, and pepper into the bowl of a food processor. Pulse to combine. In a large bowl, toss the cubed short ribs with the rub, and marinate in the refrigerator for at least 8 hours, and up to 2 days.

Heat the oven to 225°F (110°C). Remove the short ribs from the refrigerator and dust with flour. In a Dutch oven, heat the grapeseed oil over

medium-high heat, and sear the cubed short ribs on all sides, in batches if necessary, until golden brown. Return all of the meat to the Dutch oven, and add the coconut milk and beef brew. Top with a lid or foil and braise in the oven until fork-tender, 3 to 4 hours. Check occasionally and add water if the liquid reduces to expose the meat. Note that you will combine the meat mixture with the vegetable filling a half an hour before the braising time is complete.

FILLING

2 tablespoons coconut oil
2 tablespoons all-purpose flour
2 medium carrots, peeled and cubed

2 small sweet potatoes, peeled and cubed
24 pearl onions, trimmed, blanched,
  and peeled

MAKE A ROUX: Melt the coconut oil over medium heat in a large sauté pan. Dust the flour over the oil and toast, while stirring, until light brown, about 2 minutes. Add a splash of beef stock from the short rib braising pan to loosen the mixture. Throw in the carrots, sweet potatoes, and pearl onions, and stir over the heat until just combined, about 4 minutes. Set aside until ready to combine with the short rib.

TO ASSEMBLE

½ cup (30 g) finely chopped
  flat-leaf parsley

1 egg
2 tablespoons water

In the last half an hour of cooking the meat, fold the vegetable mixture into the braising liquid. When the meat and vegetables are done, fold in the parsley.

Increase the oven temperature to 400°F (200°C). Remove the dough from the refrigerator. Divide the meat mixture into eight 12-ounce deep ramekins or ovenproof bowls. (Alternatively, you can use one 3-quart [3-liter] baking dish to yield one large pie.) Roll out the pastry to about ¼ inch (.6 cm) thick and cut out circles that are slightly bigger than the diameter of your baking dishes. Place one circle of dough over the top of each dish, and gently press the sides to the dish. Poke a hole in the dough for steam to escape. In a small bowl, whisk the egg with 2 tablespoons water, and brush the dough tops with the egg wash. Bake for 20 to 25 minutes, or until golden brown. Serve immediately.

ON DRY-AGING AT HOME

There are many benefits to investing in large cuts of beef: often more affordable, more efficient, and very local—a handshake with your farmer likely seals the deal. An additional perk is that large cuts offer the option of dry-aging at home, a method that is expensive yet worth the value.

The reason dry-aged meat costs more is because the process concentrates flavor while losing salable weight. When placed in a temperature-controlled environment for at least two weeks, natural enzymes break down connective tissue in the muscular structure of the meat. The result is tender, rich, well-marbled meat, with moisture that is already contained within. A steak that holds its own broth!

To dry-age at home, you need a prime cut of well-sourced meat, preferably bone-in from the rib section, with the fat cap on; a refrigerator that holds temperature between 36°F and 40°F (2°C and 4°C); and a rack set on a rimmed baking sheet to hold the meat. Do not trim the fat; it will protect the interior meat during aging.

J. Kenji López-Alt, a chef and author who explains home cooking through scientific evaluation, further recommends a mini-fridge dedicated to the process (to keep odor from permeating other food) and outfitted with a small fan to aid air circulation. Alternatively, you can air-dry the beef for one full day and then loosely wrap in cheesecloth for the remaining aging process. If moisture releases from the meat into the cheesecloth, simply rewrap and continue aging on the rack.

Refrigerate the meat for fourteen to twenty-eight days, depending on the amount of funk, or forward flavor, you want the meat to have. Most butchers and steak houses cap the aging process at the end of this time frame, though some aficionados will age beef for as long as two months.

Turn the meat occasionally to promote even dehydration, and keep an eye on the beef throughout the process. The cut will shrink as it loses moisture, the fat will form a crust, and the color of any exposed meat will darken. Do not be alarmed by *small* formations of white mold; this is acceptable for aged meat. An odor similar to nutty blue cheese might develop over time; this is the aforementioned funk, and is also desirable. Do, however, observe with caution: Black mold is a bad sign.

At the end of the aging process, unwrap the meat and peel off the outer fat cap; it should be loose enough to remove with your hands. Using a sharp knife, carefully trim away the dried secondary layer of fat and any exposed meat, leaving as much fresh fat on the meat as possible. Discard the fat cap, secondary fat layer, and meat trimmings. Reserve any fresh fat from the trimmings; it is a delicious basting agent for the cooking process. Roast whole or cut into steaks, per the Aged Rib Steak recipe (page 136).

Before you try this method at home, I strongly recommend consulting Sandor Katz's *The Art of Fermentation* for a deeper exploration of how fermentation and meat work together.

Aged Rib Steak with Pink Marrow Butter and Sautéed Broccoli Rabe

This steak is coated with its own fat and gets an additional burst of flavor from marrow butter. Since it is basted in the pan with its own juices, the steak requires no additional stock for cooking. If you are feeling decadent, ask your butcher for the "tomahawk" cut, a bone-in rib steak that is especially striking on the plate. For a professional presentation, you can steam the bone clean by wrapping a sheet of moistened kitchen towel around the top and tightly covering it with aluminum foil during the cooking process.

ACTIVE TIME: 1 hour | **TOTAL TIME:** 2 hours (including resting and chilling) | **YIELD:** Makes 2 servings

PINK MARROW BUTTER

2 beef marrow bones (each about 3 inches [7.5 cm] long), preferably sliced lengthwise, soaked in water for 30 minutes to extract impurities
½ cup (120 ml) dry red wine, such as Merlot

1 small shallot, minced
1 teaspoon black peppercorns
1 sprig flat-leaf parsley
½ cup (115 g) unsalted butter, softened
½ teaspoon sea salt

Heat the oven to 425°F (220°C). Place the marrow bones on a sheet pan and roast in the oven for 25 minutes. Remove from the oven and rest until cool enough to handle. Scoop out the marrow and reserve at room temperature. (Keep the roasted bones for stock.)

In a saucepan, place the red wine, shallot, peppercorns, and parsley over medium-high heat. Reduce to a glaze, about 2 tablespoons. Remove from the heat, strain, and discard the solids. Set aside to cool.

Place the softened butter, cooled marrow, red wine reduction, and sea salt in the bowl of a mixer. Whip with the balloon attachment until the mixture is fluffy. Transfer to parchment or waxed paper and roll into a log. Chill or freeze.

STEAK

2 bone-in rib steaks (each about 3 to 4 inches
    [7.5 to 10 cm] thick), preferably dry-aged
4 cloves garlic, smashed
2 sprigs thyme
2 sprigs oregano

2 whole cloves
1 bay leaf
2 tablespoons Pink Marrow Butter (above)
Salt and pepper
1 tablespoon olive oil

Reduce the oven temperature to 350°F (175°C). An hour before you intend to eat, remove the steaks from the refrigerator. With a sharp knife, trim and reserve the fresh fat from the edges of the meat. Keep the steaks at room temperature, uncovered, while preparing the seasoned fat.

In a small saucepan, heat the reserved fat with the garlic, thyme, oregano, cloves, and bay leaf over medium heat until rendered, about 2 minutes. Mount with 2 tablespoons marrow butter and stir until incorporated. Remove from the heat to cool slightly. Generously season the steaks with salt and pepper, and brush the meat with the rendered fat on both sides.

In a cast-iron or carbon steel pan, heat the olive oil over medium-high heat. When the pan is hot, add the steak and sear, pressing firmly with a spatula, until browned on one side, about 2 minutes. Flip the steak, basting with pan juices, and repeat on the other side.

Transfer the steak to the oven and continue to cook until medium-rare (135°F [57°C]), occasionally basting, about 10 minutes. Remove the steak from the oven, loosely cover with aluminum foil, and rest, about 7 minutes. Wipe the pan clean.

VEGETABLE

2 tablespoons olive oil
1 bunch broccoli rabe, tough stems removed
¼ cup (60 ml) pan juices or Roasted Beef Stock

2 cloves garlic, minced
1 teaspoon red pepper flakes
Sea salt

While the steak is resting, heat the olive oil in a clean pan over medium-high heat, then toss in the broccoli rabe. Cook, stirring often, until wilted, about 2 minutes. Deglaze with pan juices or beef stock. Add the garlic and red pepper flakes, and continue cooking until al dente, another 2 minutes. Season with sea salt.

TO FINISH: Top the hot steak with a generous portion of broccoli rabe, and then top with a generous dollop of the marrow butter.

LAMB

Spring is an exciting season for sheep: It is a time when ewes give birth to lambs. The mild weather and abundant grass create an ideal habitat to welcome newborns to the land. Sheep take well to farm life: Watched over by shepherds on pasture, they graze mostly on grass and hay until ready for harvest in late summer.

Unlike cows, chickens, and pigs, lambs are more likely to be raised in flocks on pasture under the protective watch of a shepherd. This is, in part, because the cost of raising sheep in a factory setting is prohibitive. It belies the market demand for younger lamb, which offers a mild flavor that is favorable to many chefs and consumers, even though it yields a lesser quantity of meat. In the United States, large herds of sheep can be found grazing on public land; here, they prevent fires by managing underbrush and weeds. Sheep also supplement their grazing with leftovers—both excessive crops from farmland and scraps from large ruminants. All in all, the sheep industry is experiencing a decline in large enterprises and an increase in small flock operations.

The fatty acids in lamb are what make it distinguishable from beef: Lamb has a slightly more forward flavor, sometimes with a barnyard gaminess. Lamb stock can be used like, or in place of, beef or veal stock; it should guide the dish as a diluted base or be reduced to form a rich foundation. It is ideal for hearty ethnic stews, such as a Moroccan tagine and a Scotch broth.

There is a certain maternal passion associated with raising sheep, similar to that between a doula and mother and child. An ideal farmer is one whose adoration for lamb is palpable from land to plate, using regenerative grazing practices for the full lives of the animal. Avoid lamb that is sent to feedlots for finishing. As with veal, look for meaty bones from the neck, shank, and breast. Lamb stock does not make a good bone broth due to its forward flavor.

Basic Lamb Stock

This white lamb stock is built with white wine and finished with vinegar to balance and brighten the foundation. Unlike a classic white veal stock, the vegetables in this stock are sautéed to add sweetness and balance the slightly gamy flavor of lamb. Celery root is introduced to complement lamb's earthiness.

MEAT STOCKS, BROTHS, AND DISHES

ACTIVE TIME: 2 hours | **TOTAL TIME:** 7 hours (including heating, blanching, simmering, and initial cooling) | **YIELD:** Makes about 3 quarts (2.8 liters)

---

8 pounds (3.7 kg) meaty lamb bones (shanks, necks, and breast), preferably pastured

1 calf's foot, preferably grass-fed or pastured

8 quarts (7.5 L) filtered water, cold, plus water for rinsing and blanching

¼ cup (60 ml) grapeseed oil

½ pound (225 g) white onions, cut into large dice

1 pound (455 g) leeks, dark green parts removed, cut into large dice

¾ pound (455 g) carrots, cut into large dice

1 small celery root, peeled, coarsely chopped

2 cups (480 ml) dry white wine, such as Sauvignon Blanc

6 sprigs thyme

6 sprigs flat-leaf parsley

2 bay leaves

1 tablespoon black peppercorns

Sea salt to taste

1 tablespoon white wine vinegar

Rinse the lamb bones under cold water until the water runs clear. Place the bones and calf's foot in a large stockpot, and add enough cold water to cover the bones by a few inches. Turn the heat to medium-high, and slowly heat the liquid. Using a fine-mesh strainer, skim any scum that rises to the surface. When the liquid starts to ripple, before it breaks into a boil, remove the pot from the heat. Do not boil the liquid; boiling extracts flavor that should be preserved for the long simmer.

Drain the bones in a large colander, and rinse under cold water. Thoroughly clean the same pot. Return the bones to the pot and add the filtered water. Heat the pot over medium-high, and slowly bring the liquid to a tremble, skimming as soon as scum appears. When the liquid ripples, reduce the heat to medium-low and maintain a simmer, or smile. Never let the liquid boil, as impurities will be sucked to the bottom of the pot and emulsify into the liquid. Simmer the bones and water for 4 hours, skimming frequently.

Prepare the vegetables while the stock is simmering. In a sauté pan, heat the grapeseed oil over medium heat. When it starts to ripple, add the onions, leeks, carrots, and celery root, and sauté, stirring often, until they are cooked through but not caramelized, about 10 minutes. Deglaze the pan with the white wine and simmer for 1 minute. Turn off the heat and set aside until needed.

Once the bones have completed their initial simmering time, add the sautéed vegetables, herbs, and peppercorns, and slowly bring to a gentle boil. Reduce the heat to medium-low and maintain at a simmer, about 2 hours longer.

Turn off the heat and rest the stock on the stove, about 15 minutes. Gently ladle the stock through a China cap into a clean container; remove the bones and aromatics. Set a fine-mesh strainer over a clean stockpot. Line the strainer with cheesecloth. Carefully strain the stock into the pot, being careful not to force any solids through the mesh. Over medium-high heat, return the stock to a gentle boil, reduce the heat to medium, and continue to simmer until reduced by a third. Season with sea salt and finish with vinegar.

Place the container in an ice bath to rapidly cool the stock. When the stock no longer steams, transfer to the refrigerator. Refrigerate for up to 2 days or freeze in smaller containers for longer storage.

Roasted Lamb Stock

Tomatoes and tomato paste are incorporated into this brown lamb stock to intensify flavor and hue. Unlike a brown veal stock, the vegetables in this stock are not roasted, in order to avoid adding too much color. Roasting the lamb bones, while adding color, minimizes the slightly gamy flavor of the lamb.

ACTIVE TIME: 2 hours | TOTAL TIME: 10 hours (including roasting, heating, simmering, and initial cooling) | YIELD: Makes about 3 quarts (2.8 liters)

---

8 pounds (3.6 kg) meaty lamb bones (necks and breast), preferably pastured
1 calf's foot, preferably grass-fed or pastured
3 tablespoons grapeseed oil
8 quarts (7.5 L) filtered water, cold, plus water for rinsing
½ pound (225 g) white onions, cut into large dice
1 pound (455 g) leeks, dark green parts removed, cut into large dice

¾ pound (340 g) carrots, cut into large dice
¾ pound tomatoes (340 g), coarsely chopped
½ cup (115 g) tomato paste, preferably home-made (page 273)
6 sprigs thyme
6 sprigs flat-leaf parsley
2 bay leaves
1 tablespoon black peppercorns
Sea salt to taste

Preheat the oven to 400°F (200°C).

Rinse the lamb bones and calf's foot under cold water until the water runs clear. Make sure that all visible blood is removed from the bones. The rinsing of blood will help eliminate proteins that could cloud your stock. Pat the bones dry with kitchen towels. Place the calf's foot in the stockpot and all remaining bones in a single

layer on a large roasting pan. Coat the bones in the pan with the grapeseed oil and roast for 40 minutes. With tongs, turn the bones over and continue to roast until golden brown, another 40 minutes. Remove and transfer the excess rendered fat from the pan; reserve for another use (see chapter 14).

Transfer the roasted bones to the stockpot

with the calf's foot. Add water to the hot pan, place over medium heat, and scrape to loosen the browned bits and glazed juices. Pour into the stockpot. Cover the roasted bones with the filtered water and turn on the heat to medium-high. Slowly heat the liquid, skimming as soon as scum appears at the top, until the surface starts to ripple. Lower the heat to medium and maintain a simmer, about 5 hours, adding water if any content evaporates during the lengthy cook time. Continue to skim, especially during the first hour of simmering.

When the bones have completed their initial simmering time, add the onions, leeks, carrots, tomato, tomato paste, herbs, and peppercorns to the stockpot. Continue to simmer, another 2 hours.

Turn off the heat and rest the stock on the stove, about 15 minutes. Set a fine-mesh strainer over a container large enough to hold the liquid contents of the pot. Carefully ladle the stock from the pot into the strainer, leaving any cloudy liquid at the bottom of the pot. Skim any fat that appears at the surface.

Taste the stock to determine your desired concentration. If the stock tastes too watery, return it to a clean stockpot and simmer until reduced to a desirable consistency. Taste and season with sea salt.

Place the container in an ice bath to rapidly cool the stock. Skim any fat that congeals at the surface. When the stock no longer steams, transfer to the refrigerator. Once chilled, remove the fat cap and reserve for making cosmetics. Refrigerate for up to 2 days or freeze in smaller containers for longer storage.

Traditional Plum Pottage

Pottages, also known as stewed broth in medieval times, are similar to modern-day chicken potpies. The earliest known plum pottage featured young meat—veal, lamb, or chicken—speckled with currants, thickened with bread, and colored with sandalwood. You can find sandalwood powder, likely from India, at specialty spice stores or online vendors.

ACTIVE TIME: 1 hour | **TOTAL TIME:** 4 hours
(including braising, simmering, and baking) | **YIELD:** Makes 4 servings

2 tablespoons olive oil
2 lamb shanks (about 1½ pounds [680 g] each)
1 medium onion, diced
1 medium carrot, peeled and diced
1 quart (960 ml) Basic Lamb Stock

3 sprigs sage
4 eggs
2 cups (80 g) fresh bread crumbs
¼ cup (28 g) almond meal
½ cup (71 g) dried black currants

¼ cup (15 g) chopped flat-leaf parsley
½ teaspoon sea salt

½ teaspoon sandalwood powder (optional)
1 pinch saffron threads, toasted and ground

Preheat the oven to 325°F (165°C).

In a Dutch oven, heat the olive oil over medium heat until hot but not smoking. Season the lamb shanks with salt and pepper. Using tongs, place the lamb into the hot pan and brown on all sides. Transfer to a plate. In the same pan, add the onion and carrot and cook until the vegetables sweat, about 4 minutes. Return the lamb to the pan and add the stock and sage. Braise in the oven until tender, turning once, about 2 hours.

Remove the lamb from the oven to cool. Raise the heat to 350°F (175°C). Strain the braising liquid into a small saucepan; discard the solids. Place over medium heat and simmer until reduced by half. When the lamb is cool enough to handle, shred into small pieces.

Reserve both the sauce and lamb at room temperature. Save the shank bones for stock.

In a medium bowl, whisk the eggs until frothy. Fold in the bread crumbs and almond meal. Gradually add the reduced braising liquid, stirring until well combined. Add the shredded meat, currants, herbs, and spices. (The sandalwood, if using, will turn the mixture red.) Cover the bowl and rest until the liquid is absorbed, about 20 minutes.

Transfer the mixture to a large buttered 2-quart (2-liter) baking dish; smooth the top with a spatula. Cover the dish with a lid or aluminum foil, and bake until set, about 20 minutes. Remove from the oven and rest for a few minutes before serving in bowls.

Milk-Braised Lamb Neck with Wilted Escarole on Savory Oatmeal

The practice of braising meat in milk can be attributed to the Romans and has since been adopted by Italian and Middle Eastern cultures. A popular Lebanese lamb dish called *immos*, which means "his mother's milk," consists of a young lamb cooked in yogurt made from its mother's milk.

This dish pairs milk-braised lamb with savory oats, a combination seen in cuisines around the world. Sheep also eat oats, adding another contextual twist to this dish. You will get the best result with thick-cut oats; do not use the instant variety oats. The recipe calls for an entire neck, though sliced neck can also be used.

ACTIVE TIME: 1½ hours | TOTAL TIME: 3½ hours
(including braising and simmering) | YIELD: Makes 4 servings

LAMB

1 teaspoon cumin, toasted and ground	2 tablespoons olive oil
1 teaspoon coriander, toasted and ground	4 cloves garlic, smashed
¼ teaspoon cayenne pepper	½ cup (120 ml) heavy cream
Salt and pepper	2 cups (480 ml) whole milk
1 lamb neck (about 2 pounds [910 g]), trimmed	1 tablespoon honey
	3 bay leaves

In a small bowl, toss the cumin, coriander, cayenne pepper, salt, and pepper together until well combined. Generously season all sides of the lamb neck with the spices; reserve the lamb at room temperature.

In a large Dutch oven, heat the olive oil over medium heat. Add the smashed garlic and cook, stirring, about 1 minute. Remove the garlic and raise the heat to medium-high. Add the lamb neck and sear until golden brown, about 3 minutes per side. Transfer the lamb to a bowl and set aside to rest.

Pour the cream into the hot Dutch oven and stir to scrape up brown bits from the bottom. Add the milk, honey, and bay leaves; stir until combined. Return the lamb and its juices to the pan and reduce the heat to low. Cover and braise, stirring occasionally, until the lamb is fork-tender, about 2 hours.

Transfer the lamb to a bowl to cool. Bring the milk mixture to a boil and reduce by half, about 10 minutes. Discard the bay leaves. Using an immersion blender, carefully purée the mixture, then pass through a strainer into a bowl. Season with salt and pepper.

When the lamb is cool enough to handle, remove the meat from the neck bones. Return the meat to the sauce, cover, and hold at room temperature.

OATMEAL

2 tablespoons olive oil	1 cup (240 ml) water
1 medium onion, minced	1 cinnamon stick
1 medium carrot, diced	1 cup (115 g) thick-cut oatmeal (not instant)
1 medium parsnip, diced	2 tablespoons unsalted butter
1 cup (240 ml) Basic Lamb Stock	Salt and pepper

While the lamb is cooling, in a medium saucepan, heat the olive oil over medium heat. Add the onion and cook until translucent, about 3 minutes. Stir in the carrot and parsnip and cook until al dente, another 5 minutes.

Pour in the Basic Lamb Stock and water;

add the cinnamon stick. Bring to a boil and stir in the oatmeal. Reduce to a simmer and cook, stirring often, until the liquid has evaporated and the oatmeal is thick and creamy, about 12 minutes. Mount with butter and season with salt and pepper.

ESCAROLE

2 tablespoons olive oil

2 cloves garlic, minced

1 anchovy fillet, minced

2 to 3 small heads (about 1 pound [455 g]) escarole, each halved lengthwise, root ends intact

¼ cup (60 ml) Roasted Lamb Stock

1 teaspoon aged sherry vinegar

1 teaspoon honey

½ lemon, zest and juice

¼ cup (35 g) oil-cured olives, pitted and coarsely chopped

3 tablespoons dried black currants

Salt and pepper

2 tablespoons pine nuts, toasted

In a large sauté pan, heat olive oil over medium heat. Add the minced garlic and anchovy. Cook while stirring, about 3 minutes. Lay the escarole in one layer, cut-side down, in the pan and splash with the lamb stock. Cook the escarole until wilted, about 2 minutes. Coat the escarole with the vinegar, honey, and lemon zest and juice. Toss in the olives and currants. Continue cooking until the escarole caramelizes, another 5 minutes. Remove from the pan and season with salt and pepper. Top with the toasted pine nuts.

TO SERVE: Place the lamb meat and reduced milk sauce to a clean pan. Gently reheat. Divide the oatmeal into bowls, top with the lamb and escarole. Serve warm.

Smoked Lamb Breast with Black Garlic Crust and Coriander Sambal Cream

Though lamb breast can be difficult to locate whole—it is often butchered into riblets or offered as a boneless roll—this fatty cut is my favorite part of the animal. Lamb breast has a tender, flavorful layer of meat hidden within sinewy fat. When properly cooked, the meat falls off the bone and the fat caramelizes into delicious crunchy bits. Ask your butcher for a bone-in cut, preferably the entire breast, which will look like an oblong ribbed rectangle with a generous flap at one end.

The soft smoke in this recipe combines with the candy-like flavors of black garlic and is finished with sweet shallots and a spicy green sambal. Serve with jasmine rice and a simple salad for a complete meal.

ACTIVE TIME: 2 hours | **TOTAL TIME:** 3½ hours (including smoking and braising) | **YIELD:** Makes 4 servings

LAMB

1 bone-in lamb breast (about 2 to 3 pounds [910 to 1,360 g])
12 cloves black garlic (about 2 heads), or 1 head roasted garlic
1 tablespoon blackstrap molasses

2 tablespoons olive oil
2 teaspoons smoked paprika
Salt and pepper
Smoking chips, such as applewood
Water or Basic Lamb Stock, for misting

Heat an oven to 225°F (110°C). Place the breast on a cutting board, meat-side down. With a sharp boning knife, trim the flap from the ribs. (You can use the flap as an addition to farce in another recipe.) Bring to room temperature while preparing the crust.

In a small bowl, smash the black garlic cloves with a fork until they form a paste. (If using roasted garlic, squeeze the garlic from the head to form a paste. Discard the skins.) Mix in the blackstrap molasses, olive oil, smoked paprika, salt, and pepper. Stir to combine. Spread the crust generously on both sides of the breast.

Wrap the lamb in aluminum foil.

Place the wood chips in a stovetop smoker, and place a rack above the wood. Place the lamb on the rack, and secure the smoker with the lid. Heat over medium, until smoking, and continue to smoke, about 15 minutes. Turn the heat off, uncover the smoker, and unwrap the lamb. Transfer the lamb to a shallow roasting pan and place in the oven. Cook until the meat is tender, misting with water or stock and turning occasionally, about 2½ hours. Remove the lamb from the oven and rest while preparing the shallots and sambal. Increase the oven temperature to 450°F (230°C).

SHALLOTS

⅓ cup (80 ml) peanut oil
8 small shallots
1 teaspoon aged sherry vinegar

1 teaspoon honey
¼ teaspoon cayenne pepper
Sea salt

In a large sauté pan, heat the peanut oil over medium heat. Add the shallots and cook until caramelized, stirring often, about 15 minutes. Lower the heat, if necessary, to prevent the shallots from burning. When the shallots are golden brown, stir in the vinegar, honey, cayenne pepper, and salt. Continue to cook until the shallots are caramelized yet still hold their shape. Remove from the heat and set aside.

SAMBAL

3 caramelized shallots (above)
1 to 2 fresh hot green chilies
½ cup (30 g) coarsely chopped cilantro leaves

1 tablespoon coriander, toasted and ground
½ cup (120 ml) heavy cream
Salt and pepper

In a food processor, pulse the shallots, green chili, cilantro, and coriander until a paste forms. Add the cream and pulse until well combined. Transfer the cream mixture to a small saucepan. Bring to a boil, then lower to a simmer and reduce until thickened, about 5 minutes. Season with salt and pepper.

TO SERVE: Slice the lamb breast into clusters of three to four ribs per serving, as you would a rack of ribs. Line a baking sheet with aluminum foil, and place the lamb pieces on it, fatty-side up. Brush the ribs with fat drippings from the roasting pan. Roast until brown and crispy, about 15 minutes. If the lamb requires more browning, place under the broiler for a few minutes and monitor closely until caramelized.

Carefully arrange the ribs on plates or a platter. Drizzle the sambal over the lamb and garnish with the shallots.

Hay-Roasted Leg of Lamb with Poached Quince and Sumac Yogurt

Cooking in hay, or *dans le foin*, is a recently revived technique that has its origins in European homes of centuries past. Hayboxes, a type of efficiency-cooking tool, were employed in the early nineteenth century: Hay acted as insulation and held residual heat created through steam. Slow cooking at its best—these contraptions reduced active energy and increased passive cooking time, typically threefold.

In the modern home oven, the temperature is placed at a higher setting, which traps heat within the moist hay and creates a natural oven with enough residual heat to finish cooking the lamb. You can also prepare this dish in a gas grill during the warmer months. Ask your farmer if he can spare a handful of hay for your culinary endeavors. Keep in mind that hay is different than straw: Hay is grass that has been cut and dried, often for animal feed; whereas straw is the stalks of grain, such as barley or wheat, that remain after the harvest. In this dish, hay imparts grassy notes to the meat and sauce.

Lamb and quince is a common pairing in Middle Eastern cooking. Sharing the family but owning its genus, quince is the hardy, delicious cousin of apples and pears; the fruit adds a subtle sweetness to this dish. Sumac, readily foraged in the Northeast during early fall, incorporates a citrusy spark to the yogurt-based condiment. This is an elaborate dish that presents well on a platter and is ample enough to feed a small crowd.

ACTIVE TIME: 1½ hours | **TOTAL TIME:** 3½ hours
(including soaking, braising, and simmering) | **YIELD:** Makes 6 to 8 servings

LAMB

¼ cup (56 g) unsalted butter, plus 2 tablespoons for pan juices, softened
2 cloves garlic, minced
3 tablespoons finely chopped rosemary
Salt and pepper
1 leg of lamb (about 4 to 6 pounds [1.8 to 2.7 kg])

3 handfuls fresh, clean hay, rinsed
1 cup (240 ml) Basic Lamb Stock
½ cup (120 ml) dry white wine, such as Sauvignon Blanc
Fresh pomegranate seeds, for garnish (optional)

In a small bowl, cream ¼ cup butter with the garlic and rosemary. Generously season with salt and pepper. Rub the mixture on all sides of the lamb leg. Reserve at room temperature while preparing the oven and hay.

Heat an oven to 425°F (220°C). In a large bowl, soak the hay in the lamb stock for about half an hour. Transfer two-thirds of the soaked hay to a Dutch oven or deep roasting pan large enough to hold the lamb. Nestle the seasoned meat in the hay and cover with remaining hay. Drizzle wine over the hay-covered lamb.

Cover, making sure no hay is visible outside of the cooking vessel, and transfer to the hot oven. Braise the lamb at high heat for 30 minutes, then reduce the oven temperature to 350°F (175°C). Continue to cook the lamb until the internal temperature reaches 130°F (54°C), about 1½ hours longer. Remove from the oven and rest, covered, for 20 minutes.

QUINCE

1 cup (240 ml) dry white wine, such as
  Sauvignon Blanc
1 cup (240 ml) water
¼ cup (80 g) honey

2 tablespoons pomegranate molasses
2 strips lemon zest
3 quince, peeled, cored,
  and quartered

In a medium saucepan, bring the wine, water, honey, pomegranate molasses, and lemon zest to a boil. Reduce the heat to a simmer and add the prepared quince. Cook until quince becomes fork-tender, about 45 minutes. Remove from the heat and cool in the cooking liquid.

YOGURT

1 cup (225 g) plain whole
  Greek yogurt
2 tablespoons olive oil

½ lemon, zest and juice
1 teaspoon ground sumac
Sea salt

In a small bowl, whisk the yogurt, olive oil, lemon zest and juice, and ground sumac in a bowl. Lightly season with sea salt. Wrap and reserve in the refrigerator.

TO SERVE: Remove the lid from the roasting vessel and carefully remove the lamb from the hay. Strain the pan juices from the hay and braising vessel; discard the hay. In a small saucepan, bring the pan juices and 2 tablespoons of the quince poaching liquid to a boil, reduce to a simmer, and whisk in the remaining 2 tablespoons of butter. Season with salt and pepper; set aside.

Carve the lamb leg and pour the sauce over the meat. Arrange the poached quince slices around the meat. Sprinkle with pomegranate seeds. Serve warm with the yogurt sauce on the side.

Spring Lamb Pot au Feu

A traditional pot au feu is delivered to the table in stages: The meal begins with a simple bowl of strained broth, followed by a main course of meat and vegetables, served from the cooking vessel. Early writers on pot au feu debated the significance of elements from the dish: Is the boullion (broth) or the bouilli (braised meat) more important?

It is customary to serve marrow bones from the pot with bread, mustard, and cornichons. Here the marrow is roasted separately for improved texture and depth of flavor. Ask your butcher to cut the bones lengthwise so that a long strip of marrow is exposed on each portion. See chapter 3, "Influence of the French" (page 45), for more historical details about this iconic dish.

ACTIVE TIME: 2½ hours | **TOTAL TIME:** 4 hours
(including braising and simmering) | **YIELD:** Makes 6 servings

LAMB

1 lamb shoulder, boneless
  (about 3 to 4 pounds [1.3 to 1.8 kg])
Salt and pepper
2 tablespoons olive oil
1 small onion, coarsely chopped
1 medium leek, whites only,
  coarsely chopped
1 medium celery stalk, coarsely chopped

1 medium carrot, coarsely chopped
¼ cup (60 ml) dry sherry
1 quart (960 ml) Basic Chicken Stock
1 quart (960 ml) Basic Lamb Stock
½ head garlic, skin intact
Bouquet garni or a bundle
  of herbs
1 tablespoon unsalted butter

Heat the oven to 300°F (150°C). Generously season the lamb shoulder with salt and pepper. Reserve at room temperature.

In a large Dutch oven, heat the olive oil over medium heat. Add the onion, leek, celery, and carrot and cook, stirring often, until golden brown, about 10 minutes. Deglaze with sherry, stirring to scrape any brown bits. Stir in both stocks, then submerge the lamb shoulder in the liquid. Add the garlic and bouquet garni. Cover

and braise in the oven until very tender, about 3 hours. Remove from the oven and carefully transfer the lamb to a holding vessel. Rest the lamb, covered, for about 20 minutes.

Pour the remaining contents of the Dutch oven through a China cap, then pass the strained liquid through a fine-mesh sieve. Whisk in the butter and season with salt and pepper. You should have about 2 cups. Reserve, covered, to serve as the broth.

VEGETABLES

1 cup (240 ml) Roasted Lamb Stock
1 tablespoon unsalted butter
Salt and pepper
2 tablespoons olive oil
12 pearl onions, trimmed, blanched, and peeled
2 small fennel bulbs, thinly sliced, fronds
    reserved for marrow

6 baby carrots, scrubbed and
    halved lengthwise
6 baby turnips, scrubbed and halved
½ cup (100 g) English peas
1 tablespoon grainy mustard
2 cornichons, minced
2 tablespoons snipped chives

While the lamb is resting, heat the stock in a saucepan, bring to a boil, and lower to a simmer. Reduce by half and transfer to a bowl. Whisk in the butter and season with salt and pepper. Set aside.

In a large sauté pan, heat the olive oil over medium heat. Add the pearl onions and fennel and cook until translucent, about 5 minutes. Toss in the carrots and cook, stirring, about 2 minutes. Add the turnips and cook until al dente, about 3 minutes longer. Stir in the English peas and cook 2 minutes more. Stir in the reduced stock and mustard, cornichons, and chives. Season if necessary.

MARROW

6 marrow bones (about 3 inches [7.5 cm] each),
    preferably lamb, soaked in brine overnight
    to remove blood
Sea salt, preferably gray

3 tablespoons fennel fronds, reserved from
    above, finely chopped for garnish
1 teaspoon fennel pollen (optional)
Crusty bread

Turn the oven to 450°F (230°C). Drain the bones and pat them dry with a kitchen towel. Place the marrow bones cut-side up on a sheet pan. Roast for 15 to 20 minutes until the marrow is very hot and cooked through. Remove from the oven.

In a small bowl, toss the salt, fennel fronds, and fennel pollen, if using, together. Reserve.

TO SERVE: Place the crusty bread and fennel salt in the middle of the table. Welcome your guests with small bowls of the reserved broth. Arrange the meat, vegetables, and any remaining sauce on a platter. Top with roasted marrow bones and serve warm.

PORK

A quality pork stock follows the same careful process as veal stock—a slow simmer and adequate chilling time are necessary for concentration and clarity. Pork stock, especially when using bones from a pastured animal or heritage breed, should be light-bodied when fluid and thick when cold. Pork stock takes well to intense aromatics, such as star anise or cassia bud, and the flavor of smoke from cured cuts.

Heritage pork has a unique fat composition that requires diligent attention when being separated from the bones in the pot. Be sure to maintain a proper low temperature while skimming to prevent the fat from emulsifying into the liquid. After chilling the stock, you can remove the fat cap and use the washed lard to produce cosmetics at home (see chapter 14). Pork fat from heritage breeds has a suprising clarity and excellent consistency when rendered correctly.

Look for a farmer who selects slow-growing breeds that have access to farm fields in summer and woodlands in winter. Pork bones should be meaty and can come from the neck, shoulder, and leg of the pig; the feet—known as *trotters*— will add a significant boost of gelatin. Unlike chicken stock, you only need one trotter per pot of liquid; adding more will produce a glue-like texture.

Basic Pork Stock

This pork stock is the most neutral and can be used as an all-purpose base. You can also add it to other stocks, like chicken or rabbit, to develop a complex foundation. The initial blanching step helps remove excess fat and impurities that would otherwise cloud the stock.

ACTIVE TIME: 2 hours | **TOTAL TIME:** 7 hours (including heating, blanching, simmering, and initial cooling) | **YIELD:** Makes about 3 quarts (2.8 liters)

6 pounds (2.7 kg) meaty pork bones (from the neck, shoulder, or leg), preferably pastured and heritage

1 trotter (pig's foot), preferably pastured (optional)

8 quarts (7.5 L) filtered water, cold, plus water for rinsing and blanching

3 tablespoons grapeseed oil

½ pound (225 g) white onions, cut into large dice

1 pound (455 g) leeks, dark green parts
    removed, cut into large dice
½ pound (225 g) carrots, cut into large dice
½ pound (225 g) parsnips, cut into large dice
¼ pound (115 g) fresh mushrooms, gills
    trimmed

1 head garlic, split in half, broken into pieces
3 sprigs thyme
3 sprigs flat-leaf parsley
2 bay leaves
1 tablespoon black peppercorns
Sea salt to taste

Follow the cooking instructions for Basic Veal Stock (page 108), taking special care with blanching the bones to remove impurities before the long simmering time. Raw pork bones contain more blood, which will turn your stock brown if not removed by blanching. If a concentrated stock is desired, gently reduce the liquid after straining until the correct viscosity is achieved. If using the trotter, the stock will become more gelatinous as the liquid reduces. At the end of the cooking time, shred the meat from the trotter and reserve for another use. Once the stock is chilled, remove the fat cap and reserve as lard for cooking or making cosmetics (see chapter 14).

Roasted Pork Stock

This brown pork stock achieves a deep, golden color reminiscent of chicken stock, and yet has a richer flavor and more developed structure. The trotter reinforces gelatin in the stock that might be lost during the roasting process.

ACTIVE TIME: 2 hours | TOTAL TIME: 10 hours (including roasting, heating, simmering, and initial cooling) | YIELD: Makes about 3 quarts (2.8 liters)

6 pounds (2.7 kg) meaty pork bones (from the
    neck, shoulder, or leg), preferably pastured
    and heritage
1 trotter (pig's foot), preferably pastured
    (optional)
¼ cup (60 ml) grapeseed oil, divided
2 cups (480 ml) fruity red wine,
    such as Burgundy
8 quarts (7.5 L) filtered water, cold,
    plus water for rinsing

½ pound (225 g) white onions, cut into large dice
1 pound (455 g) leeks, dark green parts
    removed, cut into large dice
¾ pound (340 g) carrots, cut into large dice
¾ pound (340 g) tomatoes, coarsely chopped
6 sprigs thyme
6 sprigs flat-leaf parsley
2 bay leaves
1 tablespoon black peppercorns
Sea salt to taste

Follow the cooking instructions for Roasted Veal Stock (page 110). If a concentrated stock is desired, gently reduce the liquid after straining until the correct viscosity is achieved. If using the trotter, the stock will become more gelatinous as the liquid reduces. At the end of the cooking time, shred the meat from the trotter and reserve for another use. Once the stock is chilled, remove the fat cap and reserve as lard for cooking or making cosmetics (see chapter 14).

Smoked Pork Stock

Smoked ham hocks, or pork knuckles, are readily available from a quality butcher. This stock makes use of the smoke flavor that penetrates the nooks and crannies of the knobby hock to develop an intensely flavored base. You can use it to highlight other stocks, to add a cured note to wilted greens, or to simply baste meats. This stock is also a great foundation for making pork rillettes.

ACTIVE TIME: 2 hours | **TOTAL TIME:** 10 hours (including roasting, heating, simmering, and initial cooling) | **YIELD:** Makes about 3 quarts (2.8 liters)

4 pounds (1.8 kg) meaty pork bones (from the neck, shoulder, or leg), preferably pastured and heritage
2 smoked ham hocks, preferably heritage
1 trotter (pig's foot), preferably pastured (optional)
¼ cup (60 ml) grapeseed oil, divided
2 cups (480 ml) hard apple cider
8 quarts (7.5 L) filtered water, cold, plus water for rinsing
½ pound (225 g) white onions, cut into large dice

1 pound (455 g) leeks, dark green parts removed, cut into large dice
¾ pound (340 g) carrots, cut into large dice
1 small fennel bulb, coarsely chopped, fronds removed
6 sprigs marjoram
6 sprigs flat-leaf parsley
2 bay leaves
1 tablespoon black peppercorns
Sea salt to taste

Follow the cooking instructions for Roasted Veal Stock (page 110), washing and drying the bones well and deglazing the roasting pan with hard apple cider instead of wine. If a concentrated stock is desired, gently reduce the liquid after straining until the correct viscosity is achieved. If using the trotter, the stock will become more gelatinous as the liquid reduces. At the end of the cooking time, shred the meat from the ham hocks and trotter and reserve for another use, such as rillettes. Once the stock is chilled, remove the fat cap and reserve as lard for cooking or making cosmetics (see chapter 14).

Pork Bone Broth

The addition of natural ham hocks (knuckles that are not smoked), a trotter, and a lesser amount of water in the pot aids development of a more concentrated stock in less time. Trotters are especially high in collagen, which renders into gelatin to develop an almost solidified foundation.

Due to its naturally thick viscosity, this bone broth is intended less for sipping, as you might a chicken or beef bone broth, and more as a gelatin-heavy addition to your cooking. You can add it to other types of stocks, dilute it for use on its own, or simply employ in small quantities as you would glace de viande. Be sure to select a pastured heritage breed for this stock. Soaking the bones in vinegar is optional.

ACTIVE TIME: 3 hours | TOTAL TIME: 2 days (including roasting, heating, simmering, and chilling) | YIELD: Makes about 2 quarts (1.9 liters)

---

4 pounds (1.8 kg) meaty pork bones (from the neck, shoulder, or leg), preferably pastured and heritage

2 ham hocks, not smoked, preferably heritage

1 trotter (pig's foot), preferably pastured

¼ cup (60 ml) grapeseed oil, divided

¼ cup (60 ml) apple cider vinegar (optional)

6 quarts (5.7 L) filtered water, cold, plus water for rinsing and blanching

½ pound (225 g) white onions, cut into large dice

1 pound (455 g) leeks, dark green parts removed, cut into large dice

½ pound (225 g) carrots, cut into large dice

½ pound (225 g) parsnips, cut into large dice

1 small fennel bulb, coarsely chopped, fronds removed

6 sprigs thyme

6 sprigs flat-leaf parsley

2 bay leaves

1 tablespoon black peppercorns

Sea salt to taste

Follow the cooking instructions for Beef Bone Broth (page 126), washing and drying the bones in two batches of water to remove surface impurities. The bones will render a considerable amount of gelatin into the liquid; additional reduction is unlikely. At the end of the cooking time, shred the meat from the ham hocks and trotter and reserve for another use. Once the stock is chilled, remove the fat cap and reserve as lard for cooking or making cosmetics (see chapter 14). Don't be alarmed if there is a lot of fat that rises to the top; this is common in many heritage breeds.

Heritage Pork Scrapple with Spiced Plum Jam

Scrapple as we know it today—a crispy slab of meat scraps—is a Pennsylvania Dutch recipe that has made its way onto roadside diner menus. Scrapple, called *panhaas* ("pan rabbit") in Dutch, combines pork trimmings with cornmeal and buckwheat flour to form a loaf; when set, sliced, and fried, a crisp exterior develops while the interior remains succulent and creamy.

Though scrapple is delivered on our breakfast plates, usually alongside toast and jam, there is evidence that suggests its origins are from the Middle Ages, associated with the autumnal slaughter of hogs in preparation for winter. The wealthy would reserve the prime cuts for their own consumption, and the poor would receive scraps to make sausage and stew, often thickened with meal and allowed to set like pudding.

The head is an ideal part of the pig for making scrapple. A savory broth forms while the head is simmered, and then combined with meal as the thickening agent. The use of tongue and brain is encouraged; these parts help form the foundation of the dish and ensure that nothing goes to waste. Ask your butcher to split the head and remove the tongue and brain whole.

ACTIVE TIME: 3 hours | **TOTAL TIME:** 2 days (including soaking, braising, chilling, and simmering) | **YIELD:** Makes three 2-pound loaves

SCRAPPLE

½ cup (70 g) kosher salt
½ cup (115 g) loosely packed brown sugar
2 teaspoons black pepper
2 bay leaves
1 bunch flat-leaf parsley, divided

1 small fennel bulb, roughly chopped, fronds reserved
1 pig head (about 15 pounds [6.8 kg]), split lengthwise, with tongue and brain
¼ cup (56 g) lard
2 medium onions, roughly chopped

4 medium parsnips, peeled and roughly chopped
1 cup (240 ml) dry white wine or dry hard cider
8 sprigs thyme, divided
4 sprigs marjoram, divided

1 cup (140 g) cornmeal
½ cup (60 g) buckwheat flour
½ teaspoon cayenne pepper
Salt and pepper

In the bowl of a food processor, pulse the kosher salt, brown sugar, black pepper, bay leaves, half the parsley, and fennel fronds until a green paste is formed. Rinse the head and tongue under cold water, and pat dry with paper towels. Rub the mixture on the head and tongue and place in an airtight container. Refrigerate, at least 8 hours and up to 1 day.

In a separate container, place the brain in filtered water, and soak in the refrigerator, replacing the water twice, about 8 hours total.

Heat the oven to 190°F (85°C). In a large sauté pan, melt the lard over medium-high heat. Add the onions, fennel bulb, and parsnip, and cook, stirring often, until softened, about 6 minutes. Deglaze with the white wine. Transfer the mixture to a large roasting pan.

Drain the head and tongue, rinse under cold water, and place in the roasting pan. Add half the thyme and half the marjoram. Fill the pan with water until the head is nearly submerged. Cover and cook for 8 to 10 hours, until fork-tender. Remove from the oven, uncover, and cool the meat in the liquid.

When cool enough to handle, remove the pig head and tongue from the liquid and place in a large bowl. Strain the braising liquid through a fine-mesh sieve, twice if necessary. Place in the refrigerator and chill until the fat rises to the top.

While the stock is chilling, pick the meat off the skull, being careful to remove and discard large pieces of cartilage and any glands. Remove excess skin and fat, leaving the softer parts. With your hands or two forks, shred the tongue into relatively uniform bite-sized pieces, and combine with the head meat. Chop the remaining parsley, thyme, and marjoram. Mix the herbs into the meat mixture and refrigerate, covered, until needed.

Remove the braising liquid from the refrigerator; skim off the fat cap and reserve for another use. In a stockpot, slowly bring the liquid to a boil, then lower the heat to maintain a simmer. Reduce the liquid by half. Stir in the cornmeal and buckwheat flour and cook until tender, stirring often, about 20 to 30 minutes.

While the cornmeal mixture is thickening, remove the brain from the soaking water. Pat dry with kitchen towels and push through a fine-mesh sieve. Slowly add the brain to the hot cornmeal mixture, stirring constantly until tempered, about 3 minutes. Remove the porridge from the heat, and stir in the reserved pork mixture. Mix in the cayenne pepper and season with salt and pepper.

Divide the pork mixture among three terrine molds or loaf pans, tapping the molds on the counter to tightly pack in the meat. Cover with plastic wrap, and rest the lid or a weight on top. Refrigerate until set, at least 4 hours or overnight.

JAM

1 pound (455 g) purple plums,
   pitted and chopped
1 cup (225 g) sugar

1 lemon, zest and juice
1 teaspoon ground cloves
Dash sea salt

While the terrine is setting, make the plum jam. In a medium saucepan, combine all the jam ingredients and heat over medium-high, stirring to combine, until it reaches a boil. Immediately lower the heat and cook at a low simmer for about 45 minutes, stirring often, until the mixture coats a wooden spoon. Remove from the heat and let cool.

TO SERVE: When ready to eat, unmold the terrines and cut the scrapple into thick slices. In a cast-iron skillet, heat some lard or butter and fry until crispy and golden brown, about 2 minutes on each side. Serve with buttered sourdough toast and spiced plum jam.

German Barley Soup with Fried Trotters

In Germany, barley soup, or *graupensuppe eintopf,* is a satisfying one-pot meal that is popular in the cold months. While delicious on its own, the dish is elevated here with the addition of fried trotters. You can sprout barley for this recipe, which preserves nutrients and aids digestion, or simply stir in cooked pearled barley. Either way this soup will keep you warm in winter!

This recipe calls for the use of two stocks—3 parts vegetable stock to 1 part cured pork stock. If you only have vegetable stock on hand, you can fry *lardons*—bacon cut into small strips—in butter and olive oil to impart a cured flavor. (Set the bacon aside after it is cooked and use it for garnish or another recipe.) I don't recommend using only cured pork stock, as the concentration of smoke and gelatin will be too overpowering.

ACTIVE TIME: 3 hours | **TOTAL TIME:** 3 days (including sprouting, chilling, and simmering) | **YIELD:** Makes 4 to 6 servings, plus extra trotter terrine

SPROUTED BARLEY

¼ cup (35 g) unhulled barley

Begin the process 3 days before you intend to eat. Follow the sprouting guidelines in "Soaking versus Sprouting," page 160. Store between kitchen towels in the refrigerator until ready to use. If you choose to use pearled barley, you can skip this step and cook the grains closer to serving time.

TROTTERS

2 trotters (pig's feet)
1 quart (960 ml) Roasted Chicken Stock
2 tablespoons grapeseed oil
1 medium onion, finely chopped
1 medium carrot, peeled and finely chopped
½ small celery root, peeled and finely chopped
½ cup (120 ml) dry white wine, such as Sauvignon Blanc
¼ cup (15 g) finely chopped flat-leaf parsley
4 cornichons, finely chopped
2 tablespoons grainy mustard
Salt and pepper

One day before you serve the soup, place the trotters and chicken stock in a medium stockpot, adding water as necessary to cover the feet. Bring to a gentle boil, skimming often, and then reduce to a simmer until the meat is fork-tender, about 3 hours. Remove from the heat and cool the trotters in the liquid. When cool enough to handle, remove the feet and pick off the meat. Set aside in a large bowl.

In a large sauté pan, heat the oil over medium-high, then sweat the onion, about 5 minutes. Add the carrot and celery root, and cook, stirring often, until al dente, about 7 minutes. Deglaze with the white wine. Add the vegetables to the bowl with the meat. Stir in the parsley, cornichons, and mustard. Season with salt and pepper.

Pack the meat mixture into a terrine mold or loaf pan. Alternatively, you can roll the meat into a tight cylinder using plastic wrap. Refrigerate until firm, at least 4 hours and preferably overnight.

SOUP

2 tablespoons olive oil

2 tablespoons unsalted butter

1 medium onion, finely chopped

2 medium leeks, finely chopped

12 fingerling potatoes, sliced lengthwise

2 medium carrots, peeled and finely diced

½ small celery root, peeled and finely diced

4 cups (1 L) Basic Vegetable Stock

1½ cups (360 ml) Smoked Pork Stock

4 sprigs thyme

¼ teaspoon cayenne pepper

Freshly grated nutmeg, to taste

Salt and pepper

Sprouted barley (above) or 2 cups (400 g) cooked pearled barley

Heat the oil and butter in a large sauté pan over medium-high heat. Add the onion and leeks and cook, stirring often, until slightly caramelized, about 10 minutes. Stir in the potatoes and continue to cook, about 7 minutes. Add the carrots and celery root and cook until al dente, about 4 minutes.

Stir in both stocks with the thyme and bring to a boil, then lower the heat to maintain a simmer. Cook until the potatoes are tender but not mushy. Stir in the cayenne pepper and nutmeg. Season with salt and pepper. Remove from the heat, stir in the sprouted or cooked barley, and cover to gently heat through. Boiling the sprouted barley will harm the nutrients, but if using pearled barley, you can continue to simmer over low heat to distribute flavors.

TO ASSEMBLE

¼ cup (30 g) all-purpose flour

1 egg, lightly beaten

½ cup (55 g) dried bread crumbs

2 tablespoons grapeseed oil

Salt and pepper

¼ cup (15 g) flat-leaf parsley leaves, for garnish

Unwrap the trotter mixture and portion into ½-inch (1.25 cm) thick slices, one per serving. Dust with flour, dip into the beaten egg, and coat in bread crumbs. In a medium sauté pan, heat the oil and fry the slices until golden brown, about 3 minutes per side. Remove and drain on a kitchen towel.

Ladle the soup into serving bowls, place one fried trotter slice in the center of each bowl, and garnish with parsley leaves.

SOAKING VERSUS SPROUTING

Most recipes that call for grains and legumes begin by soaking them in water—sometimes a quick rinse, but more often a multi-hour submersion. This step removes anti-nutrients, such as phytic acid, and improves ease of absorption, reducing digestive ills such as heartburn and bloating. Soaking also reduces simmering time in the pot.

Notwithstanding the benefits of soaking grains and legumes before cooking, a recent trend has emerged among the more health-conscious: Soaking seeds to the point of germination, called *sprouting*. Sprouting from seed not only neutralizes enzyme inhibitors and aids digestion, but also preserves nutrients that can be lost during the cooking process. When seeds are moistened and kept in the dark, they begin to ferment: The enzymes and sugars break down to release probiotics. They also soften enough to be consumed without the need to apply heat, which could destroy nutrients made available through fermentation. Even more, *rejuvelac,* the tangy soaking liquid, can be imbibed as a digestive aid or used as a starter culture for other fermented foods, such as yogurt.

The variety of grains and legumes you can sprout is endless—even nuts will sprout! Popular grains include barley, spelt, buckwheat, and rye; legumes include beans, lentils, peas, and soy. In this book, there are three recipes that encourage you to start from seed, using barley (German Barley Soup, page 157), adzuki beans (Adzuki Bean Stew, page 307), and a minestrone bean blend (Sprouted Minestrone Soup, page 312).

Here's how to sprout grains and legumes: Three days before you intend to eat them, place ¼ cup seeds of your choice in a quart-sized mason jar. Fill with warm water. Place two layers of cheesecloth over the mouth of the jar, and secure tightly with a rubber band. Soak for six hours. Pour off the soaking water, fill with fresh water, and drain. Rest the jar on its side at room temperature. Rinse and drain once or twice a day. In two days, you should see tails on the seeds. The sprouts are ready when the tails are about one and a half times as long as the seeds. Store the sprouted seeds between kitchen towels in the refrigerator until ready to use.

Three Fennel Cassoulet

Kate Hill, the venerated author and educator from Kitchen at Camont, taught me that the secret to a good cassoulet is the bean broth. Tarbais (or Coco) beans, if you can find them, are well worth the expense. Rich and creamy, this large runner bean holds up to the twice-cooked practice when making cassoulet— cooked once on their own and again in their broth, along with pork and duck meat—with their respective fats—nestled within, and crisped on top. Runner beans, a reference to how the pods grow on tall, climbing plants, are the best variety for cassoulet. If Tarbais beans are unavailable, look for scarlet runner beans or runner cannellini beans.

I've taken some liberty with this dish, starting with a Spanish-style *sofrito* for the base. This recipe also acknowledges a general French dislike for celery in broth by replacing it with a good dose of fennel. In this recipe, fennel is used from seed to frond, and if that's not enough, feel free to finish with a sprinkle of fennel pollen before serving. This indulgence placates my love for fennel in sausage—the subtle anise flavor acts as a sublime foil to the richness of the meat.

Cassoulet comes from the word *cassole*, a conical earthenware pot that is made specifically for the dish. Unfortunately, these clay pots do not travel well and aren't commonly found outside of France. A wide Dutch oven is an acceptable substitute.

ACTIVE TIME: 3½ hours | **TOTAL TIME:** 2 days
(including soaking, braising, and baking) | **YIELD:** Makes 6 to 8 servings

---

RAGOUT

1 pound (455 g) boneless pork shoulder, cut into 1½-inch (3.8 cm) cubes
¼ pound (115 g) fresh pork skin, rolled into bundles, tied with butcher's twine
½ teaspoon fennel seeds, toasted and ground
½ tablespoon smoked paprika
1 tablespoon brown sugar
Salt and pepper
¼ cup (60 ml) olive oil
2 medium onions, minced
2 medium tomatoes, grated

¼ cup (50 g) duck fat
1 small fennel bulb, diced, fronds reserved for garnish
2 medium carrots, diced
2 medium parsnips, diced
8 cloves garlic, thinly sliced
1 cup (240 ml) dry white wine, such as Sauvignon Blanc
1 quart (960 ml) Basic Duck Stock or Basic Chicken Stock
1 cup (240 ml) Roasted Pork Stock
Bouquet garni or a bundle of herbs

BEANS

1 pound (455 g) dried white runner beans, preferably Tarbais, picked over and rinsed
1 smoked ham hock, preferably heritage
1 medium carrot, peeled

1 medium onion, peeled
2 tablespoons maple syrup
2 bay leaves
1 dried chili

TOPPING

1 pound (455 g) garlic pork sausage,
  halved on the bias
6 duck confit legs

Reserved fennel fronds, for garnish
Fennel pollen, for garnish (optional)

TWO NIGHTS BEFORE SERVING: In a large bowl, season the pork shoulder and pork skin rolls with ground fennel, smoked paprika, brown sugar, salt, and pepper. Cover and refrigerate, at least 4 hours or overnight. Cover the beans with water; soak for the same amount of time as the pork.

While the beans are soaking, heat the olive oil in a heavy-bottomed sauté pan over medium heat. Add the minced onions and cook, stirring often, until caramelized, about 30 minutes. Stir in the grated tomato and continue to cook, stirring often, until the liquid has evaporated and the mixture is well incorporated, another 30 minutes. Season with salt and pepper. Remove from the heat, cover, and reserve in the refrigerator.

THE DAY BEFORE SERVING: Drain and rinse the beans. Place the beans in a large saucepan or medium stockpot, and nestle the smoked ham hock in the middle. Place the peeled carrot and onion in the pot. Add enough water to cover the contents of the pan, and stir in the maple syrup, bay leaves, and dried chili pepper. Bring to a gentle boil over medium heat. Reduce the heat to maintain a simmer and cook until the beans are tender but hold their shape, about 1 hour. Add water if the beans become dry. Remove from the heat and set the beans aside to cool in their liquid.

When the beans are cool enough to handle, remove the ham hock and pick off the meat. Drain the beans, reserving the cooking liquid but discarding the spices. Fold the hock meat and reserved onion-tomato mixture into the beans. Chill the liquid and the bean mixture.

Remove the pork from the refrigerator and pat dry with a kitchen towel. In a large Dutch oven, heat the duck fat and add half the pork shoulder in one layer, cooking until lightly browned on all sides. Transfer to a bowl and repeat with the remaining pork. Add the fennel and cook, stirring occasionally, until slightly caramelized, about 7 minutes. Stir in the carrots and parsnips and cook until al dente, about 5 minutes. Add the garlic and cook until softened, about 3 minutes more. Deglaze with the white wine. Pour in both stocks and add the pork skin rolls, browned pork shoulder, and bouquet garni. Cover with a tight-fitting lid and gently simmer until the pork is tender and the liquid is slightly thickened, about 1½ to 2 hours. Remove from the oven, cool slightly, and chill in the refrigerator.

THE DAY OF SERVING: Heat the oven to 325°F (165°C). In a large cast-iron skillet over medium heat cook the sausages until browned on both sides. Remove from the heat and set aside while you prepare the cassoulet.

Remove the pork from the refrigerator. Skim the fat from the top, and strain the liquid into a separate bowl. Remove the beans and their liquid from the refrigerator. Remove and untie the rolls of pork fat, chop fine, and gently fold into the bean mixture.

In a large Dutch oven, spoon half of the beans in an even layer on the bottom. Spread the pork shoulder on top, and finish with the rest of the beans. Pour the pork broth over the beans and finish with some of the bean liquid; the total liquid should be level with the beans. Nestle the sausage and confit evenly over the beans. Bake the cassoulet, uncovered, about 1 hour.

Reduce the oven temperature to 275°F (135°C). Bake for 1 hour longer, until the surface is a deep brown and liquid is bubbling against the side of the pan. Remove from the oven and rest 15 minutes before serving. Garnish with fennel fronds and sprinkle with fennel pollen, if desired.

Choucroute Garnie

Choucroute garnie translates to "dressed sauerkraut," the dressing a reference to how cured cabbage is braised with wine, aromatics, pork, and potatoes. Originally a German dish, choucroute garnie was adopted by the French when the territory of Alsace-Lorraine was returned to France after World War I. It has many variations and yet a notable tradition in how the pig is served: a selection of cured and fresh, always, and with three types of sausage.

One of my earliest New York experiences was enjoying choucroute garnie at DB Bistro Moderne, where every fall the chef breaks down a suckling pig to its respective parts while the sauerkraut cures. A later taste of choucroute garnie in Paris confirmed my adoration for this dish: The sour note of fermented cabbage complements unctuous chunks of fatty pork. Every bite evokes a craving for the next.

If you are ambitious, try starting with a whole pig. Adam Danforth's *Butchering Poultry, Rabbit, Lamb, Goat, and Pork* is a great photographic reference that will show you how to respectfully break down a hog from snout to trotter.

ACTIVE TIME: 2½ hours | **TOTAL TIME:** 2 days (including curing and baking) | **YIELD:** Makes 8 servings

---

3 tablespoons kosher salt
1½ tablespoons brown sugar
½ teaspoon ground cloves

½ teaspoon ground black pepper
1 raw ham hock, preferably from heritage pork
1 pound (455 g) bone-in country ribs

1 pound (455 g) uncured pork belly

1 ounce (28 g) salt pork without rind,
   blanched and cubed

¼ cup (56 g) unsalted butter

2 medium onions, thinly sliced

2 medium apples, peeled and cubed

4 cloves garlic, minced

2 cups (480 ml) dry white wine, such as an
   Alsatian Riesling, divided

2 pounds (910 g) sauerkraut, drained

1 teaspoon dried juniper berries

1 teaspoon black peppercorns

2 bay leaves

½ pound (225 g) slab bacon, cut into 8 equal pieces

1 cup (240 ml) Basic Pork Stock

12 small waxy potatoes, peeled

2 Knackwurst sausages, or long pork, veal, and
   garlic sausages

2 Frankfurt sausages, or hot dogs from a
   reliable source

2 Montbeliard sausages, or mildly smoked
   spiced pork salami

Salt and pepper

Whole-grain mustard, for serving

TWO DAYS BEFORE SERVING: In a small bowl, mix the kosher salt, brown sugar, cloves, and black pepper. Rub the ham hock, country ribs, and pork belly with the mixture. Wrap in an airtight container and cure in the refrigerator for at least 1 day and up to 2 days before cooking.

THE DAY OF SERVING: Remove the pork from the refrigerator. Rinse and pat dry with a kitchen towel. Set aside while preparing the sauerkraut.

Heat a large Dutch oven over medium heat, add the cubed salt pork and cook until rendered and golden. Remove the salt pork and set aside in a small bowl. To the rendered fat, add the butter and swirl the pan to incorporate. Add the onions and cook, stirring often, until slightly caramelized, about 15 minutes. Stir in the apples and garlic and cook until fork-tender, about 4 minutes. Deglaze with ½ cup white wine.

Gently stir in the sauerkraut, juniper berries, peppercorns, and bay leaves. Nestle the ham hock, country ribs, and pork belly into

the sauerkraut. Surround the meat with the portioned slab bacon and salt pork. Pour in the remaining wine and top with pork stock. Bring to a boil and reduce to maintain a simmer. Cover the pan and cook until the meat is fork-tender, about 3 hours. Add water to the pan if the sauerkraut becomes dry.

An hour before the meat is done, place the potatoes in a medium saucepan, and fill with salted water. Simmer the potatoes until nearly tender, about 12 minutes. Remove and reserve. Add the sausages to the same water, and simmer until plump, about 8 minutes. Remove and reserve with the potatoes.

About 10 minutes before serving, preheat the broiler on high. Place the potatoes and sausages around the other meat in the Dutch oven. Transfer to the oven and broil until the sausages brown, about 3 to 4 minutes. To serve, portion the sauerkraut and top with a generous selection of meat. Season with salt and pepper. Serve with grainy mustard.

CHAPTER NINE

Poultry Stocks, Broths, and Dishes

As with stocks and broths made with ruminants and swine, stocks made with poultry are fundamental and distinctive. This chapter reviews stocks and broths created from a range of birds, including chicken, turkey, and duck. Rabbit, identified as poultry by the USDA due to its size, is also included. The spectrum of flavor provided by poultry is considerable—from the neutrality of chicken stock to the richness of duck stock—each with its own purpose in the kitchen.

Arguably the most used base in a home kitchen, chicken stock blends into the background of a dish while adding a magical quality—a salinity and minerality that is pleasing to the palate and soothing on the throat. Turkey stock, especially when made from the carcass of a heritage or rare breed, offers a slightly more savory and forward note to food. With its heightened seasonality—available closest to the holidays—turkey stock is best made in bulk and frozen for later use. Duck stock has the most assertive flavor of all the birds, making it an ideal sauce for game dishes. Rabbit, with its pale pink bone structure, is the most delicate animal in this section; like veal bones, rabbit bones are full of cartilage. As a foundation, rabbit stock is clear and silky, lending itself to elegant applications in the kitchen.

Stocks and broths made from poultry are among the most versatile foundations you can make at home. They come together quickly, offer a range of flavors, and often represent the entire animal. Providing both meat and foundation, their purpose extends well beyond the bone.

CHICKEN

The beauty of chicken stock: It is venerable as an ingredient as well as satisfying on its own. Chicken stock is good to have at the ready in any kitchen. Use it to cook grains, sauté vegetables, baste meats, or make a simple pan sauce; or throw it in a thermos as a sipper throughout your day. Chicken stock blends into a dish, adding essence—a soothing salinity—without overwhelming other elements. A rich chicken stock should take on a golden hue, and yet be clear enough to allow you to see the bottom of the pot.

As with all other meat, it is crucial to locate a farmer who raises chickens on pasture, preferably on a rotational grazing schedule alongside cattle. Seek out slow-growing heritage breeds that are suited for your climate—these chickens have a physique that ensures a more fulfilling life and results in better bone composition. For example, the Dominique, America's first chicken breed, is a beautiful bird with intricate black and white plumage and is known to be calm and friendly. This breed, valued for both eggs and meat, does exceptionally well in the cold climate of the Hudson Valley. See appendix A for more information about heritage chicken breeds.

If not using the whole bird, look for backs and necks to provide most of the bone content for stocks and broths. The addition of chicken feet is key to a foundation full of body. Feet are optional but recommended for stock—both basic and roasted—and required for bone broth.

Basic Chicken Stock

This basic chicken stock should be light in flavor and texture. It is intended as an all-purpose base—you can even use it in place of vegetable stock. If you require a richer white chicken stock, simply reduce the liquid until it attains a deep yellow-orange hue.

ACTIVE TIME: 2 hours | **TOTAL TIME:** 5 to 6 hours (including heating, blanching, simmering, and initial cooling) | **YIELD:** Makes about 4 quarts (3.8 liters)

6 pounds (2.7 kg) chicken bones (necks and
    backs), preferably pastured
1 pound (455 g) chicken feet, preferably
    pastured (optional)
4 quarts (3.8 L) filtered water, cold, plus water
    for rinsing and/or blanching
2 quarts (1.3 kg) ice cubes
½ pound (225 g) white onions, cut into large dice

1 pound (455 g) leeks, dark green parts
    removed, cut into large dice
½ pound (225 g) carrots, cut into large dice
4 sprigs thyme
4 sprigs flat-leaf parsley
1 bay leaf
8 black peppercorns
Sea salt to taste

Rinse the chicken bones and chicken feet under cold water until the water runs clear. Make sure that all visible blood is removed from the bones. Check the bones to locate and remove any organs that might still be attached. The rinsing of blood and removal of organs will help eliminate proteins that could cloud your stock.

If the water does not become clear from rinsing, blanch the bones before proceeding. To do this, place the chicken bones, not including the feet, in a large stockpot, and add enough cold water to cover the bones by a few inches. Turn the heat to medium-high, and slowly heat the liquid. Using a fine-mesh strainer, skim any scum that rises to the surface. When the liquid starts to ripple, before it breaks into a boil, remove the pot from the heat. Do not boil the liquid; boiling in this first stage will extract flavor that should be preserved for the long simmer.

Drain the bones in a large colander and rinse under cold water. Thoroughly clean the same pot. Return the bones to the pot and add the chicken feet. Top with filtered water. Heat the pot over medium-high, and slowly bring the liquid to a tremble, skimming as soon as scum appears. When the liquid ripples, reduce the heat to medium-low and maintain a simmer, or smile. Never let the liquid boil, as impurities will be sucked to the bottom of the pot and emulsify into the liquid during the long simmering time.

Continue to skim as necessary while the water is rising in temperature. When the liquid comes to a gentle boil, reduce the heat to medium-low, add the ice, and skim to remove the thickened fat. Continue to skim while the bones are simmering; the first hour of simmering is when most of the impurities will be apparent. A well-skimmed liquid will prevent impurities from emulsifying the stock. Simmer for 2 hours, skimming often.

When the bones have completed their initial simmering time, add the onions, leeks, carrots, thyme, parsley, bay leaf, and peppercorns to the pot, and slowly return the liquid to a simmer. The aromatics will rise to the top, making it more difficult to skim, though it is important to continue the clarifying process. Skim by capturing particles that gather near the bubbling part of the liquid, leaving the vegetables to simmer mostly undisturbed.

Simmer until the vegetables are cooked through but not broken down, skimming often, about 90 minutes. Turn off the heat and leave the pot on the stove to rest, about 10 minutes. Any floating particles will settle to the bottom of the pot during this resting period.

Set a fine-mesh strainer over a container large enough to hold the liquid contents of the pot. Line the strainer with cheesecloth. Carefully ladle the stock from the pot into the strainer, stopping short of, and discarding, any cloudy stock toward the bottom of the pot. Periodically remove the solids that accumulate in the basket to minimize impurities that could be forced through the strainer. Taste and season with sea salt.

Chill the stock in the refrigerator, stirring occasionally to expedite the cooling process. Refrigerate for up to 2 days or freeze in smaller containers for longer storage.

Roasted Chicken Stock

This brown chicken stock develops a depth of flavor that should be matched with bold ingredients—a mature rooster or game meat, for instance. You can start with bones from a store-bought roasted chicken, where they have been touched by indirect heat, but nothing beats the flavor achieved from roasting the actual carcass yourself.

ACTIVE TIME: 2 hours | **TOTAL TIME:** 6½ hours (including roasting, heating, simmering, and initial cooling) | **YIELD:** Makes about 4 quarts (3.8 liters)

6 pounds (2.7 kg) chicken bones (necks and backs), preferably pastured
1 pound (455 g) chicken feet, preferably pastured (optional)
½ pound (225 g) white onions, cut into large dice
1 pound (455 g) leeks, dark green parts removed, cut into large dice
¾ pound (340 g) carrots, cut into large dice
1 small fennel bulb, coarsely chopped, fronds removed
3 tablespoons grapeseed oil
6 quarts (5.7 L) filtered water, cold, plus water for rinsing
4 sprigs thyme
4 sprigs flat-leaf parsley
2 bay leaves
12 black peppercorns
Sea salt to taste

Preheat the oven to 425°F (220°C).

Rinse the chicken bones and chicken feet under cold water until the water runs clear. Make sure that all visible blood is removed from the bones. Check the bones to locate and remove any organs that might still be attached. The rinsing of blood and removal of organs will help eliminate proteins that could cloud your stock.

Place the chicken feet in a large stockpot; the feet are not roasted in order to maximize extraction of gelatin. Pat the chicken bones dry with a kitchen towel and place in a single layer on a large roasting pan. On another sheet pan, arrange the onions, leeks, carrots, and fennel in a single layer. Toss both the bones and the vegetables with grapeseed oil. Roast until the bones and vegetables are golden brown, stirring occasionally, about 40 minutes. Remove and transfer the excess rendered fat from the pan into a small bowl; set aside for another use. Transfer the bones to the stockpot with the feet; place the vegetables in a bowl and set aside.

Add water to the hot pans, place over medium heat, and scrape to loosen the browned bits and glazed juices. Pour into the stockpot. Cover the roasted bones and feet with filtered water. Heat the pot over medium-high, and slowly bring the liquid to a tremble, skimming as soon as scum appears. When the liquid ripples, reduce the heat to medium-low and maintain a simmer, or smile. Never let the liquid boil, as impurities will be sucked to the bottom of the pot and emulsify into the liquid during the long simmering time.

Continue to skim as necessary while the water temperature rises and the liquid simmers. The first hour of simmering is when most of the impurities will be apparent. A well-skimmed liquid will prevent impurities from emulsifying the stock. Simmer for 2 hours, skimming often.

Once the bones have completed their initial simmering time, add the vegetables, herbs, and spices, and slowly return the liquid to a simmer. The aromatics will rise to the top, making it more difficult to skim, though it is important to continue the clarifying process. Skim by capturing particles that gather near the bubbling part of the liquid, leaving the vegetables to simmer mostly undisturbed. Simmer for another 2 hours, skimming as necessary. Turn off the heat and leave the pot on the stove to rest, about 10 minutes. Any floating particles will settle to the bottom of the pot during this resting period.

Gently ladle the stock through a China cap; remove the bones and aromatics. Set a fine-mesh strainer over a clean stockpot. Carefully strain the stock into the pot, being careful not to force any solids through the mesh. Over medium-high heat, return the stock to a gentle boil, reduce the heat to medium, and continue to simmer until reduced by a third. Taste and season with sea salt.

Chill the stock in the refrigerator, stirring occasionally to expedite the cooling process. Refrigerate for up to 2 days or freeze in smaller containers for longer storage.

Chicken Bone Broth

This bone broth begins with a whole chicken—preferably with its head and feet intact. Don't be dissuaded if your bird has neither; you can fortify the liquid with feet from another bird. Chicken feet mostly comprise tendons and cartilage surrounding bone, which render into a lovely gelatin in the pot. As with all bone broths in this book, soaking in vinegar is optional.

ACTIVE TIME: 2½ hours | **TOTAL TIME:** 8 to 12 hours (including soaking, heating, simmering, and initial cooling) | **YIELD:** Makes about 3 quarts (2.8 liters)

---

1 whole chicken (about 4 to 6 pounds [1.8 to 2.7 kg]), preferably pastured, skin on

2 chicken feet, if whole chicken has no feet attached (required)

4 quarts (3.8 L) filtered water, cold, plus water for rinsing and/or blanching

2 tablespoons apple cider vinegar (optional)

1 quart (680 g) ice cubes

½ pound (225 g) white onions, cut into large dice

1 pound (455 g) leeks, dark green parts removed, cut into large dice

¾ pound (340 g) carrots, cut into large dice

4 sprigs thyme

4 sprigs flat-leaf parsley

1 bay leaf

8 black peppercorns

Sea salt to taste

Rinse the whole chicken and chicken feet under cold water until the water runs clear. Make sure that all visible blood is removed from the cavity of the bird. Check the cavity to locate and remove any organs that might still be attached. The rinsing of blood and removal of organs will help eliminate proteins that could cloud your stock.

In a large stockpot, cover the chicken and feet with filtered water. Add vinegar to the water, if desired. Let the chicken rest in the water for 1 hour. Heat the pot over medium-high, and slowly bring the liquid to a tremble, skimming as soon as scum appears. When the liquid ripples, reduce the heat to medium-low and maintain a simmer, or smile. Never let the liquid boil, as impurities will be sucked to the bottom of the pot and emulsify into the liquid during the long simmering time.

Continue to skim as necessary while the water is rising in temperature. When the liquid comes to a gentle boil, reduce the heat to medium-low, add the ice, and skim to remove the thickened fat. Continue to skim while the bones are simmering; the first hour of simmering is when most of the impurities will be apparent. A well-skimmed liquid will prevent impurities from emulsifying the stock.

After simmering for 1 hour, remove the chicken from the pot while the broth remains on low heat. When cool enough to handle, remove the meat from the chicken and set aside. Place the carcass back in the pot, and continue to simmer for another 4 hours.

Add the onions, leeks, carrots, thyme, parsley, bay leaf, and peppercorns, and simmer until the vegetables are cooked through but not broken down, about 90 minutes. Follow the remainder of the Basic Chicken Stock recipe (page 166) to rest, strain, season, and chill the broth.

If a more concentrated broth is desired, return the stock to a clean pot and simmer until reduced. If a more viscous broth is desired, repeat the simmering process with additional chicken feet until the gelatin is extracted from the joints, about 3 hours. The feet will ensure that the stock achieves a gelatinous state.

You can add the chicken meat to the broth or reserve for another recipe. Refrigerate for up to 2 days or freeze in smaller containers for longer storage.

Twice-Cooked Chicken and Braised Leek Soup with Fregula

A book about stocks would be incomplete without a chicken noodle soup recipe. This seems consistent with maternal lore and logic about the cold-curing effects of this revered dish.

One of my favorite stock recipes is Mark Bittman's Twice-Cooked Chicken Stock—a method that intensifies a basic stock by poaching a second bird in the liquid. The result, called a *compound stock*, lends itself to many uses; the same as a basic stock, only with the added value of having cooked meat alongside a more flavorful base.

This recipe also makes use of the unused chicken fat—rendered into schmaltz as a starting point for braising the leeks. This method reintroduces some fat to the soup in a way not usually encouraged in stock, instead as a clarified version that works as a flavorful substitute for oil or butter.

If you cannot locate *fregula*, a type of small toasted pasta from Sardinia, you can use Israeli couscous or orzo in its place. Simply toast the alternative in schmaltz, oil, or butter before adding to the broth.

ACTIVE TIME: 2 hours | **TOTAL TIME:** 3 hours (including simmering and chilling) | **YIELD:** Makes 6 to 8 servings

---

2 quarts (1.9 L) Basic Chicken Stock
1 whole chicken (about 4 to 6 pounds
  [1.8 to 2.7 kg]), preferably pastured,
  skin removed and reserved,
  cut into sixths
2 medium carrots, divided
1 small fennel bulb, divided, fronds reserved
1 clove garlic

2 sprigs flat-leaf parsley
4 medium leeks, quartered, root ends intact
2 tablespoons schmaltz or olive oil
1 teaspoon sherry vinegar
2 cups (455 g) fregula, or Israeli couscous
  or orzo, cooked
Salt and pepper
Fennel or dill fronds

In a large stockpot, combine the chicken stock and chicken over medium-high heat. Do not add the chicken skin. Add 1 chopped carrot, ½ chopped fennel bulb, garlic, and parsley. Bring to a gentle boil, then lower the heat and simmer, partially covered, until the chicken is cooked through, about 30 minutes. Skim any scum from the surface while the chicken cooks.

While the chicken is poaching, make the schmaltz. With a sharp knife, chop the chicken skin into small pieces. Set a cast-iron pan over medium-high heat, and add the skin and a couple of tablespoons water to the pan. Cook until the moisture from the fat and water evaporates. Continue rendering the fat, while stirring, until the skin and fat scraps are lightly browned. Set the temperature to low and cook until the skin is fully rendered and a clear oil rests on top. Strain the schmaltz into a small bowl; reserve the solids for another use. Cool the schmaltz.

Remove the cooked chicken from the pot and cool slightly. When cool enough to handle, remove the meat from the bones. Shred the meat by hand and set aside. Strain the stock twice, once through a China cap and then through a strainer, and place it back into the clean stockpot. Set aside.

While the chicken is cooling, braise the leeks. In a large sauté pan, melt 2 tablespoons schmaltz over medium-high heat. Lay the quartered leeks across the length of the hot pan in one layer, and sear for 2 minutes, turning once halfway. Lower the heat and continue cooking until the leeks are soft, about 5 minutes longer. Deglaze the pan with ½ cup of the strained chicken stock and the sherry vinegar. Cook until the liquid reduces, leaving the leeks glazed and golden brown. Turn off the heat, cover the pan, and reserve while finishing the soup.

Place the stock over medium-high heat until the liquid comes to a gentle boil, then lower the temperature and maintain at a simmer. Cut the remaining carrot and fennel into small, uniform dice, and add to the pot. Add the cooked fregula and simmer until incorporated, about 5 minutes. Return the shredded chicken to the pot. Season with salt and pepper.

To assemble, layer one or two braised leeks in the middle of a bowl. Ladle the soup over the leeks. Garnish with the fennel fronds or fresh dill. Serve hot.

Seared Moroccan Chicken with Peppered Turmeric Broth

A bright memory from my childhood is coming home to the smell of chicken simmering in a rich aromatic broth. My father would often prepare what he called Yellow Chicken—a one-pot meal of an entire chicken, skin on, coarsely cut into eighths and slowly stewed with onions and turmeric, his simplified version of a Moroccan favorite. Here the dish is revised by searing the seasoned chicken before stewing it in a spiced broth; a method that adds texture to the skin and enhances color in the final dish.

Turmeric has recently been touted among nutritionists for its medicinal qualities. The main active ingredient in turmeric is *curcumin*, which acts as an anti-inflammatory and a strong antioxidant, though it is poorly absorbed into the bloodstream through the consumption of the spice alone. The black pepper in this recipe is used to enhance absorption, as well as flavor, and chicken schmaltz assists with the fat solubility of the curcumin.

ACTIVE TIME: 1½ hours | **TOTAL TIME:** 3+ hours
(including marinating and simmering) | **YIELD:** Makes 4 to 6 servings

SPICE RUB

2 teaspoons cumin seeds
1 teaspoon coriander seeds
½ teaspoon black peppercorns
2 teaspoons sea salt
2 teaspoons brown sugar

1 tablespoon smoked paprika, preferably sweet
½ teaspoon ground ginger
½ teaspoon ground turmeric
½ teaspoon ground cinnamon
Pinch cayenne pepper

In a small, dry skillet, combine the cumin and coriander seeds with the peppercorns. Cook over moderate heat, stirring occasionally, until the seeds are toasted and fragrant, about 2 minutes. Transfer to a plate and cool completely. Place the cooled spices in a spice grinder, and grind to a powder. In a small bowl, add the toasted spices with the remaining spice rub ingredients. Set aside.

CHICKEN STEW

1 whole chicken (about 4 to 6 pounds
    [1.8 to 2.7 kg]), preferably pastured,
    skin on, cut into eighths
3 tablespoons olive oil, divided
1 pinch saffron threads, toasted
½ cup (120 ml) dry white wine, such as
    Sauvignon Blanc, or water
2 medium onions, coarsely chopped
3 cloves garlic, thinly sliced

1 tablespoon grated ginger
1 serrano chili, seeded and minced
1 tablespoon peeled and grated fresh turmeric,
    or 1 teaspoon ground turmeric
1 teaspoon black pepper, coarsely cracked
1 quart (960 ml) Basic Chicken Stock or
    Chicken Bone Broth
¼ cup (85 g) honey
1 cinnamon stick

2 bay leaves
1 lemon, thinly sliced
½ cup (70 g) oil-cured olives, pitted

Salt and pepper, to taste
Cilantro, chopped

Generously coat the chicken pieces with the spice rub. Place in the refrigerator, covered, for at least 2 hours and up to 1 day. In a large Dutch oven, heat half of the olive oil until hot but not smoking. Add the chicken, skin down, in batches if necessary, and cook until lightly browned, about 10 minutes. Turn the chicken once while it sears. Remove the browned chicken from the pan, and set aside to rest while building the stew.

While the chicken cooks, soak the saffron in the white wine. Set aside to bloom.

Wipe the Dutch oven with a paper towel to remove any browned chicken bits, and then heat the remaining olive oil over medium-high heat. Add the onions and cook, stirring, until slightly caramelized, about 8 minutes. Stir in the garlic, ginger, and chili, and cook for another 2 minutes. Add the turmeric and black pepper; stir to coat the onions, cooking for another 2 minutes.

Add the reserved saffron mixture, stock, and honey to the pot. Stir to combine. Add the cinnamon, bay, lemon, and olives. Place the chicken back in the pot, and simmer, partially covered, for 20 minutes. Remove the cinnamon and bay. Season with salt and pepper, and garnish with chopped cilantro. Serve with couscous or rice.

Farmhouse Rooster Coq au Vin

This recipe is a classic among farmers for good reason: It makes use of tough, old birds. Though a young chicken can be used, the red wine sauce benefits from being made with a rooster—its age adds depth of flavor—and the combination improves with time in the pot. The rooster, also known as a *bull cock*, is mature; those that are pastured have had a chance to develop stronger bones, lending to a darker, richer sauce.

The origins of this recipe have a fabled start with Julius Caesar, who was bestowed a chicken of dubious quality from a conquered territory. He thusly instructed his chef to cook it at length. Nevertheless, the practical implications of the recipe are inherent within its original ingredients. A French classic, coq au vin was revived in the American farmhouse as a way to make use of spent birds, later popularized by Julia Child.

If using rooster, be prepared for a lengthy braise. The butchering method here is designed to use the dry white meat for the stock and the moist dark meat for the stew. The slow cooking time ensures a sumptuous blend of tender meat and flavorful sauce. If using a young chicken, the cooking time is reduced.

ACTIVE TIME: 2½ hours | TOTAL TIME: 2 days
(including marinating and braising) | YIELD: Makes 6 to 8 servings

---

1 whole rooster (or chicken) (about 4 to 6
    pounds [1.8 to 2.7 kg]), preferably pastured,
    cut into eighths, giblets and carcass reserved
2 quarts (1.9 L) Roasted Chicken Stock
3 whole cloves
1 bottle (750 ml) fruity red wine,
    such as Burgundy
3 tablespoons Calvados (apple brandy), plus a
    splash for the pan
Salt and pepper
6 slices thick-cut bacon
2 medium onions, chopped

1 small fennel bulb, sliced
2 cloves garlic, thinly sliced
2 medium carrots, chopped
2 tablespoons all-purpose flour
Bouquet garni or a bundle of herbs
2 tablespoons unsalted butter, divided,
    plus more for finishing
20 pearl onions, trimmed, blanched, and peeled
1 cup (85 g) fresh wild mushrooms,
    such as morel or chanterelle
1 tablespoon fresh lemon juice
1 tablespoon Classic Demi-Glace (optional)

TWO DAYS BEFORE SERVING: Follow the recipe for Roasted Chicken Stock, using the carcass of a rooster if available. Add the breast meat and giblets when you place the roasted bones in the stockpot. Add the cloves when you add the herbs to the pot. Reserve the finished stock in the refrigerator until needed.

ONE DAY BEFORE: Marinate the dark meat. In a nonreactive container, cover the legs and thighs with the red wine and 2 tablespoons of the Calvados. Season with salt and pepper. Place in the refrigerator, preferably overnight.

THE DAY OF SERVING: Slice the bacon into lardons, strips about ¼ inch (.6 cm) wide. In a heavy casserole, melt 1 tablespoon butter and cook the bacon, stirring occasionally, until golden. Remove the bacon, leaving the fat in the pan, and set aside.

Remove the dark meat from the marinade; set the marinade aside. Place the meat in the hot pan with the bacon fat; do not overcrowd the pan. Add a splash of Calvados to the pan. Sear, turning once, until golden brown on both sides. Transfer the chicken to a bowl.

In the same pan, add the onions and fennel and cook over medium-high heat. As you stir, scrape the brown bits from the bottom of the pan into the mixture. When the vegetables are translucent, add the garlic and carrots, and continue to cook until lightly browned. Meanwhile, heat the stock in a small stockpot.

Sprinkle the onion mixture with the flour, and cook for 2 minutes, stirring, until browned. Add the reserved marinade and bouquet garni to the pan. Add the seared chicken and cover with reserved stock. Bring the mixture to a gentle boil, lower the heat, and hold at a simmer. Cook, partially covered, about 1½ hours for rooster and 1 hour for chicken.

While the bird is simmering, cook the vegetables for the final assembly. In a cast-iron pan, melt 1 tablespoon butter; add the pearl onions and mushrooms. Season with salt and pepper. Cook, stirring often, until lightly browned, about 12 minutes. Toss with the reserved bacon and fresh lemon juice. Set aside.

When the bird is tender, transfer it from the pan to a covered dish. Strain the cooking liquid into a saucepan, and bring to a boil. Stir the demi-glace into the liquid until dissolved. Reduce the liquid until it is slightly thickened; it should coat the back of a spoon. Mount a small slice of butter into the sauce to render a nice gloss. Place the rooster back in the pan, and coat with the sauce.

TO SERVE: Plate a piece of the bird with the vegetable mixture and a healthy spoonful of sauce. This dish goes especially well with Brown Butter Kamut Spaetzle (page 259) or wide, flat noodles, such as pappardelle.

Hay-Smoked Brick Chicken

The method in this recipe messes with the principle of a haybox through clever butchery and basic heat diffusion. Here we spatchcock a young chicken by removing the breastbone and searing it flat; hay moistened with stock is introduced during the final cooking stage, acting as insulation in a very hot oven. Hay imparts a distinctive bouquet and infuses the chicken with subtle flavors of cured blades of grass. Make an effort to use grass-fed butter here, as the quality of the source makes a notable difference.

ACTIVE TIME: 1½ hours | **TOTAL TIME:** 7+ hours
(including marinating and cooking) | **YIELD:** Makes 4 servings

1 young chicken (about 3 pounds [1.4 kg])
4 cloves garlic, skin on, smashed
½ cup (120 ml) olive oil, plus 2 tablespoons
    for the pan
2 tablespoons cider vinegar
4 sprigs thyme, divided
1 lemon, thinly sliced, divided

Salt and pepper
1 handful fresh, clean hay, rinsed
⅓ cup (80 ml) Basic Chicken Stock
3 tablespoons unsalted butter,
    preferably grass-fed
Special equipment:
    2 bricks, each wrapped in aluminum foil

On a work surface, place the whole chicken breast-side down. Starting at the thigh, use kitchen shears to cut along one side of the backbone. Repeat on the other side of the backbone; remove and reserve for stock. Firmly press down on the wings to break the breastbone. Flip the chicken over and lay it flat on the surface. Snip the wing tips; reserve for stock.

Combine the garlic, olive oil, and cider vinegar in a bowl large enough to fit the chicken. Add 2 sprigs thyme and half of the lemon slices. Generously season the marinade with salt and pepper. Thoroughly coat the chicken with the marinade; refrigerate for a minimum of 4 hours or overnight.

Remove the chicken from the marinade, shaking off excess. If time permits, refrigerate the chicken, uncovered, for 2 hours. Air-drying helps crisp the skin during cooking.

Heat the oven to 450°F (230°C). Remove the chicken from the refrigerator; season with salt and pepper. Set a large cast-iron skillet over medium-high heat; coat with olive oil. When hot, place the chicken, skin-side down, in the pan. Immediately place a brick on top of each half. Reduce the heat to medium and cook until the skin is golden brown, about 15 minutes. Remove the bricks, turn the chicken over, place hay around the chicken, sprinkle with chicken stock, and finish roasting the chicken in the oven, another 20 to 25 minutes. The chicken is done when an instant-read thermometer reads 165°F (75°C), or the juices run clear from the thickest part of the thigh. Remove the chicken from the oven and rest for 5 minutes.

While the chicken is resting, melt the butter, preferably grass-fed (it stands out in this dish), with the remaining thyme and lemon. Throw in a few blades of hay and infuse for a few minutes. Strain and serve with the chicken.

TURKEY

For many home cooks, making turkey stock is a seasonal affair, the result of roasting a large bird for a family gathering around the holidays. Turkey stock can be made and used in the same manner as other poultry stocks. It adds a slightly gamier note than chicken stock while being less forward than duck stock.

Acquiring a pastured turkey can be tricky: One well-raised turkey can cost five times the price of a factory bird. When you invest in one, however, you are supporting a farmer who provides the animals with continual access to land and pays for higher-quality grain and additional processing fees. The price of organic feed alone can match that of a finished conventional turkey.

A commitment to these birds—and the farmers who raise them—will yield a more nutritious plate while supporting humane animal husbandry and biodiversity on the land. Over the past five decades, the conventional turkey has been selectively bred to develop a large breast in a short amount of time. This means the bird is paralyzed in natural flight and reproduction. Heritage breeds, however, thrive outdoors and live longer lives—reflected in their smaller breasts and robustly flavored meat. Farmers who maintain endangered breeds are perpetuating the stock; in turn, those birds are enriching the soil and land around them.

While a good turkey stock employs the same types of bones as other poultry—backs, necks, and feet—individual turkey bones can be difficult to locate. Most often turkey stock is made with a leftover carcass, especially around the holidays. The wings on a turkey—larger than those of a chicken—are a meaningful addition to the stockpot. Substitute chicken feet if your farmer cannot supply turkey feet.

Basic Turkey Stock

This white turkey stock begins with bones from an unroasted bird—best made when you are deboning a whole animal before cooking or you know a turkey farmer who breaks down fowl for sale. The addition of fennel, apple, and marjoram lends a floral sweetness to the gaminess of the stock.

ACTIVE TIME: 2 hours | **TOTAL TIME:** 6 to 7 hours (including heating, blanching, simmering, and initial cooling) | **YIELD:** Makes about 4 quarts (3.8 liters)

6 pounds (2.7 kg) turkey bones, not roasted
    (including neck, wing and leg bones),
    preferably pastured or heritage
1 pound (455 g) turkey feet or chicken feet,
    preferably pastured or heritage (optional)
4 quarts (3.8 L) filtered water, cold, plus water
    for rinsing and/or blanching
2 quarts (1.3 kg) ice cubes
½ pound (225 g) white onions,
    cut into large dice

1 pound (455 g) leeks, dark green parts
    removed, cut into large dice
¾ pound (340 g) carrots, cut into large dice
1 small fennel bulb, coarsely chopped,
    fronds removed
1 medium apple, peeled, cored, and chopped
4 sprigs marjoram
4 sprigs flat-leaf parsley
1 bay leaf
8 black peppercorns
Sea salt to taste

Follow the cooking instructions for Basic Chicken Stock (page 166), lengthening the initial simmering time to 3 hours. If a concentrated stock is desired, gently reduce the liquid after straining until the correct viscosity is achieved. If using feet, the stock will become more gelatinous as the liquid reduces.

Roasted Turkey Stock

This recipe is ideal for your turkey carcass leftover from holiday celebrations. The addition of cognac adds a festive touch—a richness that complements savory autumnal flavors. For an all-purpose brown stock, omit the spirit.

ACTIVE TIME: 2 hours | **TOTAL TIME:** 7½ to 8½ hours (including roasting, heating, simmering, and initial cooling) | **YIELD:** Makes about 4 quarts (3.8 liters)

1 turkey carcass (from a 15-pound [6.8 kg]
    bird), roasted (including neck, wing, and leg
    bones), preferably pastured or heritage
1 pound (455 g) turkey feet or chicken feet,
    preferably pastured or heritage (optional)
6 quarts (5.7 L) filtered water, cold,
    plus water for rinsing
½ pound (225 g) white onions, cut into large dice

1 pound (455 g) leeks, dark green parts
    removed, cut into large dice
½ pound (225 g) carrots, cut into large dice
½ pound (225 g) parsnips, cut into large dice
1 small fennel bulb, coarsely chopped,
    fronds removed
3 cloves garlic, unpeeled, crushed
3 tablespoons grapeseed oil

¼ cup (60 ml) cognac (optional)

4 sprigs marjoram

4 sprigs flat-leaf parsley

2 bay leaves

12 black peppercorns

Sea salt to taste

Using kitchen shears, cut the turkey carcass into smaller pieces; the bones should fill the stockpot about halfway. Follow the cooking instructions for Roasted Chicken Stock (page 168), lengthening the initial simmering time to 3 hours. For a festive touch, deglaze the hot roasted vegetable pan with the cognac, scraping to gather brown bits, and add to the simmering liquid. If a concentrated stock is desired, gently reduce the liquid after straining until the correct viscosity is achieved. If using feet, the stock will become more gelatinous as the liquid reduces.

Turkey Bone Broth

This bone broth begins with less water and requires the addition of feet to render a more concentrated stock in less time. Soaking the bones in vinegar is optional.

ACTIVE TIME: 2½ hours | **TOTAL TIME:** 10 to 12 hours (including soaking, heating, simmering, and initial cooling) | **YIELD:** Makes about 3 quarts (2.8 liters)

1 turkey carcass (from a 25-pound [11.3 kg] bird), or 2 turkey carcasses (from two 10-pound [4.5 kg] birds), not roasted (including neck, wing, and leg bones), preferably pastured or heritage

1 pound (455 g) turkey feet or chicken feet, preferably pastured or heritage (required)

¼ cup apple cider vinegar (optional)

4 quarts (3.8 L) filtered water, cold, plus water for rinsing and/or blanching

2 quarts (1.3 kg) ice cubes

½ pound (225 g) white onions, cut into large dice

1 pound (455 g) leeks, dark green parts removed, cut into large dice

¾ pound (340 g) carrots, cut into large dice

1 small fennel bulb, coarsely chopped, fronds removed

4 sprigs marjoram

4 sprigs flat-leaf parsley

1 bay leaf

8 black peppercorns

Sea salt to taste

Using kitchen shears, cut the turkey carcasses into smaller pieces; the bones should fill the stockpot about halfway. Follow the cooking instructions for Chicken Bone Broth (page 169), excluding the poaching and shredding step and lengthening the initial simmering time to 6 hours. If a more concentrated broth is desired, return the stock to a clean pot and simmer until reduced. If a more viscous broth is desired, repeat the simmering process with additional chicken or turkey feet until the gelatin is extracted from the joints, about 3 hours. The feet will ensure that the stock achieves a gelatinous state.

Turkey Giblet Stock

Giblets refers to the offal of fowl—the gizzard, heart, liver, and other organs. For this stock, use the gizzard only and add the neck to reinforce bone content, so that you can prepare it while roasting the turkey. This foundation is an ideal starting point for gravy, leaving the whole carcass for a more formal stock.

ACTIVE TIME: 2 hours | **TOTAL TIME:** 5 hours (including heating, simmering, and initial cooling) | **YIELD:** Makes about 1½ quarts (1.4 liters)

Neck and gizzard, from 1 turkey, preferably pastured and/or heritage
2 tablespoons grapeseed oil
¼ pound (115 g) white onions, cut into large dice
½ pound (225 g) leeks, dark green parts removed, cut into large dice
½ pound (225 g) carrots, cut into large dice
½ small fennel bulb, coarsely chopped, fronds removed

1 clove garlic, smashed with skin on
1 cup (240 ml) dry white wine, such as an unoaked chardonnay
2 quarts (1.9 L) filtered water, cold, plus water for rinsing
4 sprigs marjoram
4 sprigs flat-leaf parsley
1 bay leaf
8 black peppercorns
Sea salt to taste

Rinse the neck and gizzard under cold water until the water runs clear. Make sure that all visible blood is removed from the bones. The rinsing of blood will help eliminate proteins that could cloud your stock. Pat the neck and giblets dry.

In a medium stockpot, heat the grapeseed oil over medium-high heat. When it starts to ripple, add the neck and gizzard and cook, turning occasionally, until golden brown, about 5 minutes. Add the vegetables and sauté until they begin to caramelize, about 7 minutes longer. Deglaze the pan with the white wine and simmer for 1 minute. Add the filtered water, herbs, and peppercorns, and slowly bring to a gentle boil. Reduce the heat to medium-low and maintain at a simmer, about 2 hours.

Turn off the heat and leave the pot on the stove to rest, about 10 minutes. Any floating particles will settle to the bottom of the pot during this resting period. Set a fine-mesh strainer over a container large enough to hold the liquid contents of the pot. Line the strainer with cheesecloth. Carefully ladle the stock from the pot into the strainer, stopping short of and discarding any cloudy liquid at the bottom of the pot. Periodically remove the solids that accumulate in the basket to minimize impurities that could be forced through the strainer. Taste and season with sea salt.

Once strained, chop and add the gizzard to the broth or use for another recipe; necks are great for dog food. Chill the stock in the refrigerator, stirring occasionally to expedite the cooling process. Once chilled, scrape off any solidified fat and use as a substitute for schmaltz or thickener for dog food. Refrigerate for up to 2 days or freeze in smaller containers for longer storage.

Savory Turkey Breakfast Sausage with Grilled Cider Apples

Grinding your own meat is one of the most satisfying ways to make use of scraps, and making breakfast sausage is one of the simplest ways to use ground meat. Turkey is lean and takes well to the addition of pork fat; enriched here with savory herbs and mushrooms, sweetened with maple and fruit. Breakfast sausage is not cured and should be eaten fresh or portioned and frozen for later use.

ACTIVE TIME: 1 hour | **TOTAL TIME:** 2 hours (including chilling) | **YIELD:** Makes 4 to 6 servings

SAUSAGE

2 pounds (910 g) turkey meat, mostly breast, diced

½ pound (225 g) pork fatback, diced

2 tablespoons Roasted Turkey Stock or Turkey Bone Broth

2 teaspoons sea salt

1 teaspoon black pepper

2 tablespoons finely chopped sage leaves

1 tablespoon minced fresh garlic

1 tablespoon maple sugar or light brown sugar

½ teaspoon freshly grated nutmeg

½ teaspoon cayenne pepper

¼ cup (56 g) unsalted butter

2 medium cider apples, cored and diced

½ cup (42 g) fresh wild mushrooms, preferably chanterelles, diced

In a large bowl, combine all ingredients except butter, apples, and mushrooms and chill for 1 hour.

While the meat and spice mixture is chilling, melt the butter in a sauté pan over medium heat. Add the diced apples and mushrooms and cook until golden brown, about 4 to 5 minutes. Remove from the heat and place into a large bowl.

Using the fine blade of a grinder, grind the meat mixture into the bowl with the apples and mushrooms. Mix until thoroughly combined. Form into patties and sauté over medium heat until brown on both sides. Refrigerate any remaining sausage mixture and use within 3 days or freeze for up to 3 months.

APPLES

½ ounce (14 g) dried mushrooms, ground
1 tablespoon maple sugar or
    light brown sugar
Pinch sea salt

3 cider apples, cored and sliced into eighths
¼ cup (56 g) unsalted butter
2 tablespoons maple syrup
Splash Roasted Turkey Stock

In a small bowl, mix the dried mushroom powder with the maple sugar and salt. Toss the apple slices with the mixture.

In a large cast-iron skillet, heat the butter over medium-high heat. When hot, add the apple slices in a single layer and cook for 2 minutes. Add the maple syrup and a splash of turkey stock to the pan. Flip the apples to cook on the other side, until the liquid has evaporated and the apples are golden brown, about another 3 minutes. Serve with the sautéed sausage and a glug of maple syrup.

Sobaheg with Sunchokes and Chestnuts

Sobaheg is a traditional stew of the Wampanoag nation, a native people that resided in North America long before Europeans arrived. Their main diet consisted of beans, maize, and squash, the trinity of native food often referred to as the *three sisters*. Wild turkey and other fowl, such as swans, ducks, and geese, were plentiful to these easterners. The ground nuts in this dish are used to thicken the stew during the final simmer.

ACTIVE TIME: ¾ hour | TOTAL TIME: 3 hours (including simmering) |
YIELD: Makes 4 to 6 servings

½ pound (225 g) dried heirloom beans, such as
Jacob's cattle, soaked in water overnight
½ pound (225 g) coarse semolina
1 pound (455 g) turkey, preferably heritage,
bone-in cuts
1 teaspoon sea salt
2 quarts (1.9 L) Basic Turkey Stock

1 quart (960 ml) water
1 small winter squash, peeled and cubed
1 cup (150 g) scrubbed and cubed sunchokes
¼ cup (56 g) roasted and ground chestnuts
2 tablespoons maple syrup
½ cup (30 g) chopped flat-leaf parsley
Pumpkin seed oil, for garnish

In a large heavy-bottomed stockpot or clay cooking vessel, combine the soaked beans, turkey, coarse grits, sea salt, turkey stock, and water. Over medium heat, bring the mixture to a gentle boil, cover, then reduce the heat and hold the stew at a simmer, about 2 hours. Stir occasionally to prevent the mixture from sticking. Skim the top of the liquid periodically.

When the beans are al dente, break up the turkey meat and remove the bones. (You can wash and reuse the bones for stock.) Add the squash and sunchokes, and simmer until tender and incorporated into the stew, about 30 minutes.

Add the chestnuts and maple syrup, stirring to combine and simmering to thicken, about 5 minutes. Garnish with chopped parsley and drizzle with pumpkin seed oil. Season with sea salt as necessary. Serve immediately.

Dry-Brined Turkey Leg Confit

When roasting a whole turkey, the legs, if exposed to dry heat, cook first and are at risk of becoming dry. This recipe takes a different approach, requiring the legs from your whole bird (or in this case, four birds, suggesting a communal affair) and cooking them separately as confit.

Turkey is a lean bird—here, the legs are first cured and then slowly cooked in duck fat, a technique that ensures moist, flavorful meat. The initial dry brine works by drawing juices out of the meat, which are reabsorbed over time, allowing natural enzymes to break down muscle proteins. The result is tender meat that does not contract while cooking, especially when bathed and slow-roasted in duck fat.

Confiting is a classic preservation technique that takes time; begin this recipe at least two days in advance. Stock is introduced at the end of this recipe to create a simple sauce.

ACTIVE TIME: 1½ hours | **TOTAL TIME:** 2 days (including curing and cooking) | **YIELD:** Makes 8 servings

---

8 whole turkey legs, skin on
½ cup (58 g) coarse sea salt
2 tablespoons brined green peppercorns, divided
1 bunch sage, coarsely chopped, divided
4 turkey gizzards (optional)

4 cups (910 g) duck fat, or enough to cover turkey parts
½ cup (120 ml) dry white wine, such as an unoaked chardonnay
¾ cup (180 ml) Turkey Giblet Stock or Roasted Turkey Stock

For each turkey leg, score the skin at the top of the leg, just below the knob. This helps shrink the meat and clean the bone during the long cooking time.

In the bowl of a food processor, combine the sea salt with half of the green peppercorns and half of the sage leaves. Pulse until the mixture is thoroughly combined. Rub the green salt on the turkey legs and gizzards, and pack them in an airtight container. Refrigerate overnight.

The next day, remove the turkey parts from the refrigerator and rinse to remove the salt. Pat the turkey dry with a kitchen towel. Place the legs on a sheet pan or a rack and air-dry in the refrigerator, about 3 hours. Refrigerate the gizzards in an airtight container and hold in the refrigerator.

Preheat the oven to 190°F (85°C). In a medium saucepan, heat the duck fat over low heat until it melts. Position the turkey legs and gizzards in a single layer in a large cast-iron

pan and cover the meat with the duck fat. Place in the oven, uncovered, for 6 to 8 hours. Remove and let the turkey cool in the fat at room temperature.

When you are ready to eat, remove the legs and gizzards from the fat, shaking off excess. Sear, in batches, in a cast-iron skillet over medium-high heat, until browned, about 4 minutes per side for each leg and 2 minutes per side for each gizzard. Strain all but 2 tablespoons fat from the pan and reserve for future use.

Deglaze the pan with the white wine, stirring for 1 minute. Add the stock and remaining green peppercorns and sage leaves. Lower the heat to medium-low and simmer until reduced by half, about 5 minutes. Strain and serve with the confit.

To preserve, refrigerate the turkey confit until the fat solidifies. Poke a hole in the fat and drain the liquid. Cover tightly and store in the refrigerator or freezer, up to 6 months.

STOCKS AND BROTHS IN THE KITCHEN

Spatchcocked Bourbon Red Turkey

If you are short on time, spatchcocking a turkey is a fast and convenient way to grill a heritage bird. With the backbone removed, there is no cavity for stuffing. Instead, place the bird on a rack, and bake the dressing and vegetables on a baking sheet settled underneath the rack to catch the drippings. A dry brine is included here as a way to crisp the skin—it's highly recommended, if time permits.

This recipe calls for a Bourbon Red turkey, a heritage breed named for its Kentucky origin and the partial coloring of its plumage. The Livestock Conservancy acknowledges this breed for the size of its breast and rich flavor of its meat. Look for a turkey that weighs in between 18 and 20 pounds (8.2 and 9.1 kilograms), which is midweight for the breed. If you can't locate a Bourbon Red, endeavor to find another heritage breed, such as the American Bronze and lesser-seen White Holland.

ACTIVE TIME: 1 hour | **TOTAL TIME:** 8+ hours
(including curing, roasting, and simmering) | **YIELD:** Makes 4 to 6 servings

TURKEY

1 whole heritage turkey (around 18 to 20 pounds [8.2 to 9.1 kg]), preferably Bourbon Red
½ cup (70 g) kosher salt
½ teaspoon baking soda
¼ cup (56 g) unsalted butter, softened
1 tablespoon black pepper
2 green-skinned apples, sliced, cores reserved

2 small fennel bulbs, roughly chopped, fronds removed
2 medium onions, roughly chopped
4 medium carrots, peeled and roughly chopped
4 sprigs thyme
4 sprigs marjoram
2 bay leaves

Rinse the bird, inside and out, and pat dry with kitchen towels. Place it breast-side down on a cutting board. Holding the turkey firmly with one hand, cut along one side of the backbone with kitchen shears, from tail to neck. After you snip through all the ribs, use your hands to

—186—

partially open the cavity. Repeat the cut on the other side of the backbone, holding it to gain leverage as you cut. Trim the fat around the neck area as necessary.

Turn the turkey over, and using both hands, press down on the breastbone to flatten the bird. One or two cracks will indicate that the turkey is complying. Tuck the wing tips behind the breast. Place the turkey on a rack, and place the rack over an aluminum-foil-covered sheet pan.

Time permitting, mix the kosher salt with the baking soda, and rub the turkey with the mixture, slipping some under the skin where possible. Chill the turkey, loosely covered, for 4 hours or overnight. Remove the turkey, pat dry with kitchen towels, and bring to room temperature, about 2 hours.

Heat the oven to 450°F (230°C). Rub the softened butter under the skin of the turkey. Season the outside with black pepper. Lift the rack with the turkey on it, and scatter the fruit, vegetables, and herbs on the sheet pan. Rest the rack with the turkey over the vegetables on the sheet pan.

Transfer the turkey to oven and roast, rotating the pan every 20 minutes or so, until an instant-read thermometer registers 150°F (65°C) at the breast and 165°F (75°C) at the thigh, about 90 minutes. During the last half an hour of cooking time, baste the turkey with the glaze (below) every 10 minutes or so.

GLAZE

1 cup (240 ml) sweet apple cider
1 cup (240 ml) Roasted Turkey Stock
½ cup (155 g) maple syrup
¼ cup (56 g) unsalted butter

½ teaspoon sea salt
¼ teaspoon cayenne pepper
Freshly grated nutmeg

While the turkey is roasting, make the glaze. In a small saucepan, heat the apple cider, turkey stock, maple syrup, butter, and spices over medium-high heat. Bring the mixture to a gentle boil, and then lower the heat to maintain a simmer. Reduce the mixture by half.

TO SERVE: When fully cooked, remove the turkey from the oven and transfer the rack to a new baking sheet, allowing the bird to rest for about 15 to 20 minutes before carving. Reserve any juices that collect on the new baking sheet. On a large platter, place the roasted vegetables in the center and top with the carved turkey. Drizzle some of the pan juices over the turkey to keep it moist. Serve with glaze on the side.

DUCK

My first job in New York City was selling duck for Hudson Valley Duck Farm at Greenmarkets across most boroughs. By the end of my tenure, I was developing recipes for the farm, which required the procurement of a chest freezer for my small Brooklyn loft. It doubled as an office desk, covered with a cloth and a mess of papers, hiding gems of whole ducks and delicious duck parts. I hold a certain culinary bias for duck in my kitchen.

Duck is a divine bird—dense with nutrients and a host of good fats, it carries deeply developed texture and flavor to the plate. Duck stock has a forward taste and complements recipes with game meats, either as a base or reduced to a glaze. It serves as an excellent foundation for cold-weather dishes, or it can be clarified for a light, rich soup.

Of the popular mallard breed, *Birds of North America* claims that the historical persistence of duck "reflects its adaptability to varied habitats, its hardiness in cold climates, its catholic food tastes, and its tolerance to human activities." Farmland benefits from the resilience of a duck's character: They graze on rotational pasture and near ponds; their natural behavior helps regenerate soil. Locate a farmer who allows ducks to roam without confinement; a good substitute is a farmer who raises ducks outside of a cage.

As with chicken, duck stock makes use of neck and backbones and relies on feet for a boost of gelatin. You can substitute chicken feet if duck feet are unavailable. Due to its gamy flavor, I do not recommend using duck bones to make bone broth.

Basic Duck Stock

This white duck stock follows the same technique as a basic lamb stock, sautéing the vegetables, adding parsnips and more savory herbs, and finishing with a touch of vinegar to mellow the game. It is good for light soups or as a foundation for risotto.

ACTIVE TIME: 2 hours | **TOTAL TIME:** 6 to 7 hours (including heating, blanching, simmering, and initial cooling) | **YIELD:** Makes about 4 quarts (3.8 liters)

5 pounds (2.3 kg) duck bones (necks and
  backs), preferably pastured
1 pound (455 g) duck or chicken feet,
  preferably pastured
4 quarts (3.8 L) filtered water, cold, plus water
  for rinsing and/or blanching
2 quarts (1.3 kg) ice cubes
3 tablespoons grapeseed oil
½ pound (225 g) white onions, cut into large dice
¾ pound (455 g) leeks, dark green parts
  removed, cut into large dice

½ pound (225 g) carrots, cut into large dice
½ pound (225 g) parsnips, cut into large dice
1 cup (240 ml) dry white wine, such as
  Sauvignon Blanc
4 sprigs marjoram
4 sprigs sage
4 sprigs flat-leaf parsley
1 bay leaf
8 black peppercorns
Sea salt to taste
1 teaspoon white wine vinegar

Rinse the duck bones and duck or chicken feet under cold water until the water runs clear. Make sure that all visible blood is removed from the bones. Check the bones to locate and remove any organs that might still be attached. The rinsing of blood and removal of organs will help eliminate proteins that could cloud your stock.

If the water does not become clear from rinsing, blanch the bones before proceeding. To do this, place the duck bones, not including the feet, in a large stockpot, and add enough cold water to cover the bones by a few inches. Turn the heat to medium-high, and slowly heat the liquid. Using a fine-mesh strainer, skim any scum that rises to the surface. When the liquid starts to ripple, before it breaks into a boil, remove the pot from the heat. Do not boil the liquid; boiling in this first stage will extract flavor that should be preserved for the long simmer.

Drain the bones in a large colander, and rinse under cold water. Thoroughly clean the same pot. Return the bones to the pot and add the duck or chicken feet. Top with filtered water. Heat the pot over medium-high, and slowly bring the liquid to a tremble, skimming as soon as scum

appears. When the liquid ripples, reduce the heat to medium-low and maintain a simmer, or smile. Never let the liquid boil, as impurities will be sucked to the bottom of the pot and emulsify into the liquid during the long simmering time.

Continue to skim as necessary while the water is rising in temperature. When the liquid comes to a gentle boil, reduce the heat to medium-low, add the ice, and skim to remove the thickened fat. Continue to skim while the bones are simmering; the first hour of simmering is when most of the impurities will be apparent. A well-skimmed liquid will prevent impurities from emulsifying the stock. Simmer for 3 hours, skimming often.

Prepare the vegetables while the stock is simmering. In a sauté pan, heat the oil over medium heat. When it starts to ripple, add the onions, leeks, carrots, and parsnips, and sauté, stirring often, until they are cooked through but not caramelized, about 10 minutes. Deglaze the pan with the white wine and simmer for 1 minute. Turn off the heat and set aside until needed.

Once the bones have completed their initial simmering time, add the sautéed vegetables, herbs, and peppercorns, and slowly bring to a gentle boil. Reduce the heat to medium-low and maintain at a simmer, about 2 hours longer.

Turn off the heat and rest the stock on the stove, about 15 minutes. Gently ladle the stock through a China cap into a clean container; remove the bones for another use and discard the aromatics. Set a fine-mesh strainer over a clean stockpot. Line the strainer with cheesecloth. Carefully strain the stock into the pot,

being careful not to force any solids through the mesh. Over medium-high heat, return the stock to a gentle boil, reduce the heat to medium, and continue to simmer until reduced by a third. Season with sea salt and finish with vinegar.

Place the container in an ice bath to rapidly cool the stock. When the stock no longer steams, transfer to the refrigerator. Refrigerate for up to 2 days or freeze in smaller containers for longer storage.

Roasted Duck Stock

This roasted duck stock is concentrated to achieve depth of flavor. Similar to a brown lamb stock, the vegetables are not roasted, relying on color achieved from roasting the bones and the addition of tomato paste. Juniper berries, which add an herbal pungency, match well with wintry meat dishes.

ACTIVE TIME: 2 hours | **TOTAL TIME:** 8 hours (including roasting, heating, simmering, and initial cooling) | **YIELD:** Makes about 2 quarts (1.9 liters)

---

5 pounds (2.3 kg) duck bones (necks and backs), preferably pastured

1 pound (455 g) duck or chicken feet, preferably pastured

⅓ cup (80 ml) grapeseed oil

6 quarts (5.7 L) filtered water, cold, plus water for rinsing

½ pound (225 g) white onions, cut into large dice

¾ pound (340 g) leeks, dark green parts removed, cut into large dice

½ pound (225 g) carrots, cut into large dice

¾ pound (340 g) tomatoes, coarsely chopped

¼ cup (58 g) tomato paste, preferably homemade (page 273)

4 sprigs thyme

4 sprigs flat-leaf parsley

1 bay leaf

5 dried juniper berries

8 black peppercorns

Sea salt to taste

Preheat the oven to 425°F (220°C).

Rinse the duck bones and duck or chicken feet under cold water until the water runs clear. Make sure that all visible blood is removed from the bones. Check the bones to locate and remove any organs that might still be attached. The rinsing of blood and removal of organs will help eliminate proteins that could cloud your stock.

Place the feet in a large stockpot; the feet are not roasted, in order to maximize extraction of gelatin. Pat the remaining duck bones dry with kitchen towels and place in a single layer on a large roasting pan. Toss with the grapeseed oil. Roast until the bones are golden brown, turning about halfway through the cooking process, about 40 minutes total. Remove and transfer the excess rendered fat from the pan into a small bowl; set aside for another use. Transfer the bones to the stockpot with the feet.

Add water to the hot pan, place over medium heat, and scrape to loosen the browned bits and glazed juices. Pour into the stockpot. Cover the roasted bones and feet with filtered water. Heat the pot over medium-high, and slowly bring the liquid to a tremble, skimming as soon as scum appears. When the liquid ripples, reduce the heat to medium-low and maintain a simmer, or smile. Never let the liquid boil, as impurities will be sucked to the bottom of the pot and emulsify into the liquid during the long simmering time.

Continue to skim as necessary while the water is rising in temperature and as the liquid simmers. The first hour of simmering is when most of the impurities will be apparent. A well-skimmed liquid will prevent impurities from emulsifying the stock. Simmer for 3 hours, skimming often.

Once the bones have completed their initial simmering time, add the onions, leeks, carrots, tomatoes, tomato paste, herbs, juniper berries, and peppercorns, and slowly return the liquid to a simmer. The aromatics will rise to the top, making it more difficult to skim, though it is important to continue the clarifying process. Skim with aromatics by capturing particles that gather near the bubbling part of the liquid, leaving the vegetables to simmer mostly undisturbed. Simmer for another 2 hours, skimming as necessary.

Turn off the heat and rest the stock on the stove, about 15 minutes. Gently ladle the stock through a China cap; remove the bones for another use and discard the aromatics. Set a fine-mesh strainer on the lip of a clean stockpot. Carefully strain the stock a second time into the pot, being careful not to force any solids through the mesh. Over medium-high heat, return the stock to a gentle boil, reduce the heat to medium, and continue to simmer until reduced by half. Taste and season with sea salt.

Chill the stock in the refrigerator, stirring occasionally to expedite the cooling process. Refrigerate for up to 2 days or freeze in smaller containers for longer storage.

Country Duck Pâté with Dried Cherries

This pâté requires patience yet yields a result that will feed you for days. Duck and cherries are a natural combination, further enhanced with dry sherry and rich spices and moistened with reduced duck stock. Caul fat—the lacy membrane that encases the organs of pigs, cows, and sheep—is used here to wrap the pâté. It creates a beautiful web around the finished terrine and carries a pleasant mouthfeel.

ACTIVE TIME: 2½ hours | **TOTAL TIME:** 2 to 4 days (including marinating, baking, and chilling) | **YIELD:** Makes two 1-quart (910 g) terrines

---

1 small duck (about 3 pounds [1.4 kg]), skinned and deboned, with liver

4 cloves garlic, minced, divided

2 bay leaves

2 teaspoons sea salt, divided

1 teaspoon ground black pepper, divided

¼ cup (60 ml) olive oil, divided

½ cup (120 ml) dry sherry, divided

1 cup (140 g) dried cherries

3 small shallots, minced

2 cups (480 ml) Roasted Duck Stock

1 pound (455 g) pork shoulder, cubed and chilled

¼ pound (115 g) pork fatback, cubed and chilled

1 teaspoon fennel seed, toasted and ground

½ teaspoon smoked paprika

½ teaspoon ground allspice

¼ teaspoon ground nutmeg

2 tablespoons fresh thyme

1 tablespoon orange zest

2 eggs, lightly beaten

1 pound (455 g) caul fat, soaked in water

Cut the duck breasts into small strips and place in a medium bowl. Mix in 1 minced garlic clove, bay leaves, ½ teaspoon sea salt, and ¼ teaspoon black pepper. Drizzle 2 tablespoons olive oil and 2 tablespoons sherry over the mixture. Stir to combine. Wrap well and refrigerate at least 24 hours and up to 2 days. Coarsely chop the remaining duck meat; reserve in the refrigerator.

In a small bowl, combine the remaining sherry with the dried cherries. Macerate at least 30 minutes; reserve, covered, at room temperature.

In a small saucepan, heat the remaining olive oil, and sauté the shallots with the remaining garlic until translucent. Set aside to cool. In a small saucepan, bring the duck stock to a boil over medium-high heat, lower to a simmer, and reduce by half. Set aside to cool.

In the bowl of a food processor, purée the duck liver, then add the chilled chopped duck meat (not the breast), pork shoulder, and fatback. Pulse until combined; the mixture should be coarse. Transfer to a large bowl; stir in the reserved shallot mixture and reduced duck stock. Stir in the fennel, paprika, allspice, nutmeg, thyme, and orange zest with the remaining salt and pepper. Stir in the eggs. With your hands or a wooden spoon, mix until well combined. Reserve in the refrigerator while you prepare the terrine molds.

Heat the oven to 325°F (165°C). Drain the macerated cherries; toss with the marinated duck breast strips, discarding the bay leaves. Line two terrine molds (about 1-quart [1-liter] capacity each) with caul fat, leaving a 2-inch (5 cm) overhang. Place a quarter of the meat mixture in each of the molds, pressing firmly with the back of a spoon. Cover the meat mixture with the duck breast mixture. Top with remaining meat mixture and gently pack down with a spoon. Fold the caul fat over and press

to seal the terrine, trimming if necessary. Cover with aluminum foil.

Place both terrines in a roasting pan, making sure the sides are clear for air movement. Pour boiling water into the roasting pan to come halfway up the sides of the terrine molds. Bake until an instant-read thermometer comes to 140°F (60°C), about 1½ hours. Remove from the oven and uncover the terrines. Place a weight on top of each terrine; rest in the water bath, about 1 hour.

Transfer the weighted terrines to the refrigerator and chill overnight or up to 2 days. Unmold and serve with crusty bread, grainy mustard, and pickled vegetables.

Pan-Seared Duck Breast with Duck Liver Butter on Le Puy Lentils

Duck liver is often associated with foie gras—a delicacy that requires the enlargement of the liver through controversial handling of the animal. Regardless of your position, the liver of common-sized ducks is delicious on its own accord. Here duck livers are cooked and blended with seasoned butter to create a compound fat that melts into the seared meat and lentils in broth. The key to a properly seared duck breast is cooking it fat-side down in a hot pan, and then finishing on the other side until medium rare.

ACTIVE TIME: 1 hour | TOTAL TIME: 2 hours
(including chilling, resting, and simmering) | YIELD: Makes 2 servings

BUTTER

½ teaspoon sea salt
¼ teaspoon black pepper
Pinch ground cloves

2 duck livers
½ cup (115 g) unsalted butter, preferably grass-fed, divided

2 small shallots, minced
1 clove garlic, minced

Splash port or brandy

Mix the sea salt, black pepper, and cloves in a bowl. Season the livers with the spice mixture. Set aside.

In a small sauté pan, heat 2 tablespoons of the butter over medium heat. Add the shallots and garlic and sauté until they just begin to caramelize, about 5 minutes. Add the seasoned livers and sear until golden, about 2 minutes on

each side. Deglaze with port. Remove from the heat and set aside to cool completely.

In a food processor, pulse the duck liver mixture with the remaining butter until combined. Continue to pulse until smooth. Press the mixture through a sieve onto parchment paper. Roll the mixture into a log, twisting the parchment at the ends. Reserve in the refrigerator or freezer.

LENTILS

1 cup (225 g) Le Puy lentils
2 cups (480 ml) Basic Duck Stock
2 tablespoons unsalted butter
2 teaspoons aged sherry vinegar
1 small red onion, finely diced

1 medium carrot, peeled and finely diced
1 small tomato, finely diced
½ cup (30 g) finely chopped
   flat-leaf parsley
Salt and pepper

Rinse the lentils in cold water and place in a saucepan. Cover with duck stock. Over medium-high heat, bring the mixture to a boil, then reduce the heat and simmer until the lentils are al dente, about 20 minutes. Drain the lentils, reserving the liquid, and set aside.

Return the lentil cooking liquid to the saucepan. Bring to a boil, lower to a simmer, and reduce the liquid to 2 tablespoons. Mount with the butter, stirring until melted and combined. Pour over the lentils and stir until combined. Toss with vinegar, red onion, carrot, tomato, and parsley. Season with salt and pepper.

DUCK

1 large or 2 small boneless duck breasts
   (about 1 pound [455 g] total),
   skin on

Kosher salt
24 red pearl onions, trimmed, blanched,
   and peeled

Score the skin of each breast, cutting into ½-inch (1.25 cm) interval crosshatches, being careful to avoid puncturing the meat. Generously season with kosher salt. Rest at room temperature for 30 minutes.

Pat the duck breasts with a kitchen towel to remove excess moisture. In a large, dry, cold sauté pan, place the duck breasts skin-side down, leaving room between each breast, then turn the heat to medium-high. As the pan heats, the skin will begin to render. Continue to sear the duck, fat-side down, pressing down to ensure even contact on the pan, about 4 to 5 minutes.

When the duck is nearly done, flip it over and cook another 2 to 3 minutes, until medium rare. Using tongs, hold the sides of the breast to the pan, quickly searing, about 20 seconds each side. Remove the breasts from the heat, reserving the fat in the pan. Tent the meat with aluminum foil and rest at room temperature, about 10 minutes.

In the same pan, return the heat to medium-high and add the prepared pearl onions. Cook, stirring often, until caramelized, about 10 minutes. Remove from the heat.

TO SERVE: Thinly slice the meat at an angle against the grain. Serve the sliced duck breast on a bed of lentils with the caramelized onions and topped with a slice of the duck liver butter.

Roasted Duck Thigh on Fennel Hearts with Barolo Chinato Sauce

Due to the thick layer of fat on duck, the thigh takes longer to cook. This method is convenient—layering the seared thigh atop oil-coated vegetables and roasting in the oven until both are done. The gaminess of duck takes well to rich sauces, as showcased here. This dish is simple to prepare and elegant on the plate, making it an ideal presentation for your loved one on Valentine's Day.

Barolo Chinato, an Italian fortified wine, blends with a concentrated duck stock to form a decadent sauce for this dish. This liqueur is classified as a *quinquina*—a variety of apéritif that includes cinchona bark, the source of quinine. Combined with rich duck stock, warm spices, and dark chocolate, Barolo Chinato is an exquisite base for this dish. If you cannot locate Barolo Chinato, you can use ruby port or Byrrh as acceptable substitutes.

ACTIVE TIME: ¾ hour | **TOTAL TIME:** 2 hours
(including resting, roasting, and simmering) | **YIELD:** Makes 2 servings

DUCK

2 duck thighs (about 1 pound [455 g] total),
   skin on
Kosher salt
2 small fennel bulbs, fronds reserved
2 medium carrots, preferably Kyoto, scrubbed
6 fingerling potatoes, halved

2 tablespoons olive oil
Salt and pepper
2 tablespoons Roasted Duck Stock
4 sprigs thyme
¼ cup (15 g) chopped flat-leaf parsley
1 tablespoon lemon zest

Generously season the duck thighs with kosher salt. Rest at room temperature, about 30 minutes.

While the duck is resting, heat the oven to 400°F (200°C). Slice the fennel into ¾-inch (2 cm) slices, leaving the root end intact. Slice the carrots on the bias into 2-inch (5 cm) logs. In a large bowl, toss the fennel, carrots, and potatoes with olive oil. Season with salt and pepper. Set aside.

Using kitchen towels, pat the duck thighs to remove excess moisture. Heat a large cast-iron skillet and sear the thighs, skin-side down, until browned, about 4 minutes per side. Deglaze with the stock. Remove from the heat. Evenly distribute the vegetables around the duck; top with the thyme sprigs. Roast in the oven until the fat is rendered, the vegetables are caramelized, and the duck is cooked through, about 1 hour. Juices should run clear when the thigh joint is punctured.

In a small bowl, combine the parsley, lemon zest, and reserved fennel fronds. Set aside for garnish.

SAUCE

1 cup (240 ml) Barolo Chinato (or ruby port
   or Byrrh)
1 cup (240 ml) Roasted Duck Stock
1 cardamom pod, crushed

½ teaspoon aged sherry vinegar
2 tablespoons unsalted butter
2 ounces (56 g) dark chocolate, grated
Salt and pepper

In a medium saucepan, heat the Barolo Chinato (or other wine), duck stock, and cardamom pod over medium-high heat. Bring to a boil, then lower the heat to maintain a simmer. Reduce by half. Strain into a small bowl; stir in the vinegar. While hot, mount the sauce with butter and chocolate, stirring until combined.

Season with salt and pepper.

TO SERVE: Spoon some sauce onto a plate and top with roasted vegetables. Place a roasted duck thigh on the vegetables, brush with more sauce, and garnish with the reserved lemon-herb mixture.

Moulard Duck Galantine

Galantines, an elaborate poultry dish that requires a deft hand, have been around since the French Revolution. The process begins by deboning a whole bird, which is then stuffed with cured forcemeat, wrapped in its skin, and poached in stock. When pressed and chilled, the galantine sets into a natural aspic, ready to be served cold.

The encyclopedia of gastronomy, *Larousse Gastronomique*, suggests that *galantine* comes from an old French word for "chicken." Contemporary historians purport the meaning derives from the word *gelatin*. Regardless of its etymology, this dish is a superb exercise in getting the most from a bird; an advanced recipe for the ambitious cook. For detailed instructions on how to butcher the duck, see "Deboning a Bird" on page 199.

ACTIVE TIME: 5 hours | **TOTAL TIME:** 2 days (including marinating, poaching, and chilling) | **YIELD:** Makes 12 to 14 servings

---

1 large duck (about 6 pounds [2.7 kg]), preferably Moulard, deboned except for wing and leg bones

¼ pound (115 g) boneless pork shoulder, cubed

¼ pound (115 g) pork fatback, cubed

¾ cup (180 ml) tawny port

½ teaspoon ground ginger

½ teaspoon ground clove

¼ teaspoon ground nutmeg

1 teaspoon ground black pepper

1 tablespoon kosher salt

2 teaspoons pink curing salt (Prague Powder #1 or Insta Cure #1)

1 egg

1 cup (240 ml) heavy cream

⅛ pound (56 g) pancetta, diced

2 small shallots, minced

1 cup (85 g) chopped fresh mushrooms, preferably morel

4 leaves Swiss chard, chopped

¼ cup (32 g) walnuts, toasted and chopped

1 quart (960 ml) Basic Duck Stock

2 sprigs thyme

2 bay leaves

TO SEPARATE SKIN FROM MEAT: Place the duck breast-side down on a cutting board. With the tip of a sharp knife, gently separate skin from meat, starting at the back of the neck and moving toward the tail. Move slowly to avoid tearing the skin; the tip of your knife will help release the skin from the meat. The goal is to remove the skin from the entire duck in one piece, leaving the end joints (wing and leg) intact.

Cover a sheet pan with plastic wrap. Lay the skin on the pan, gently stretching so it lies flat and covers as much surface area as possible. (Be careful not to puncture the skin; holes will expand when heated.) Scrape off any excess fat on the interior of the skin. Double wrap with plastic wrap; reserve in the refrigerator.

TO MAKE THE FARCE: Cube all the loose duck meat and place in a large bowl. Combine with the pork shoulder and fatback. Add the port, ginger, clove, nutmeg, black pepper, kosher salt, and pink salt. With your hands or a wooden spoon, mix until well combined. Cover and marinate in the refrigerator overnight or up to 1 day.

In a grinder set to medium, grind the spiced meat mixture into the bowl of an electric mixer. Attach the paddle attachment, add the egg, and beat on low speed until combined. Gradually add the cream and continue beating until smooth.

TO MAKE THE FILLING: Heat a large, dry sauté pan over medium-high heat. Add the diced pancetta and stir until the fat is rendered and the meat is cooked through, about 4 minutes. Transfer the pancetta to a bowl, leaving the rendered fat in the pan. Add the shallots to the hot pan and cook until translucent, about 3 minutes. Stir in the mushrooms and sauté until dry and slightly caramelized, about 5 minutes. Add the chopped Swiss chard and stir until wilted. Transfer the mixture to the bowl with the pancetta; mix in the toasted walnuts and stir until well combined. Season with salt and pepper. Set aside to cool.

TO ASSEMBLE: Remove the prepared duck skin from the refrigerator. Spread half the farce down the center of the skin, leaving space between the farce and joints. Spoon the mushroom mixture in an even layer over the farce. Top with remaining farce. Fold the side skin over so it meets in the middle; fold the neck skin down and tuck between the legs. Using butcher's twine, tie the duck to hold the skin and contents in place. Reserve.

Heat a large, dry sauté pan over medium-high heat. Carefully transfer the duck to the pan and sear until the skin browns, about 4 minutes on each side. Using tongs, turn the bird so the sides touch the heat, about 30 seconds per side. Lay a piece of cheesecloth large enough to contain the duck on the sheet pan or a cutting board, and transfer the duck to the cheesecloth. Wrap and secure with additional twine; hold at room temperature.

In a stockpot large enough to fit the duck, slowly heat the stock to a quiver. Add the thyme and bay leaves. Submerge the wrapped duck and poach until an instant-read thermometer inserted into the center reads 160°F (70°C), approximately 20 minutes per pound. Remove the pot from the heat and set aside to cool, about 1 hour. Transfer to the refrigerator, leaving the bird in the liquid, and chill overnight.

TO SERVE: Remove the duck from the poaching liquid. Reserve the stock for another use. Remove the cheesecloth and butcher's twine; discard both. Slice the cold galantine from the neck end; the joints will help the duck stay together. Serve cold with a bitter green salad and champagne vinaigrette.

DEBONING A BIRD

This butchering technique yields a whole bird—chicken, turkey, or duck—without the majority of its bones. If you have never deboned poultry, give yourself ample time to explore the process. Each step will ensure clean removal of meat and skin from the carcass, leaving only the leg and wing bones for elegance of presentation. Throughout the process, do your best to avoid cutting through the skin.

On a large cutting board, place the bird breast-side down; the ridge of the backbone will face upward. With a sharp knife, carefully cut through the skin along the entire length of one side of the spine. Starting at the neck, use the tip of the knife to separate meat from frame. Follow along the rib cage with your knife, cutting as close to the bone as possible. When you come across the wishbone, bend until it breaks free from the carcass. Continue to cut along the rib cage, working toward the breast and stopping short of the leg and wing joints.

Grasp a wing with one hand and stabilize the bird with the other. Twist the wing until it pops free from the joint. Using your fingers, locate the gap between the wing bone and the socket.

Carefully cut through the joint and tendons with the tip of the knife, avoiding the skin. Using the same technique, pop out the leg joint with your hands and cut through the joint and tendons with your knife. Continue separating meat from frame until you reach the area of the breastbone that comes closest to skin.

Rotate the bird and repeat the entire process on the other side. Beginning at the spine, disjoint the wing and leg and end at the cartilage breastbone. Using one hand, lift the rib cage and gently cut away any remaining meat attached to bone. Move slowly—this area is where the skin is the thinnest. Arrange the meat flat on the cutting board, skin-side down. Run your fingertips over the meat and cut away any small bones or cartilage that poke through.

At this point, you have a bird with meat and skin; only the leg and wing bones remain. These bones are kept intact to preserve the tautness of the skin, which is typically tied for a professional presentation. Should a recipe call for an entirely boneless bird, simply cut around the thighbone and pop the joint between the leg bones to remove; cut at the released wing joints to remove the wings.

RABBIT

Rabbit was a common food for early Americans. There was such a natural abundance when the Dutch arrived that the Manhattan peninsula came to be known as Coney Island. Over time, however, rabbits lost their appeal as a popular food source and became a common household pet—their fluffy coats and floppy ears endearing them to kids around the world.

In recent years, food activists have pointed to rabbit as an ideal animal to raise for local consumption. Rabbits grow quickly, eat plants, and flourish in clean habitats without disease. They are easier to harvest than chickens. As delicate as their meat, rabbits are fragile creatures, and are startled easily, which means they are better suited for the gentle habitat of a small farm.

The taste of rabbit meat is often compared to chicken—mild in flavor, with only a hint of game. With its smaller anatomy, rabbit yields lean meat, a silkier mammalian version of domesticated poultry. It is elegant when served on the bone, yet hearty enough to hold up in a hunter's stew. Rabbit bones are dense with cartilage and yield a stock full of body.

Look for farmers in your area who is transparent about their operation: Baby rabbits should feed on their mother's milk; rabbits might have the luxury of living in colonies, or at the very least, within clean and spacious enclosures; and they should have access to fresh air in summertime. Their food supply should include supplemental feed, such as alfalfa or rich, leafy clover hay, with no hormones or antibiotics. A clean kidney is a good sign of health in a rabbit; some farmers will be happy to show you. You can use the entire carcass, including the head, for stock.

Basic Rabbit Stock

This white rabbit stock will yield a light, silken stock that works well in soup or a simple pan sauce. It is ideal for sophisticated dishes that require a delicate foundation. Fennel is an excellent foil to the subtle game. You can use this base in place of basic chicken stock.

ACTIVE TIME: 2 hours | **TOTAL TIME:** 5 to 6 hours (including heating, blanching, simmering, and initial cooling) | **YIELD:** Makes about 2 quarts (1.9 liters)

3 rabbit carcasses (about 4 pounds [1.8 kg]total)

2 quarts (1.9 L) filtered water, cold, plus water
    for rinsing and/or blanching

1 quart (680 g) ice cubes

½ pound (225 g) white onions, cut into
    large dice

1 pound (455 g) leeks, dark green parts
    removed, cut into large dice

½ pound (225 g) carrots, cut into large dice

½ small fennel bulb, coarsely chopped,
    fronds removed

4 sprigs thyme

4 sprigs flat-leaf parsley

1 bay leaf

8 black peppercorns

Sea salt to taste

Using kitchen shears, cut the rabbit carcasses into smaller pieces; the bones should fill the stockpot about halfway. Follow the cooking instructions for Basic Chicken Stock (page 166). Keep in mind that rabbit bones are a good source of collagen; the addition of chicken feet is not necessary. If a concentrated stock is desired, gently reduce the liquid after straining until the correct viscosity is achieved.

Roasted Rabbit Stock

This brown rabbit stock is rich and hearty, an excellent foundation for a hunter's stew. Dry sherry adds a rounded depth to the foundation; tomatoes incorporate color and lengthen the texture. You can use it in place of roasted chicken stock.

ACTIVE TIME: 2 hours | **TOTAL TIME:** 6½ hours (including roasting, heating, simmering, and initial cooling) | **YIELD:** Makes about 2 quarts (1.9 liters)

3 rabbit carcasses (about 4 pounds [1.8 kg]total)

3 quarts (2.8 L) filtered water, cold,
    plus water for rinsing

½ pound (225 g) white onions, cut into
    large dice

1 pound (455 g) leeks, dark green parts
    removed, cut into large dice

½ pound (225 g) carrots, cut into
    large dice

½ small fennel bulb, coarsely chopped,
    fronds removed

¼ cup (60 ml) dry sherry (optional)

¾ pound (340 g) tomatoes, coarsely chopped

4 sprigs thyme

4 sprigs flat-leaf parsley

1 bay leaf

8 black peppercorns

Sea salt to taste

Using kitchen shears, cut the rabbit carcasses into smaller pieces; the bones should fill the stockpot about halfway. Follow the cooking instructions for Roasted Chicken Stock (page 168). For additional flavor, deglaze the hot roasted vegetable pan with the sherry, scraping up the brown bits, and add to the simmering liquid. If a concentrated stock is desired, gently reduce the liquid after straining until the correct viscosity is achieved.

Rabbit Bone Broth

This bone broth uses a ratio of more bones to less water and suggests adding chicken feet to fortify gelatin content.

ACTIVE TIME: 2½ hours | **TOTAL TIME:** 8 to 12 hours (including soaking, heating, simmering, and initial cooling) | **YIELD:** Makes about 1½ quarts (1.4 liters)

2 whole rabbits (about 6 pounds [2.7 kg] total)
½ pound (225 g) chicken feet, preferably pastured (optional)
2 tablespoons apple cider vinegar (optional)
3 quarts (2.8 L) filtered water, cold, plus water for rinsing and/or blanching
1 quart (680 g) ice cubes
½ pound (225 g) white onions, cut into large dice

1 pound (455 g) leeks, dark green parts removed, cut into large dice
½ pound (225 g) carrots, cut into large dice
½ small fennel bulb, coarsely chopped, fronds removed
4 sprigs thyme
4 sprigs flat-leaf parsley
1 bay leaf
8 black peppercorns
Sea salt to taste

Follow the cooking instructions for Chicken Bone Broth (page 169). The use of chicken feet here fortifies the stock, strengthening the liquid. If a more concentrated stock is desired, gently reduce the broth after straining until the correct viscosity is achieved.

Rabbit Rillettes with Pistachios and Sorrel Aspic

Similar to pâté, rillettes are a type of potted meat served generously throughout central France. The name derives from the Old French word *reille*, meaning "strip of wood," referring to the rails of meat that develop from the slow cooking method. Rillettes are a great way to use extra bits of meat and fat. They also make great gifts when packed in jars.

Aspic, otherwise known as meat jelly, adds texture, flavor, and color; most importantly, it helps to preserve the spread. Rillettes will hold in your refrigerator for at least 2 weeks. You can make your own grass-fed gelatin powder from fresh or spent pork bones (see chapter 14, page 336).

ACTIVE TIME: 1½ hours | **TOTAL TIME:** 1 day
(including marinating, braising, and chilling) | **YIELD:** Makes 8 to 12 servings

RILLETTES

1 rabbit (about 3 pounds [1.4 kg]),
    cut into 8 pieces
Salt and pepper
1 pound (455 g) lard
½ cup (120 ml) Basic Rabbit Stock
2 ounces (58 g) pancetta
4 cloves garlic
2 medium shallots, minced

2 bay leaves
1 teaspoon mustard seeds
2 allspice berries
2 dried juniper berries, smashed
½ teaspoon red pepper flakes
½ cup shelled pistachios, toasted and
    coarsely chopped

Season the rabbit with salt and pepper. Place in a container, cover, and refrigerate overnight or up to 1 day.

Heat the oven to 250°F (120°C). Select a heavy-bottomed pot wide enough to hold the rabbit in a single layer. Over medium heat, melt the lard and rabbit stock, then add the pancetta, garlic, shallots, and bay leaves. Once

melted but not hot, remove from the heat and add the rabbit in one layer. Wrap the spices in cheesecloth or a spice bag and add to the pot. Cover and braise in the oven until very tender, about 4 hours. Remove and cool in the pot.

When the rabbit is cool enough to handle, remove from the fat with a slotted spoon, discard the spice bag, and pick the meat from the bones. Place the meat in a bowl; reserve the bones for Basic Rabbit Stock (page 200) or Dog Food (page 356). Strain the fat and set aside.

Shred the meat with your hands and add enough of the reserved fat to hold the meat together. Toss in the pistachio nuts. Season with salt and pepper if necessary. Pack the rillettes in ramekins or sterilized jars, smoothing with the back of a spoon to eliminate air bubbles, and refrigerate while making the aspic.

ASPIC

½ cup (120 ml) Basic Rabbit Stock
¼ cup (15 g) coarsely chopped flat-leaf parsley
¼ cup (15 g) coarsely chopped sorrel
2 tablespoons Gelatin Powder or 6 gelatin sheets

2 tablespoons water
2 tablespoons dry white wine, such as
    Pinot Grigio
Sea salt

In a blender, blend the rabbit stock with the parsley and sorrel until the liquid turns green. Strain into a small saucepan. Discard the solids. Over medium heat, gently warm the stock; remove from the heat.

While the stock is heating, soften the gelatin in water, about 2 minutes, then dissolve in the hot stock. Stir in the white wine. Season with sea salt if necessary. Cool for 5 minutes.

Pour the aspic over the rillettes and refrigerate until set, about 1 hour. Serve the rillettes with crusty bread, grainy mustard, and cornichons.

Roasted Cardoon and Rabbit Consommé

Every good French chef knows how to make consommé. The technique exemplifies how a concentrated bouillon can be delicate and flavorful at the same time. This method first appeared in Francois Pierre de la Varenne's cookbook *Le Cuisinier Francois* (1651).

The signs of a quality consommé are translucence, intense flavor, and rich mouthfeel; classically achieved by clarifying concentrated stock with a protein raft. As the stock heats up, the protein in the egg white and ground meat develops a web that captures impurities from the liquid and gathers solids at the surface. See chapter 2, "Consommé," page 23, for more about consommé.

Here a gentle rabbit consommé is infused with the flavor of cardoon, a flowering plant that looks like overgrown celery but shares a botanical family with artichokes. This recipe begins by stripping the cardoons of bitterness—by soaking in vinegar and then blanching quickly—a key step toward matching the sophistication of a respectable consommé.

ACTIVE TIME: 2 hours | **TOTAL TIME:** 3 hours (including soaking and simmering) | **YIELD:** Makes 4 servings

CONSOMMÉ

2 stalks cardoon

1 tablespoon apple cider vinegar

Sea salt

2 tablespoons olive oil

1 pound (455 g) cooked rabbit meat (poached or baked), finely shredded

1 medium onion, chopped

1 medium leek, chopped

2 medium carrots, chopped

2 egg whites

1 quart (960 ml) Roasted Rabbit Stock, chilled

4 sprigs flat-leaf parsley

2 sprigs tarragon

2 bay leaves, preferably fresh

8 black peppercorns

Heat the oven to 425°F (220°C). Trim the bottom of the cardoon stalks; remove any leaves or thorns. Using a sharp vegetable peeler, remove any tough, stringy fibers from the stalks. Cut into 2-inch (5 cm) pieces. In a medium bowl, combine the vinegar with enough water to cover the cardoons; soak for 30 minutes.

Fill a small saucepan with water, season with sea salt, and bring to a boil over medium-high heat. Add the cardoons and blanch until tender, about 3 minutes. Drain the cardoons and pat dry with a kitchen towel.

Toss the cardoons with the olive oil and layer on a baking sheet. Roast in the oven until golden and caramelized, about 25 minutes. Remove and set aside to cool.

In a large mixing bowl, combine the rabbit, onion, leek, carrots, and cardoons. Stir in the egg whites until well combined.

In a medium stockpot, combine the stock with the parsley, tarragon, bay leaves, and black peppercorns. Add the rabbit mixture to the stock. Over medium heat, slowly bring the mixture to a simmer and allow the proteins and vegetables to form a raft on top of the stock. Reduce the heat to low and simmer for 20 minutes.

Line a strainer with cheesecloth, and place it over a large bowl. Carefully ladle the stock mixture through the strainer. Repeat the straining process with clean cheesecloth. The liquid should be free of solids and crystal clear. Season with sea salt.

GARNISH

1 stalk cardoon, trimmed (see Consommé),
    cut into ⅛-inch (.3 cm) batons
2 small carrots, cut into ⅛-inch (.3 cm) batons

4 fingerling potatoes, quartered lengthwise
Chervil, to finish

Blanch the cardoon in boiling salted water, about 2 minutes. With a slotted spoon, transfer the cardoon to a bowl of ice water. Return the water to a boil, and blanch the carrots, about 2 minutes. Transfer the carrots to the ice water. Once more, return the water to a boil and add the potatoes, simmering until fork-tender, about 8 minutes.

TO SERVE: Gently reheat the consommé over medium heat. Place four potato quarters in a shallow bowl and top with cardoons and carrots. Ladle the consommé over the vegetables. Garnish with chervil leaves.

Cured Rabbit Chasseur with Charred Leeks

This dish is a hunter's-style stew that features a rich compound sauce as its base. *Chasseur* is associated with game meats and derives from the French word for "hunter." The rabbit in this recipe is cured to enhance its color and texture. Chasseur is traditionally served with mushrooms, which would have been gathered by hunters returning from their pursuit.

ACTIVE TIME: 2½ hours | **TOTAL TIME:** 1+ day
(including curing, drying, and braising) | **YIELD:** Makes 6 servings

RABBIT

1 quart (960 ml) water
½ cup (70 g) kosher salt
¼ cup (50 g) cane sugar
1 tablespoon pink curing salt (Prague Powder
    #1 or Insta Cure #1)

3 cloves garlic, smashed
10 black peppercorns
1 rabbit (about 3 pounds [1.4 kg]),
    cut into 6 parts, head reserved for
    broth (below)

In a pot large enough to hold the rabbit, combine the water, salt, sugar, pink salt, garlic, and peppercorns. Bring to a boil and stir to dissolve the salt and sugar. Remove from the heat and cool to room temperature.

When the brine is cool, add the rabbit and refrigerate at least 8 hours and up to 1 day. Remove the rabbit from the brine, rinse under cold water, and pat dry with kitchen towels. Place the rabbit pieces in a single layer in a glass dish and refrigerate, uncovered, about 4 hours.

BROTH

2 tablespoons grapeseed oil
Rabbit head (above)
1 medium onion, chopped
1 medium leek, chopped
1 medium carrot, chopped
½ small fennel bulb, chopped

½ head garlic
½ cup (120 ml) dry white wine, such as
    Pinot Grigio
2 cups (480 ml) Roasted Rabbit Stock
Bouquet garni or a bundle of herbs
Salt and pepper

While the rabbit is curing, make the broth. In a medium stockpot, heat the grapeseed oil over medium, then add the reserved rabbit head. Cook until brown on both sides, about 6 minutes. Add the onion, leek, carrot, fennel, and garlic; cook while stirring, another 6 minutes. Deglaze with white wine, scraping the brown bits from the bottom of the pot. Stir in the rabbit stock, add the bouquet garni, and simmer over medium-low heat, about 45 minutes. Discard the bouquet garni. Season with salt and pepper. Refrigerate overnight; remove the fat from the chilled stock before proceeding.

STEW

2 tablespoons all-purpose flour
Salt and pepper
Rabbit (above)
2 tablespoons unsalted butter
2 tablespoons olive oil
3 medium shallots, thinly sliced

2 cups (170 g) mushrooms, such as chanterelles
    or hen of the woods
1 small tomato, diced
3 cloves garlic, thinly sliced
Broth (above)

Heat the oven to 350°F (175°C). Season the flour with salt and pepper; dust the rabbit with the flour. In a large skillet, melt the butter with the olive oil over medium-high heat. Add the rabbit, being careful not to overcrowd the pan, and sear until golden brown, about 3 minutes per side. Transfer the rabbit to a plate.

Add the shallots to the pan, and cook over medium heat, stirring occasionally, until translucent, about 7 minutes. Stir in the mushrooms and cook until softened, about 4 minutes. Add the tomato and garlic and stir until combined.

Nestle the rabbit pieces over the mushroom mixture and pour 1½ cups broth over the rabbit. Braise in the oven, covered, for 30 minutes; uncover and baste with juices, adding water if the liquid is low. Continue to braise for another 30 minutes, or until the rabbit is fork-tender.

Carefully remove the skillet from the oven. Using tongs, transfer the rabbit and vegetables to a plate; cover with aluminum foil to keep warm. Strain the remaining liquid into a bowl; reserve for the leeks.

LEEKS

2 tablespoons unsalted butter
4 small leeks, trimmed and halved with
　roots intact
2 tablespoons cognac
½ cup (120 ml) heavy cream
½ cup broth (reserved from stew)

2 tablespoons grainy mustard
1 tablespoon minced tarragon
¼ teaspoon smoked paprika,
　preferably bittersweet
Salt and pepper

In a large sauté pan, melt the butter over medium-high heat. Add the leek halves to the pan and cook until they begin to caramelize, about 3 minutes per side. Deglaze with cognac. Add the cream, broth, and mustard. Bring to a simmer and reduce until slightly thickened, about 6 minutes. Stir in the tarragon; season with smoked paprika, salt, and pepper.

Serve the rabbit with the mushroom mixture and top with leeks and cream sauce.

Spit-Roasted Whole Rabbit
with Grilled Figs and Elderberry Sauce

The inspiration for this dish is from Gabrielle Hamilton of Prune, where I had the fortune of sharing a perfectly executed, spit-roasted rabbit with a friend. Pan drippings form the base of the glaze in this recipe, another example of how a foundation can be built without additional stock. The elderberry sauce, also known as *pontack*, has its origins in seventeenth-century England and improves with age. If you don't have a rotating spit on your grill, you can roast the marinated rabbit over indirect heat, flipping occasionally, until fully cooked.

ACTIVE TIME: 2½ hours | **TOTAL TIME:** 6½+ hours
(including simmering, marinating, and grilling) | **YIELD:** Makes 4 to 6 servings

SAUCE

2 cups (160 g) fresh elderberries, or 1 cup
(140 g) dried elderberries, destemmed
1 cup (240 ml) apple cider vinegar
4 small shallots, minced

5 allspice berries
10 black peppercorns
½ teaspoon sea salt
Fresh grated nutmeg

In a heavy-bottomed saucepan, bring the elderberries and vinegar to a boil, then lower the heat to maintain a very low simmer. Cook the mixture over low heat until the fruit and liquid are combined, about 1 hour. Strain the mixture, pressing on the berries to extract all the liquid. Discard the solids.

Return the sauce to the pan, add the shallots and spices, and heat over medium heat until it comes to a boil. Turn off the heat and steep for 15 minutes. Strain and reserve ¾ cup (180 ml) or the rabbit. You can heat-seal the remaining sauce in jars and store in your pantry. This sauce mellows with age.

RABBIT

3 sprigs marjoram
3 sprigs thyme
3 sprigs flat-leaf parsley or chervil
2 cloves garlic, smashed
1 lemon, zest and juice
¼ cup (60 ml) olive oil, divided
1 rabbit (about 3 pounds [1.4 kg]),
    whole

Salt and pepper
2 tablespoons unsalted butter, softened
2 tablespoons honey
¾ cup Elderberry Sauce (above)
8 fresh figs, halved
Special equipment:
    Grill with spit-roast attachment, and natural
    hardwood charcoal if using outdoor grill

In a container large enough to hold the rabbit, combine the marjoram, thyme, parsley or chervil, garlic, lemon zest and juice, and 2 tablespoons olive oil. Season the rabbit with salt and pepper and submerge in the marinade. Seal the container and refrigerate at least 4 hours or overnight.

Remove the rabbit from the marinade; reserve the marinade. Thread one long or two short metal skewers through the length of the rabbit. Whip the butter and honey together until well combined. Brush most of the honey butter on the rabbit, reserving some for the figs.

In a grill, light some charcoal and let it burn until it turns to embers. Carefully suspend the rabbit over the hot coals. Place a pan under the rabbit to catch the drippings as it rotates. Pour some water into the pan. Roast the rabbit, basting with the marinade and rotating the spit every 10 minutes or so, until golden brown

and cooked through, about 45 to 60 minutes, depending on the heat from the grill. An instant-read thermometer should read 150°F (65°C) when inserted into the thigh joint. When done, carefully remove the rabbit from the heat and rest on the spit, about 15 minutes.

While the rabbit is resting, pass the pan drippings through a fine-mesh strainer into a small saucepan. Bring to a simmer over medium heat and reduce to 2 tablespoons. Stir in the Elderberry Sauce, return to a simmer, and reduce until slightly thickened, about 5 minutes.

A few minutes before the meal, place the figs on the hot grill. Baste with remaining honey butter and grill until cooked through but not falling apart, about 2 minutes per side.

Remove the rabbit from the spit and carve into pieces. Serve with the grilled figs and warm Elderberry Sauce.

CHAPTER TEN

Seafood Stocks, Broths, and Dishes

Stocks made from fish and shellfish are a classification of their own, with an aromatic quality unlike any made from land animals. Seafood bases speak of origin waters. The structural components of fish reflect where in the ocean they reside, whether on the surface or the floor, and this comes through in the pot. Shellfish, too, represent their habitat, acting as ecosystem engineers by clarifying the water around them through a unique filtering system. When cooking with fish and seafood, these characteristics are imparted to the liquid—from the neutrality that comes from flatfish to the briny nature of clams and oysters.

As with land animals, the types of bones you select will make a difference in the excellence of your foundation. Consider buying whole fish and filleting it at home—the meat will provide one meal, leaving the skeleton to be used immediately or frozen for later. Alternatively, ask your fishmonger to package the bones and head separate from the fillets; otherwise, they might toss them. Mollusks, on the other hand, must be alive when extracting their essence; this leaves the meat from mussels, clams, and oysters to be enjoyed on their own or in a dish with their liquor. I recommend stockpiling lobster shells in the freezer after the meat is removed. In all cases, making stocks with the bones and shells of seafood is an efficient and delicious way to make your food go further.

The water systems of the world are an ever-changing environment, susceptible to man-made pollution and symptomatic of climate change. To protect this precious resource, it is important to understand how your seafood is harvested, and better yet, to know your fisherman. This chapter identifies types of seafood that are either abundant in natural waters or cultivated to enhance their habitat; in all cases, the fish and shellfish identified are heavily monitored for population control and harvest methodology across the globe. This section also provides resources to consult when you need more information about the quality of your source.

FISH

There is a long-held rule in French cooking about fish fumet: Never simmer it for longer than 40 minutes; any more time in the pot will introduce bitterness. This guideline likely derived from the type of fish that was often used in old French restaurants. Bones from flatfish, such as halibut, flounder, and sole, can impart bitterness when overcooked; whereas bones from white bony fish, or those from the dominant vertebrate order, take well to a long, slow simmer. This includes snapper, grouper, and cod.

Small amounts of bones from other fish types can also be used to infuse flavor and texture into stock. The monkfish tail imparts an oyster-like note; the cartilaginous skate wing adds significant body. If skate wing is unavailable—or momentarily appears on the Do Not Harvest list—use cartilage-rich fish collars for a similar effect. Fish heads help make a delicious stock. Remove the eyes and gills before placing them in the pot. Avoid making stock from oily fish, such as mackerel and salmon, unless a particular recipe calls for an intense flavor profile.

When selecting sustainably harvested fish, consult guides that are frequently updated by a reputable conservation group, such as the Monterey Bay Aquarium Seafood Watch. These monitors keep track of the environmental conditions of global waters and how each type of fish is being managed within those waters. They will also apprise you of fish farming methods that are good for, or have less impact on, the environment.

Basic Fish Fumet

The key to this fumet is soaking the bones in successive batches of water overnight to remove blood and impurities. Make sure the water is clear before bringing a fresh pot to a simmer. Since this fumet has a short simmering time, you can use any type of white fish—either flatfish or bony fish—provided the water movement does not go beyond a smile.

ACTIVE TIME: 2 hours | **TOTAL TIME:** 9+ hours (including soaking, heating, simmering, and initial cooling) | **YIELD:** Makes about 4 quarts (3.8 liters)

---

5 pounds (2.3 kg) fish bones, tails, skin, and fins removed

½ quart (340 g) ice cubes

2 tablespoons grapeseed oil

½ pound (225 g) white onions, cut into large dice

1 pound (455 g) leeks, dark green parts removed, cut into large dice

¾ pound (340 g) carrots, cut into large dice

½ small fennel bulb, coarsely chopped, fronds removed

1 cup (240 ml) dry white wine, such as Sauvignon Blanc

6 sprigs thyme

6 sprigs flat-leaf parsley

2 bay leaves

1 tablespoon black peppercorns

6 quarts (5.7 L) filtered water, cold, plus water for soaking

Sea salt to taste

Using kitchen shears, cut the fish bones into 3- to 5-inch (7.5 to 12.5 cm) pieces. Remove and discard any gills or organs that might still be attached, including the eyes. Rinse the bones under cold water until the water runs clear. If any veins are apparent, cut them out with a knife and rinse thoroughly under cold water. The removal of organs and rinsing of blood will help eliminate proteins that could cloud your stock.

Place the bones in a large container, and add enough water and ice to cover them. Place in the refrigerator and soak for 8 hours, or overnight, changing the water a few times to continually remove blood. You should end up with bones in

clear water. Drain the bones in a large colander, and rinse under cold water.

In a large stockpot, heat the grapeseed oil over medium heat. When it starts to ripple, add the onions, leeks, carrots, and fennel, and sauté, stirring often, until they are cooked through but not caramelized, about 7 minutes. Deglaze the pan with the white wine and simmer for 1 minute.

Add the bones, herbs, and peppercorns to the pot and fill with the filtered water. Turn the heat to medium-high, and slowly heat the liquid. Using a fine-mesh strainer, skim any scum that rises to the surface. When the liquid begins to ripple, reduce the heat to medium-low and maintain at a simmer for about 40 minutes.

Turn off the heat and rest the stock on the stove, for about 15 minutes. Line a fine-mesh strainer with cheesecloth and set it over a container large enough to hold the liquid contents of the pot. Carefully ladle the stock from the pot into the strainer, leaving any cloudy liquid at the bottom of the pot. Skim any fat that appears at the surface and discard.

Taste the stock to determine your desired concentration. If the stock tastes too watery, return it to a clean stockpot and simmer until reduced to a desirable consistency. Taste and season with sea salt.

Place the container in an ice bath to rapidly cool the stock. Skim any fat that congeals at the surface. When the stock no longer steams, transfer to the refrigerator. Refrigerate for up to 2 days or freeze in smaller containers for longer storage.

Roasted Fish Stock

Wash the bones thoroughly before roasting them; the water should run clear. Select white bony fish—such as snapper, grouper, or cod—for this stock; bones from flatfish might impart a bitterness to the liquid due to the longer simmering time.

ACTIVE TIME: 2 hours | **TOTAL TIME:** 4 hours (including roasting, heating, simmering, and initial cooling) | **YIELD:** Makes about 4 quarts (3.8 liters)

---

3 pounds (1.4 kg) fish bones, tails, skin, and fins removed

2 pounds (910 g) fish heads, eyes and gills removed

½ pound (225 g) white onions, cut into large dice

1 pound (455 g) leeks, dark green parts removed, cut into large dice

¾ pound (340 g) carrots, cut into large dice

½ small fennel bulb, coarsely chopped, fronds removed

2 tablespoons grapeseed oil

2 cups (480 ml) dry white wine, such as Sauvignon Blanc, divided

6 quarts (5.7 L) filtered water, cold, plus water for rinsing

6 sprigs thyme

6 sprigs flat-leaf parsley

2 bay leaves

1 tablespoon black peppercorns

Sea salt to taste

Preheat the oven to 350°F (175°C).

Using kitchen shears, cut the fish bones into 3- to 5-inch (7.5 to 12.5 cm) pieces. Remove and discard any gills or organs that might still be attached, including the eyes. Rinse the bones under cold water until the water runs clear. If any veins are apparent, cut them out with a knife and rinse thoroughly under cold water. The removal of organs and rinsing of blood will help eliminate proteins that could cloud your stock. Pat the bones dry with kitchen towels.

In a large roasting pan, scatter the onions, leeks, carrots, and fennel in a single layer and nestle the fish bones into the vegetables. Toss with grapeseed oil and roast for 30 minutes. Transfer the vegetables and bones to a large stockpot. Add ½ cup wine to the hot pan, place over medium heat, and scrape to loosen the browned bits and glazed juices. Pour into the stockpot.

Cover with the filtered water and remaining white wine; add the herbs and peppercorns. Slowly heat the liquid over medium-high, skimming as soon as scum appears at the top, until the surface starts to ripple. Lower the heat to medium and maintain a simmer, about 2 hours. Continue to skim throughout the full simmering time.

Turn off the heat and rest the stock on the stove, about 15 minutes. Line a fine-mesh strainer with cheesecloth and set it over a container large enough to hold the liquid contents of the pot. Carefully ladle the stock from the pot into the strainer, leaving any cloudy liquid at the bottom of the pot. Skim any fat that appears at the surface and discard.

Taste the stock to determine your desired concentration. If the stock tastes too watery, return it to a clean stockpot and simmer until reduced to a desirable consistency. Taste and season with sea salt.

Place the container in an ice bath to rapidly cool the stock. Skim any fat that congeals at the surface. When the stock no longer steams, transfer to the refrigerator. Refrigerate for up to 2 days or freeze in smaller containers for longer storage.

Fish Bone Broth

This bone broth uses fish collar and skate wing, which add a silky, gelatinous texture to the stock. Use mild, white bony fish—snapper, grouper, or cod—for the bones; a small amount of monkfish tail adds a delicious note, too. Less water in the pot helps achieve a thicker viscosity in less time. Vinegar is used in place of wine to brighten flavors during the reduction.

ACTIVE TIME: 2 hours | **TOTAL TIME:** 12+ hours (including soaking, heating, simmering, and initial cooling) | **YIELD:** Makes about 3 quarts (2.8 liters)

3 pounds (1.4 kg) fish bones (tails, skin, and
  fins removed)

1 pound (455 g) fish collar, preferably
  grouper or cod

¼ pound (115 g) skate wing bones

2 tablespoons grapeseed oil, divided

½ pound (225 g) white onions, cut into large dice

1 pound (455 g) leeks, dark green parts
  removed, cut into large dice

¾ pound carrots (340 g), cut into large dice

½ small fennel bulb, coarsely chopped,
  fronds removed

1 tablespoon apple cider vinegar

4 quarts (3.8 L) filtered water, cold, plus water
  for soaking

6 sprigs thyme

6 sprigs flat-leaf parsley

2 bay leaves

1 tablespoon black peppercorns

Sea salt to taste

Follow the cooking instructions for Basic Fish Fumet (page 213), using the bone types listed above, decreasing the amount of water and deglazing the pan with vinegar instead of wine. Lengthen the simmering time to 4 hours. If the final broth is too thick, simply add additional water and heat until it reaches the desired viscosity.

HOW TO CLEAN AND DEBONE A FISH

Start with a whole fish that has not yet been cleaned. If it has scales, remove them by grasping the tail with one hand and using the back of a knife to scrape them off in one direction. Run the fish under water to loosen and detach any remaining scales.

Pat the fish dry with a kitchen towel. On a cutting board, lay the fish flat with its belly facing you. With the tip of a knife, make an incision at the anal opening and cut along the belly to the head. Do not cut too deep in order to avoid the intestines.

Carefully spread the body open and scoop out the entrails with your hands. Discard. With a small spoon, remove the kidney by the backbone.

Discard. Rinse the cavity of the fish under fresh water. The fish is ready to be cooked whole.

To debone the fish: Place the fish on a cutting board with its spine facing you. Using a fillet knife, and starting at the head, make an incision along one side of the backbone and cut until you reach the tail. Gently detach the meat from the bone as you follow the rib cage. Repeat on the other side of the backbone.

With a pair of kitchen shears, cut the backbone free at both ends of the fish. Lift the backbone and rib cage from the fish. The fish is ready to be stuffed and cooked; the bones, of course, can be used for stock.

HOW TO SOFTEN FISH BONES

On a recent road trip from the Hudson Valley through the Blue Ridge Parkway, I happened upon an excellent restaurant in North Carolina. Built to the vision of Chef Nathan Allen, Knife and Fork is located in Spruce Pine, an old mining town, and is dedicated to Appalachian cooking. Trout are as abundant in the North Toe River surrounding his restaurant as they are in the streams of New York's Catskill Mountains. The chef uses every bit of the fish, featured in all manners on his menu, including a delicious spread made by pressure-cooking trout

bones until they are soft enough to eat. The efficiency of his process intrigued me.

As it turns out, this method of softening fish bones is common to commercial canning: Whole fish or fish fillets, with their pinbones intact, are packed into cans and cooked under enough pressure to soften bones to a degree desirable for consumption. This technique works well with fish that have small to medium pinbones, such as trout, salmon, mackerel, and sardines. You can substitute fillets or whole small fish for the trout in this recipe.

CANNED TROUT

ACTIVE TIME: ½ hour | TOTAL TIME: 2 hours (including packing and canning) |
YIELD: Makes 2 pint jars (about 960 ml)

---

3 small trout (about 2 to 3 pounds [910 to 1,360 g] total), heads, tails, and fins removed, cut into thick strips
1 tablespoon kosher salt

1 tablespoon pink peppercorns, crushed
2 bay leaves
Special equipment: Pressure canner

In a bowl, coat the trout with kosher salt and crushed pink peppercorns. Distribute the fish between two sterilized pint (500 ml) mason jars, packing the fish and leaving 1 inch (2.5 cm) of headspace. Slide one bay leaf into each jar. Place the lids on the jars; do not seal too tightly to allow for expansion under pressure.

Before you begin the canning process, consult the manufacturer's guide for instructions about how to use your pressure canner. The size and model of the canner will determine how much water to add and how long to pressurize the trout. You might also need to contact your local extension service to determine the correct pressure to apply based on the altitude of your location.

Place the jars on a wire rack set inside a pressure canner. Fill with 3 inches (7.5 cm) of water. Lock

the pressure canner and set over high heat until fully pressurized. Set to 10 pounds of pressure and reduce the heat to low. Maintain pressure for 1 hour and 40 minutes. Turn the heat off and rest the cooker until fully depressurized. Allow the entire pressure canner to cool before opening. *Do not remove the lid before the canner is cool; improper handling can cause severe burns.*

When the display shows 0, carefully unlock the pressure canner and remove the lid with your face aimed away from the steam. With canning tongs, remove the pint jars and place on kitchen towels. Rest until cool, then check the lids to confirm they are properly sealed. If the lids are firm, the jar can be stored in a pantry. If the lid pops, keep in the refrigerator and eat within 4 days.

Monkfish Liver Torchon
with Pressed Cabbage-Apple Salad

Also known as the anglerfish, monkfish is a large bottom-feeder that boasts an enormous liver. Once considered bycatch by fishermen, monkfish is now considered a delicacy, especially to the Japanese. The French refer to monkfish liver as *foie gras de la mer*, or "goose liver of the sea," a reference to its smooth texture and unctuous flavor when prepared in the same manner as goose or duck liver.

Monkfish is a controversial catch, typically relying on a trawling method that can damage the seabed. In recent years, responsible fisheries have experimented with benthic release panels that reduce impact on the environment. When procuring the liver, make sure it comes from a fish of mature size (at least 28 inches [70 cm]). This is further assurance of responsible harvesting.

ACTIVE TIME: 2 hours | **TOTAL TIME:** 1 day
(including soaking, brining, chilling, and poaching) | **YIELD:** Makes 8 servings

TORCHON

1 small monkfish liver (about 1 pound [455 g])
1 cup (240 ml) whole milk
¼ cup (34 g) kosher salt
1 tablespoon pink curing salt
   (Prague Powder #1 or Insta Cure #1)
2 teaspoons sugar

1 teaspoon black pepper
1 quart (960 ml) filtered water, cold
1 cup (240 ml) dry white wine, preferably Riesling
1 cup (240 ml) Basic Fish Fumet
1 cup (240 ml) Dashi
¼ cup (60 ml) apple cider

In a small bowl, cover the monkfish liver with the milk. Cover and soak in the refrigerator overnight. In a medium saucepan, combine the kosher salt, curing salt, sugar, pepper, and water, stirring to combine, and heat until dissolved. Remove from the heat and cool to room temperature. Transfer the brine to a sealed container and chill overnight.

The next day, remove the liver from the milk, rinse under cold water, and place in the brine. Return to the refrigerator and chill for 3 hours. Remove from the brine, rinse under cold water, and pat dry on kitchen towels.

On a work surface, lay the monkfish liver bottom-side up. With a sharp boning knife, remove the veins and connective tissue, taking care to leave the liver in one piece. Cut a piece of cheesecloth into a rectangle that is large enough to wrap around the liver twice. Place the liver onto the cheesecloth and roll it into a log. Secure the ends with butcher's twine. Place the log on a small sheet pan and chill while preparing the poaching liquid, at least 30 minutes.

In a saucepan large enough to hold the torchon, heat the wine, fumet, dashi, and apple cider until it boils. Lower the heat to medium, submerge the torchon, and poach until firm, about 10 minutes. Remove from the poaching liquid, keeping the liquid in the pan, and immediately transfer to an ice bath until cool. Chill until firm, about 2 hours. Continue to simmer the poaching liquid until reduced by half. Reserve.

SALAD

2 tablespoons lemon juice
2 Fuji apples, peeled and
    quartered
1 cup (240 ml) dry white wine, preferably Riesling
2 cups (480 ml) water
2 cups (320 g) thinly sliced napa cabbage

1 teaspoon sea salt
¼ cup (60 ml) umeboshi vinegar or
    apple cider vinegar, divided
1 tablespoon coconut oil
1 teaspoon tahini
6 shiso leaves, julienned

Sprinkle the lemon juice over the apples. In a medium saucepan, heat the wine and water until boiling, add the apples, and reduce the heat to maintain a simmer. Poach until fork-tender, about 10 minutes. Remove from the heat and cool the apples in the poaching liquid.

In a large bowl, toss the sliced cabbage with sea salt and 2 tablespoons of the vinegar. Massage the cabbage with your hands until it begins to wilt, about 1 minute. Top with a plate or a press and let sit until the liquid from the cabbage is released, about 30 minutes.

Meanwhile, in a small bowl, whisk the remaining vinegar, 2 tablespoons of the reduced poaching liquid, coconut oil, and tahini until emulsified. Drain the cabbage thoroughly, pressing with your hands to release the liquid. Toss with the sliced apples, shiso leaves, and dressing. Serve with slices of the chilled torchon.

Grilled Fish Collar with
Fried Radish Cake and Chile Coconut Oil

Fish collars have long been popular in Asian cuisine: a rich, knobby cut often reserved by chefs for themselves. Collars aren't tidy, yet the tender, fatty fish chunks that lie under the gills and within the pectoral fins are worth the effort. There are two collars per fish, and larger fish—such as striped bass, lingcod, halibut, salmon, or if you're lucky, yellowtail (a type of amberjack)—yield the best results. Don't be shy at the table: Some of the best bits are hiding beneath bone and skin!

In Japanese restaurants, grilled fish collars (called *kama-yaki*) are typically served with grated daikon radish and a citrusy ponzu sauce. Here the radish is turned into fried rice cakes and served with a spicy coconut-lime dipping sauce.

ACTIVE TIME: 1½ hours | **TOTAL TIME:** 1 day
(including marinating and chilling) | **YIELD:** Makes 6 servings

FISH COLLAR

¼ cup (51 g) white miso paste
¼ cup (60 ml) sake
2 teaspoons light soy sauce
2 tablespoons mirin
2 tablespoons maple syrup

1 tablespoon grapeseed oil
3 scallions, thinly sliced on the bias
6 fish collars (from 3 fish, about 3 pounds
    [1.4 kg] total), such as striped bass, lingcod,
    halibut, salmon, or yellowtail

In a large bowl, whisk the miso, sake, soy sauce, mirin, maple syrup, and oil until well combined. Stir in the scallions. Add the fish collars, coating well with the mixture. Cover and marinate in the refrigerator, at least 1 hour or overnight.

RADISH CAKE

1 medium daikon radish (about 1½ pounds
  [680 g]), grated
¼ cup (60 ml) Fish Bone Broth
1½ cups (240 g) rice flour (not glutinous)
1 teaspoon sea salt

¾ cup (180 ml) water
1 teaspoon honey
2 tablespoons olive oil, for browning cake
  in final step

While the fish collar is marinating, heat the oven to 325°F (165°C). Line an 8-inch (20 cm) square pan with parchment.

In a small saucepan, heat the grated radish and broth over medium heat. Simmer until the radish is tender, about 30 minutes. Remove from the heat and let cool.

In a small bowl, whisk the rice flour and sea salt with the water until smooth. Stir in the cooled radish and juices. Spread the mixture in the prepared pan; cover with parchment paper. Place the filled pan in a larger roasting pan; pour hot water into the roasting pan to reach halfway up the square pan. Bake until firm, about 45 minutes. Remove from the oven and cool slightly, then place in the refrigerator and chill overnight.

DIPPING SAUCE

½ cup (120 ml) coconut oil
½ cup (120 ml) olive oil
1 tablespoon dried Thai chilies,
  crushed

½ teaspoon coarse sea salt
¼ teaspoon black pepper
1 tablespoon honey
2 tablespoons lime juice

In a small saucepan, heat the coconut oil and olive oil until melted. Add the crushed chilies, salt, and pepper and cook until toasted, stirring often, about 3 minutes. Remove from the heat and whisk in the honey and lime juice. Set aside to cool.

TO FINISH: Heat the broiler on low. Place the fish collars, skin-side down, on a sheet pan in a single layer. Broil until the fish begins to brown and the marinade caramelizes, about 5 to 6 minutes. With tongs, flip the collars and continue to broil until the skin becomes crispy, about 6 minutes longer.

While the fish collars are broiling, heat the remaining 2 tablespoons olive oil in a sauté pan over medium heat. Slice the radish cake into cubes and fry, stirring, until golden, about 2 minutes per side. Serve the fish collars with fried radish cakes and dipping sauce on the side.

Bourride with Sea Urchin Aioli

Bourride is a classic fish stew from Provence. Though its components are similar to bouillabaisse, its composition is quite different—the aioli is blended into the stew instead of served on the side. This nuance is enough to inspire endless arguments about historical precedent and regional preference among the French.

With origins dating back to the Phocaeans, this dish is a traditional fisherman's stew that calls for white fish, typically monkfish. Similar to the etymology of *boullion*, the meaning of *bourride* refers to the cooking process. As with stock, it is important not to boil this stew, especially when blending with the aioli, for risk of separation. A gentle simmer is key to achieving a proper creamy texture.

Unlike in bouillabaisse, shellfish are not a common addition to bourride. This recipe takes liberty with the sea urchin in the aioli. If you are a purist, simply eliminate the shellfish.

ACTIVE TIME: 1 hour | **TOTAL TIME:** 1½ hours (including simmering) | **YIELD:** Makes 4 to 6 servings

STEW

3 tablespoons olive oil

2 medium leeks, chopped

1 small fennel bulb, chopped

6 cloves garlic, minced

4 small carrots, chopped

2 Yukon gold potatoes, cubed

1 cup (240 ml) dry white wine, such as Sauvignon Blanc

1 quart (960 ml) Basic Fish Fumet

3 sprigs thyme

2 bay leaves

2½ pounds (1.1 kg) monkfish or grouper fillets, skinned and deboned, cut into 1-inch (2.5 cm) pieces

¼ cup (15 g) flat-leaf parsley leaves, for garnish

1 lemon, quartered, for garnish

In a large Dutch oven, heat the olive oil over medium heat. Add the leeks, fennel, and garlic; cook, stirring, until translucent, about 4 minutes. Add the carrots and potatoes; continue to cook, stirring, 4 minutes longer. Deglaze the pan with white wine.

Pour the fish stock into the pot; add the thyme and bay leaves. Bring the mixture to a boil, then lower the heat to maintain a simmer. Simmer for 10 minutes to soften the carrots and potatoes. Add the fish, cover, and poach until cooked through, about 4 minutes.

With a slotted spoon, carefully remove the fish and vegetables from the broth. Reserve the broth while preparing the aioli.

AIOLI

2 cloves garlic
½ teaspoon sea salt
¼ teaspoon cayenne pepper
1 egg yolk

1¼ ounces (50 g), or ½ small tray, sea urchin roe
½ cup (120 ml) light olive oil
½ lemon, juiced
Sliced baguette, for serving

With a mortar and pestle, mash the garlic, sea salt, and cayenne pepper until a paste forms. Transfer to the bowl of a food processor; pulse to combine. Add the egg yolk and sea urchin to the bowl. Pulse again to combine.

With the processor running, gradually add ¼ cup of the olive oil, drop by drop, to emulsify. Add the lemon juice to aid emulsification, then continue to slowly add the remaining olive oil. Transfer to a bowl and season with salt and pepper. If the aioli is too thick, blend in one or two drops of fish stock.

TO FINISH: In a blender, blend 2 cups of the broth with 2 tablespoons of the aioli. Stir the mixture into the warm broth, then return the fish and vegetables to the pot. Over low heat, gently heat the stew until the flavors combine, about 3 minutes. Be careful not to boil, to avoid separating the stew.

Ladle the soup into bowls and garnish with the parsley. Serve with lemon wedges, sliced baguette, and the remaining aioli on the side.

Sea Bream à la Nage with Saffron Potato Confit

There is something satisfying about poaching a whole fish—as though returning it to wild waters. As such, *à la nage* is a technique that translates to "while swimming" and refers to the marriage of whole fish briefly poached in court bouillon. Here the poaching liquid is served as part of the dish: The light broth is reduced to concentrate flavor and mounted with butter to add structure.

ACTIVE TIME: 1 hour | **TOTAL TIME:** 1½ hours
(including poaching, baking, and simmering) | **YIELD:** Makes 4 servings

CONFIT

24 small potatoes, halved
½ lemon, thinly sliced
4 cloves garlic
1 pinch saffron threads, toasted and ground
1 teaspoon sea salt
½ teaspoon black pepper
1 cup (240 ml) olive oil
2 tablespoons snipped chives

In a medium saucepan, combine the potatoes, lemon, garlic, saffron, salt, and pepper. Pour olive oil over the potatoes to cover. Turn the stove on medium and gently heat the potatoes until fork-tender, about 30 minutes.

Strain the potatoes from the oil (reserve the oil); toss with snipped chives. Tent with aluminum to keep warm while the fish is cooking.

FISH

1 whole red sea bream or porgy
   (about 3 to 4 pounds [1.4 to 1.8 kg]),
   gutted, cleaned, and scaled
¼ cup (60 ml) confit oil, from above, divided
1½ teaspoons sea salt
1 teaspoon black pepper
½ teaspoon smoked paprika
1 cup (240 ml) dry white wine,
   such as Sauvignon Blanc
1 cup (240 ml) Roasted Fish Stock
1 cup (240 ml) water
3 cloves garlic, smashed
2 sprigs lemon thyme
2 bay leaves
½ lemon, thinly sliced
2 tablespoons unsalted butter

Heat the oven to 375°F (190°C). Pat the fish dry with kitchen towels. Rub the entire fish with half of the confit oil, making sure to coat the skin. Season both the exterior and interior of the fish with sea salt, black pepper, and smoked paprika.

Select a sauté pan that is large enough to hold the fish in one layer and deep enough to contain the poaching liquid. In the pan, heat the remaining confit oil over medium-high heat until hot but not smoking. Gently place the fish in the pan and sear until the skin is crispy, about 4 minutes. Carefully turn the fish over and continue to cook, about 3 minutes. Deglaze with white wine.

Pour in the fish stock and water; stir in the garlic, thyme, and bay leaves. Place lemon slices on top of the fish. Bring the liquid to a boil, then transfer the pan to the oven. Bake until the fish is tender and flaky, about 12 to 15 minutes.

Remove the fish from the oven and carefully transfer it to a platter. Strain the liquid into a small bowl; discard the garlic and herbs. Return the liquid to the pan, and bring to a boil over medium-high heat. Reduce the heat and simmer until reduced by half. Mount with butter, whisking to combine, and season with additional salt and pepper, if necessary. Serve the sauce with the carved fish and confit potatoes.

HOW TO CARVE A WHOLE COOKED FISH

On a cutting board or platter, carefully rest the cooked fish on one side. With your fingers, remove the fin bones: There will be one on the backside (dorsal) and another on the belly side (ventral). Using a fillet knife, make an incision where the head meets the collarbone. Make another incision near the tail.

Next, observe the fillet to locate the line where the dorsal and ventral halves naturally divide. Follow this line with your knife from tail to head. Using your knife or a large spoon, gently remove the dorsal half of the fillet from the bone. Repeat with the ventral half of the fillet. Remove any bones that might remain.

With one hand, grab the tail and lift the rib cage from the bottom fillet, taking the head with it. If the head does not come off with the spine, remove it with a knife or spoon. (Don't forget to eat the delicious cheeks and other meat found within!)

Remove any bones that appear on the bottom fillet. The fish is now carved and ready to be eaten. The bones can be used for stock.

SHELLFISH

Shellfish culture, when managed responsibly, illustrates the symbiotic nature of regenerative farming: Oysters, mussels, and clams clean water where they reside. As filter feeders, bivalve mollusks remove nitrogen from the water and process residual nitrogen and phosphate in a manner that catalyzes plant growth. They also nourish us in the process.

Oysters, mussels, and clams must be alive when you set out to extract their liquor, the natural brine that resides within each shell. This means that when you buy shellfish it is whole, never cooked, and with its meat intact. All of the mollusk-based stock recipes in this book take this detail into account. The shellfish are steamed until they open and the meat is removed before it becomes rubbery, leaving the liquor in the pot to simmer through to completion.

Find shellfish farmers or cultivators who are excited about the environmental benefits of their operation. The shellfish should reside in low-density areas where ocean currents and tidal flow prevent the accumulation of waste. Unlike wild-caught mollusks, which are only recommended in cold months, farmed bivalves are good to eat year-round.

As a crustacean, lobster is slow to mature in its ocean habitat—a characteristic that makes it susceptible to overfishing. There have been temporary restrictions on lobstering in Long Island, for instance, due to dwindling populations. With its relative proximity to the Hudson Valley, the long-touted Maine lobster is what we see here. It takes the honor of many generations of lobstermen to abide by a bevy of regulations—from size restrictions to trap limits—in order to maintain reasonable populations. Acidification of ocean waters, a side effect of carbon pollution, is also slowing the growth of lobsters in Maine. It is important to source lobster from a well-managed stock and to consume it in reasonable quantities during the high season.

If you live close to the water, look for wild-caught early-season shedders—lobsters that have shed their hard shells. These soft-shelled lobsters won't survive lengthy travel once caught, making them less valuable to distributors. A recent abundance of soft-shell lobsters and a shortage of processors have lowered the direct return for lobstermen. Buying these lobsters supports local trade, provided early-season limits are adopted such that the remaining pod has time to develop hard shells. If you only have access to hard-shelled lobster, make sure it comes from lobstermen who follow strict harvesting guidelines.

While shrimp shells produce a delicious stock, I have omitted shrimp from this book due to its low population in the Northeast, as well as its exceedingly high carbon footprint around the world. Consult consortium guides to determine best choice selections for shrimp in your area. A foundation made with lobster shells is an excellent substitute for shrimp stock.

Shellfish stocks—whether combined or individual—add a distinctive oceanic note to food. The liquors from clams and oysters offer a pleasant salinity to a dish, whereas mussel stock lends minerality. Lobster stock is bright, buttery, and decadent. You can use shellfish stocks in dishes that will benefit from a taste of the sea—a rich bisque, an aromatic risotto, or a creamy sauce.

Shellfish Stock

This aromatic stock includes elements of a classic bouillabaisse—saffron, tomato, white wine, and anise liqueur. Add milk or cream to the stock for a simple soup or reduce to a glaze and mount with butter for an exquisite sauce. You can snack on the shellfish meat or use it in another recipe, say, simply tossed with pasta or grains. As always, make sure the shellfish is alive when you make the stock.

ACTIVE TIME: 1 hour | **TOTAL TIME:** 2 hours (including heating, simmering, and initial cooling) | **YIELD:** Makes about 3 quarts (2.8 liters)

---

3 tablespoons grapeseed oil

½ pound (225 g) white onions, cut into large dice

½ pound (225 g) leeks, dark green parts removed, cut into large dice

½ pound (225 g) carrots, cut into large dice

1 small fennel bulb, coarsely chopped, fronds removed

1 head garlic, halved

¾ pound (340 g) tomatoes, coarsely chopped

¼ cup (58 g) tomato paste, preferably homemade (page 273)

1 cup (240 ml) dry white wine, such as Sauvignon Blanc

2 tablespoons anise liqueur, such as Pernod

4 quarts (3.8 L) filtered water, cold

6 sprigs thyme

6 sprigs flat-leaf parsley

6 sprigs tarragon

2 bay leaves

1 tablespoon black peppercorns

1 large pinch saffron threads, toasted and ground

1 pound (455 g) mussels, scrubbed, beards removed

1 pound (455 g) clams, scrubbed

1 pound (455 g) oysters, washed

Sea salt to taste

In a large stockpot, heat the grapeseed oil over medium-high heat. When it starts to ripple, add the onions, leeks, carrots, fennel, and garlic; sauté while stirring, until the mixture sweats, about 7 minutes. Stir in the tomatoes and tomato paste and cook for another 5 minutes. Stir in the wine and liqueur and simmer until the alcohol evaporates, about 4 minutes longer.

Add the filtered water, herbs, peppercorns, and saffron, and slowly bring to a gentle boil. Add the shellfish, cover, and immediately reduce the heat to maintain a simmer. Cook for 10 to 15 minutes, or until all the shellfish have opened and released their liquor. Using tongs, transfer the shellfish to a bowl, cool slightly, and remove the meat. Reserve for another use. Return the shells to the simmering liquid and continue to cook, uncovered, another 30 minutes. Discard any shellfish that do not open.

Turn off the heat and rest the stock on the stove, about 15 minutes. Line a fine-mesh strainer with cheesecloth and set it over a container large enough to hold the liquid contents of the pot. Carefully ladle the stock from the pot into the strainer, leaving any cloudy liquid at the bottom of the pot. Skim any fat that appears at the surface and discard. Repeat the straining process two or three times to ensure that no grit from the shellfish is transferred to the clean stock.

Taste the stock to determine your desired concentration. If the stock tastes too watery, return it to a clean stockpot and simmer until reduced to a desirable consistency. Taste and season with sea salt.

Place the container in an ice bath to rapidly cool the stock. Skim any fat that congeals at the surface and discard. When the stock no longer steams, transfer to the refrigerator. Refrigerate for up to 2 days or freeze in smaller containers for longer storage.

Mussel Stock

This mussel stock can be matched with its meat to form the foundation for a delicious linguini dish. It can also be brightened with aromatics and expanded with liquid for poaching fish, or reduced to a glaze for building a sauce. Mussels go exceptionally well with the flavor of anise—fennel and absinthe, for instance. Make sure the mussels are alive when you make the stock.

ACTIVE TIME: 1 hour | TOTAL TIME: 2 hours (including heating, simmering, and initial cooling) | YIELD: Makes about 1 quart (960 ml)

2 pounds (910 g) whole mussels
2 tablespoons grapeseed oil
¼ pound (115 g) white onions, cut into large dice
½ pound (225 g) leeks, dark green parts removed, cut into large dice
½ small fennel bulb, coarsely chopped, fronds removed
2 cloves garlic, smashed
2 tablespoons dry vermouth

1 cup (240 ml) dry white wine, such as Sauvignon Blanc
1½ quarts (1.4 L) filtered water, cold, plus water for rinsing
4 sprigs thyme
4 sprigs flat-leaf parsley
2 bay leaves
2 teaspoons black peppercorns
Sea salt to taste

One at a time, examine the mussels to determine freshness: Closed mussels are fresh, and open ones need to be tested further. Place the fresh, closed mussels in a bowl. Lightly tap any mussels that are open on a surface; if they close shut, they are safe to eat. Any that remain open or appear damaged should be discarded. Pull off the beard from each mussel and rinse under cold water. Set aside.

In a large stockpot, heat the grapeseed oil over medium-high heat. When it starts to ripple, add the onions, leeks, fennel, and garlic; sauté while stirring, until the mixture sweats, about 7 minutes. Stir in the dry vermouth and scrape up the brown bits from the bottom of the pan. Simmer until the alcohol evaporates, about 1 minute.

Add the white wine, filtered water, herbs, and peppercorns, and slowly bring to a gentle boil. Add the mussels, cover, and immediately reduce the heat to maintain a simmer. Cook for 10 to 15 minutes, or until all the mussels have opened and released their liquor. Using tongs, transfer the shellfish to a bowl—being careful to leave the liquid in the pot—cool slightly, and remove the meat (reserve for another use). Return the shells to the simmering liquid and continue to cook, uncovered, another 30 minutes. Discard any mussels that do not open.

Turn off the heat and rest the stock on the stove, about 15 minutes. Line a fine-mesh strainer with cheesecloth and set it over a container large enough to hold the liquid contents of the pot. Carefully ladle the stock from the pot into the strainer, leaving any cloudy liquid at the bottom of the pot. Skim any scum that appears at the surface. Repeat the straining process two or three times to ensure that no grit from the mussels is transferred to the clean stock.

Taste the stock to determine your desired concentration. If the stock tastes too watery, return it to a clean stockpot and simmer until reduced to a desirable consistency. Taste and season with sea salt.

Place the container in an ice bath to rapidly cool the stock. When the stock no longer steams, transfer to the refrigerator. Refrigerate for up to 2 days or freeze in smaller containers for longer storage.

Clam Liquor

This recipe is a dilution of the liquid released from clamshells when they open in the pot. You can use it for chowder, grains, or even brunch cocktails. Reduce the broth to create concentrated clam nectar and add a dash to dishes, as you would fish sauce. Clams have a natural salinity; additional sea salt is likely unneeded. And as always, make sure the clams are alive when you make the stock.

ACTIVE TIME: ¾ hour | **TOTAL TIME:** 1½ hours (including heating, simmering, and initial cooling) | **YIELD:** Makes about 2 cups (480 ml)

---

6 pounds (2.7 kg) clams, preferably large, such as cherrystone

1 quart (960 ml) filtered water, cold, divided, plus water for rinsing
2 bay leaves

One at a time, assess the clams to determine freshness: Closed clams are fresh, and open ones require further examination. Place the fresh, closed clams in a bowl. Lightly tap any clams that are open on a surface; if they close shut, they are safe to eat. Any that remain open or appear damaged should be discarded. Be cautious of clams that feel heavy: They could be full of sand, which will cloud the stock. Test heavy clams by prying them open and discarding the ones that are filled with sand. Using a clean scouring pad, scrub each clam and rinse under cold water to remove surface grit. Set aside.

In a large stockpot, bring half the water to a boil over medium-high heat. Add the clams, cover, and immediately reduce the heat to maintain a simmer. Steam the clams for 5 minutes, then remove the cover. Using tongs, transfer the clams to a bowl as they pop open, being careful to leave the liquid in the pot.

Continue simmering until all the clams have opened and released their liquor, replacing the lid as needed, about 15 minutes. Discard any clams that do not open.

When the clams are cool enough to handle, remove the meat from the shell and gently squeeze excess liquid into the stockpot. Reserve the clam meat for another use. Add the remaining water and bay leaves to the stockpot. Simmer for another 15 minutes.

Turn off the heat and rest the stock on the stove, about 15 minutes. Line a fine-mesh strainer with cheesecloth and set it on the lid of a container large enough to hold the liquid contents of the pot. Carefully ladle the stock from the pot into the strainer, leaving any cloudy liquid at the bottom of the pot. Skim any scum that appears at the surface. Repeat the straining process two or three times to ensure that no grit from the clams is transferred to the clean stock.

Taste the stock to determine your desired concentration. If the stock tastes too watery, return it to a clean stockpot and simmer until the brininess of the clams comes through.

Place the container in an ice bath to rapidly cool the stock. When the stock no longer steams, transfer to the refrigerator. Refrigerate for up to 2 days or freeze in smaller containers for longer storage.

Oyster Essence

The liquor from oysters rarely makes it from oyster shell to stockpot in my kitchen; I greedily slurp all the essence each raw oyster has to offer. Should you have more restraint, this essence is excellent for stuffing and stews, or for deglazing fish and vegetables.

When selecting oysters, I recommend staying local: As much as I adore oysters from Pacific waters, for instance, when in New York I always stick with oysters plucked from beds along the eastern seaboard. They travel a shorter distance from harbor to market and tend to hold their liquor better during this shorter transit. Sea salt is a likely unnecessary addition to the essence since oysters are briny by nature.

ACTIVE TIME: ¾ hour | **TOTAL TIME:** 1 hour (including heating, simmering, and initial cooling) | **YIELD:** Makes about 2 cups (480 ml)

3 dozen raw oysters, preferably local to your region, scrubbed
2 cups (480 ml) filtered water, cold, divided
2 tablespoons grapeseed oil
¼ pound (115 g) leeks, dark green parts removed, cut into large dice

½ small fennel bulb, coarsely chopped, fronds removed
1 small celery root, peeled, coarsely chopped
½ cup (120 ml) dry white wine, such as Sauvignon Blanc
8 black peppercorns
1 bay leaf

In a large saucepan, bring 1 cup water to a boil over high heat, and then reduce the heat to medium. Add the oysters, cover, and steam, about 2 minutes. As the shells partially open, carefully tip their liquor into the pan liquid, and remove

with tongs. Keep the pan covered until all the oysters open from the steam; discard any oysters that do not open. When all the oysters have been removed from the pan, remove the pan from the heat, pour the liquid into a bowl, and set aside.

Using a shucking knife, open the steamed oysters and pour any remaining juices into the bowl. Reserve the oyster meat for another use.

In a small stockpot, heat the grapeseed oil over medium-high heat. When it begins to ripple, add the leeks, fennel, and celery root and cook, stirring occasionally, until softened, about 5 minutes. Deglaze the pan with wine, scraping any bits from the surface, and simmer for 1 minute. Return the oyster liquid and the remaining water to the pan. Add the peppercorns and bay leaf. Slowly simmer the liquid over medium heat until reduced by half, about 8 minutes.

Turn off the heat and rest the stock on the stove, about 10 minutes. Line a fine-mesh strainer with cheesecloth and set it over a container large enough to hold the liquid contents of the pot. Carefully ladle the stock from the pot into the strainer, leaving any cloudy liquid at the bottom of the pot. Strain once or twice more to ensure no sediment remains.

Chill the stock in the refrigerator, stirring occasionally to expedite the cooling process. Refrigerate for up to 2 days or freeze in smaller containers for longer storage.

Lobster Stock

A proper lobster stock will glisten with a coral-like hue and have a taste that is reminiscent of butter. This stock works well as a base for risotto or stews; also as a supplement to dishes with other seafood stocks. Lobster stock also makes a decadent substitute for shrimp stock. You can reduce it to a glaze and add a vanilla bean to round out its sea-born intensity. Unlike large bones, lobster bodies are small enough to collect in the freezer, should you only indulge on occasion.

ACTIVE TIME: 1 hour | TOTAL TIME: 3 hours (including heating, simmering, and initial cooling) | YIELD: Makes about 1 quart (960 ml)

3 lobster bodies (about 1 pound (455 g) total), meat removed

2 tablespoons grapeseed oil

½ pound (225 g) leeks, dark green parts removed, cut into large dice

½ pound (225 g) carrots, cut into large dice

½ small fennel bulb, coarsely chopped, fronds removed

2 cloves garlic, smashed

¾ pound (340 g) tomatoes, coarsely chopped

1 cup (240 ml) dry white wine, such as Sauvignon Blanc

1½ quarts (1.4 L) filtered water, cold, plus water for rinsing

4 sprigs thyme

4 sprigs flat-leaf parsley

2 sprigs tarragon

2 bay leaves

2 teaspoons black peppercorns

Sea salt to taste

Using your hands or a spoon, hollow the cavities of the lobster bodies and remove the gills and inner organs. Rinse the cleansed shells and pat dry with kitchen towels. With kitchen shears, cut the lobster bodies into smaller pieces.

In a large stockpot, heat the grapeseed oil over medium-high heat. When it starts to ripple, add the lobster shells and sear, while stirring, until they turn bright red. Continue to cook until the shells are toasted but not burnt, about 4 minutes total.

Add the leeks, carrots, fennel, and garlic; sauté while stirring, until the mixture sweats, about 5 minutes. Stir in the tomatoes and cook for another 3 minutes. Stir in the wine and scrape up the brown bits from the bottom of the pan. Simmer until the alcohol evaporates, about 3 minutes longer.

Add the filtered water, herbs, and peppercorns and slowly bring to a gentle boil. Lower the heat and maintain at a simmer, about 1 hour.

Turn off the heat and rest the stock on the stove, about 15 minutes. Line a fine-mesh strainer with cheesecloth and set it over a container large enough to hold the liquid contents of the pot. Carefully ladle the stock from the pot into the strainer, leaving any cloudy liquid at the bottom of the pot. Skim any scum that appears at the surface. Repeat the straining process to ensure that no grit from the shellfish is transferred to the clean stock.

Taste the stock to determine your desired concentration. If the stock tastes too watery, return it to a clean stockpot and simmer until reduced to a desirable consistency. Taste and season with sea salt.

Place the container in an ice bath to rapidly cool the stock. When the stock no longer steams, transfer to the refrigerator. Refrigerate for up to 2 days or freeze in smaller containers for longer storage.

Bouillabaisse Terrine

Bouillabaisse is a traditional stew from the port town of Marseille. A dish based on fisherman's catch, the type of fish it uses is what the seafood industry now calls "rough fish," or lower-valued species often neglected by chefs. These types of fish are reclaiming a place at the table amidst a contemporary movement to highlight the ocean's diversity.

Customarily served in courses, a meal of bouillabaisse begins as an appetizer of broth, served with bread and rouille, and proceeds with an entrée of fish and vegetables. Here the seafood is composed as a terrine in gelatinous layers. Serve on toast points slathered with rouille.

ACTIVE TIME: 1½ hours | **TOTAL TIME:** 12 hours
(including marinating, roasting, and chilling) | **YIELD:** Makes 12 servings

TERRINE

1 pound (455 g) rockfish or lingcod, filleted
  and sliced into strips
1 pound (455 g) sea scallops, side muscles
  removed, sliced horizontally
2 medium Japanese eggplant, thinly sliced
  lengthwise
2 medium zucchini, thinly sliced lengthwise
½ cup (120 ml) olive oil

2 teaspoons red wine vinegar
3 cloves garlic, minced
2 tablespoons minced fennel fronds
Pinch cayenne pepper
1 teaspoon kosher salt
¼ teaspoon black pepper
2 sprigs thyme
2 sprigs marjoram

Place the fish and scallops in a bowl. In another bowl, place the sliced eggplant and zucchini. Set aside while making the marinade.

In a small bowl, whisk the oil, vinegar, garlic, fennel fronds, cayenne pepper, salt, and pepper together until well combined. Evenly distribute the marinade over the fish and vegetables, and top each with a sprig of thyme and marjoram. Wrap and marinate in the refrigerator, about 2 hours.

Heat the oven to 250°F (120°C). Arrange the fish and scallops on a sheet pan in a single layer; pour some of the marinade on top and cover with foil. Bake until tender, about 10 minutes. Remove from the oven and cool.

Turn the oven to the low broiler setting. Drain the vegetables and arrange them on a sheet pan in a single layer. Broil until browned on one side, about 5 minutes. With tongs, turn the vegetables over and broil until caramelized, another 5 minutes. Remove from the oven and cool. Chill the fish, scallops, and vegetables until needed.

ASPIC

⅓ cup (80 ml) olive oil
1 medium leek, sliced
1 medium carrot, sliced
1 small fennel bulb, chopped, fronds reserved
  for above
2 cloves garlic, sliced
1 medium tomato, chopped
1 strip orange peel

1 large pinch saffron, toasted and ground
8 black peppercorns
½ teaspoon sea salt
½ cup (120 ml) dry white wine, such as
  Sauvignon Blanc
Splash Pernod or absinthe
1 cup (240 ml) Shellfish Stock
2 tablespoons Gelatin Powder or 6 sheets gelatin

Heat the oil in a large sauté pan over medium heat. When hot but not smoking, add the leek, carrot, fennel, and garlic; sauté until the vegetables sweat, about 5 minutes. Stir in the tomato, orange strip, saffron, peppercorns, and salt. Continue to cook until the tomatoes are incorporated, another 5 minutes. Deglaze with wine and Pernod, stirring, about 1 minute. Add the shellfish stock and simmer until the flavors meld, about 10 minutes. Remove from the heat and strain into a bowl. Reserve 3 tablespoons for the rouille. Set aside to cool.

When lukewarm, transfer ½ cup (120 ml) of the bouillabaisse liquid to a small saucepan. Sprinkle the gelatin over the liquid, and gently heat on low, stirring until dissolved. Remove from the heat and add to the remaining liquid (excluding the stock set aside for the rouille).

ROUILLE

3 cloves garlic, minced
1 slow-roasted Roma tomato, seeded, or
   1 sun-dried tomato, soaked
½ teaspoon smoked paprika, preferably sweet
½ teaspoon sea salt

¼ teaspoon cayenne pepper
¾ cup (85 g) dried bread crumbs
½ tablespoon lemon juice
⅓ cup (80 ml) olive oil
Fresh baguette, for serving

In a mortar and pestle, mash the garlic and tomato with the paprika, salt, and cayenne pepper until blended. Transfer to a bowl and toss with the bread crumbs; stir in the lemon juice and reserved 3 tablespoons of bouillabaisse liquid. Add the oil in a slow stream, working the pestle continuously until mixture is well combined. Wrap and chill until needed.

TO ASSEMBLE: Line a terrine mold with plastic wrap. Line with strips of eggplant, allowing an overhang on both sides. Arrange a layer of fish over the eggplant, followed by lengthwise slices of zucchini. Add a layer of scallops, and repeat with more zucchini. Repeat with another layer of fish, zucchini, and scallops. Pour the aspic over the terrine, pushing down with your hands. Fold the eggplant the over and brush with more aspic. Securely wrap with plastic wrap; weight the terrine and chill overnight to set.

The next day, unwrap the terrine and invert onto a cutting board. Slice and serve with rouille and a fresh baguette.

Oysters, Two Ways

Oysters were once found in abundance throughout the Hudson River estuary, covering some 200,000 acres, cherished by natives and settlers alike. By the early twentieth century, area oyster reefs became extinct due to overharvesting, dredging, and pollution. Recent environmental efforts have restored conditions to allow for oyster habitation, most notably the *Crassostrea virginica*, and in turn the filter-feeding activity of the oysters help clean surrounding waters.

Regenerative projects aside, oysters are delicious, whether on the half shell or with accoutrements. This recipe offers a chilled gelée and a warm spiced cream as counterpoints to the pop and pleasure of the oysters.

ACTIVE TIME: 1½ hours | **TOTAL TIME:** 1½ hours | **YIELD:** Makes 12 servings

OYSTERS

24 raw oysters, preferably local to your region, scrubbed

Using an oyster knife, carefully shuck the oysters, reserving the liquor that is released during the process. Place the oysters in an airtight container and chill until needed. Strain the liquor into a small bowl; reserve in the refrigerator. Wash and dry the oyster shells.

WATERCRESS ASPIC

1 tablespoon Gelatin Powder or
   3 sheets gelatin
Oyster liquor (above)
¼ cup (9 g) watercress leaves, rinsed

¼ cup (60 ml) Oyster Essence
1 teaspoon lemon juice
½ teaspoon sea salt
Dash cayenne pepper

In a small bowl, sprinkle the Gelatin Powder over ¼ cup of the reserved oyster liquor; set aside to soften. In a blender, purée the watercress leaves, Oyster Essence, and lemon juice. Strain the mixture into a saucepan, discarding the solids. Add the salt and cayenne pepper. Stir in the gelatin mixture and gently heat until the gelatin dissolves. Remove from the heat and cool slightly, about 5 minutes.

While the aspic is cooling, spread a kitchen towel on a sheet pan. Set twelve oyster shells on the kitchen towel to hold in place; return one oyster to each shell. When the gelatin mixture is tepid, spoon some of the aspic into each shell, glazing each oyster. Place the sheet pan in the refrigerator to set the aspic.

PINK PEPPERCORN SABAYON

2 egg yolks
2 tablespoons sparkling wine,
    such as Prosecco
1 tablespoon Oyster Essence

1 tablespoon unsalted butter, softened
1 tablespoon heavy cream
1 teaspoon pink peppercorns, crushed
¼ teaspoon sea salt

In the bowl of a double boiler, whisk the egg yolks with the sparkling wine and Oyster Essence. Add just enough water to the base saucepan to create steam when heated. Over medium heat, bring the water to a simmer; set the bowl over simmering water, making sure there is only steam between the water and bowl. Over moderate heat, continuously whisk the eggs until the sauce holds its shape, about 5 minutes. The sauce should form ribbons when done.

In a small bowl, whisk the softened butter and cream until combined. Stir in the pink peppercorns and sea salt. Mount the warm sauce with the butter mixture, 1 tablespoon at a time, until incorporated. Keep warm.

TO SERVE: Preheat the broiler on low. Arrange the remaining twelve oysters on a small sheet pan. Spoon some warm sabayon over each oyster. Broil until puffed and lightly brown, about 4 minutes.

Serve warm oysters alongside cold oysters for a nice contrast in texture and flavor. This appetizer is especially pleasant with a chilled glass of sparkling wine!

Absinthe Mussels on Braised Cardoons

There's a wonderful woman who distills absinthe in the Hudson Valley. Cheryl Lins of Delaware Phoenix is responsible for the process—from mash to ferment to delivery—and at least one of her bottles always adorns my home bar.

This recipe is a happy accident arrived at when I was chasing the green fairy while preparing a meal for friends. Mussels and absinthe are a fine pairing—the sweetness of tender mollusk highlighted by herbal notes from the spirit.

Mussels, like oysters, are bio-indicators that inform us of the water quality that surrounds them. They reproduce quickly, grow rapidly, and thrive abundantly. Look for farmed varieties, which are generally beneficial to their habitat.

ACTIVE TIME: ¾ hour | **TOTAL TIME:** 1¼ hours
(including simmering and braising) | **YIELD:** Makes 2 to 4 servings

MUSSELS

2 tablespoons olive oil
2 small shallots, minced
1 clove garlic, minced
2 cups (480 ml) dry white wine,
  such as Sauvignon Blanc
2 tablespoons absinthe

1 bay leaf
8 black peppercorns
2 pounds (910 g) fresh mussels, scrubbed
2 tablespoons unsalted butter
Salt and pepper
Fresh chervil, for garnish

In a medium stockpot or shellfish pan, heat the olive oil over medium-high heat. When the oil is hot, but not smoking, add the shallots and garlic and cook, stirring, until translucent, about 3 minutes. Pour in the wine and absinthe, add the bay leaf and peppercorns, and bring to a gentle simmer.

Place the closed mussels in the pan, cover, and steam until the mussels open and release their juices, about 7 to 10 minutes. With tongs, remove the mussels as they open and reserve in a bowl tented with aluminum.

Remove the mussel stock from the heat and gently strain into a bowl. Pour the stock through cheesecloth to remove fine sediment that may have passed through the strainer. Reserve.

CARDOONS

2 tablespoons unsalted butter
4 young cardoon stalks, washed and peeled

2 medium leeks, halved lengthwise, roots intact
Salt and pepper

Preheat the oven to 425°F (220°C). Butter a baking dish large enough to hold the vegetables in a shallow layer. Split the cardoons lengthwise and layer with the leeks in the dish. Pour ¾ cup (180 ml) of the mussel stock over the vegetables; season with salt and pepper. Cover the

—238—

dish with aluminum foil, and bake until tender and caramelized, about 20 minutes.

TO FINISH: Place the remaining mussel stock in a small saucepan and bring to a simmer over medium heat. Reduce the stock to a glaze and mount with butter, 1 tablespoon at a time, stirring until incorporated. Season with salt and pepper.

For each serving, wrap a cardoon and leek around a fork to center in a shallow bowl. Top with warm mussels in their shells. Spoon the mussel glaze around the bowl and garnish with chervil leaves.

Littleneck Clam and Millet Grits with Saffron Emulsion

This is my take on the classic pairing of shrimp and grits, only with clams and millet as the essential ingredients. Unlike farmed shrimp, farm-raised clams can support the health of their environment; clams improve water quality in the same manner as oysters and mussels.

Millet, too, is versatile—a grain that is sturdy in texture, nutty in flavor, and full of nutrients. It is also an excellent source of magnesium and antioxidants, protein and dietary fiber. The grits here impart a rich, creamy base for the Cajun-spiced clam ragout.

ACTIVE TIME: 1 hour | **TOTAL TIME:** 1½ hours
(including heating and simmering) | **YIELD:** Makes 4 servings

GRITS

1 tablespoon olive oil
1 cup (200 g) hulled millet
1 cup (240 ml) Clam Liquor
2 cups (480 ml) water
½ teaspoon sea salt

½ cup (55 g) grated sharp cheddar
¼ cup (27 g) grated Parmesan
½ cup (115 g) crème fraîche
2 tablespoons unsalted butter

In a medium saucepan, add the olive oil and millet, and stir over medium heat until toasted, about 4 minutes. Stir in the Clam Liquor, water, and sea salt; bring to a boil. Reduce the heat to maintain a simmer, stirring occasionally, until tender, about 15 minutes. Fold in the cheeses, crème fraîche, and butter, and continue to cook over low heat until thick and creamy. Cover and keep warm.

CLAMS

2 tablespoons olive oil

2 Andouille sausages, sliced on the bias

1 cup (175 g) corn kernels, cobs reserved for emulsion (below)

½ medium red bell pepper, diced

1 cup (240 ml) Shellfish Stock

1 cup (240 ml) Basic Whey

3 pounds (1.4 kg) littleneck clams, scrubbed

2 tablespoons unsalted butter

1 teaspoon smoked paprika, preferably bittersweet

Salt and pepper

1 bunch scallions, thinly sliced on the bias, for garnish

1 lemon, quartered, for garnish

In a large sauté pan, heat the olive oil over medium-high heat until hot but not smoking. Add the sausage and cook until browned. Transfer to a plate with a slotted spoon. To the same pan, add the corn and red pepper, and cook while stirring, until charred, about 4 minutes. Add the vegetables to the sausage; cover with aluminum foil to keep warm.

Deglaze the pan with a splash of the Shellfish Stock, scraping the bottom of the pan with a wooden spoon, then add the remaining stock and whey and bring to a boil. Add the clams to the pot, cover, and reduce the heat to maintain a simmer. Cook until the clams open, about 7 to 10 minutes. As they open, transfer the clams to the holding plate.

Uncover the pan and continue simmering the liquid until reduced by half. Mount the sauce with butter and add the paprika, stirring until combined. Season with salt and pepper. Remove from the heat. Return the clams, sausage, and vegetables to the pan. Cover to keep warm.

EMULSION

2 tablespoons olive oil

½ medium leek, sliced

1 clove garlic, minced

2 large corn cobs, kernels reserved for clams (above)

½ cup (120 ml) Shellfish Stock

½ cup (120 ml) Clam Liquor

1 large pinch saffron threads, toasted and ground

¼ cup (56 g) unsalted butter

Salt and pepper

In a large sauté pan, heat the olive oil over medium-high heat, then add the leek and garlic, and cook until translucent, about 3 minutes. Toss the corn cobs into the pan and toast on each side, about another 3 minutes. In a small bowl, combine the Shellfish Stock and Clam Liquor, and crumble the saffron into the liquid. Add the saffron-infused liquid to the sauté pan. Bring to a boil, then lower the heat to maintain a simmer. Reduce the liquid until it thickens, about 5 minutes. Remove the sauce from the heat and pass through a strainer into a small bowl, pushing on the solids to extract the liquid. Mount the sauce with the butter, stirring until combined. Season with salt and pepper. Using a hand blender, froth until the sauce emulsifies. Hold over low heat.

TO SERVE: Spoon the grits into a bowl and top with clams, sausage, and vegetables. Pour the emulsion over the clams, sprinkle with sliced scallions, and serve with lemon wedges.

Lobster Eggs Sardou with Vanilla Bean Hollandaise

A few summers ago, I took a respite from New York—off the coast of Maine, staying in a coastal house run by two generations of lobstermen. It was a brief time for me—with their early mornings on the water and late evenings with the bottle, a lifestyle reserved for those with a seafaring heart. As such, I was often on my own for breakfast, which is how this recipe came about. It is a decadent adaptation of a classic New Orleans brunch dish.

While there, I learned about the challenges that lobstermen face amidst climate change. Fisheries from the Gulf of Maine and Georges Bank are managed well and maintain an abundant lobster population. Avoid lobster from southern New England, where the population has been in decline for over two decades.

ACTIVE TIME: 1 hour | **TOTAL TIME:** 1½ hours (including heating and simmering) | **YIELD:** Makes 6 servings

SARDOU

1 cup (240 ml) Lobster Stock
¼ cup (56 g) unsalted butter, divided
1 clove garlic, minced
1 medium shallot, minced
2 tablespoons all-purpose flour
1¼ cups (300 ml) whole milk
¼ teaspoon hot sauce

3 cups (90 g) fresh spinach leaves, coarsely chopped
Salt and pepper
6 whole artichoke bottoms, fresh or canned
1 lobster, gently steamed, meat removed, shells reserved for stock
6 eggs, poached

In a small saucepan, heat the Lobster Stock on medium-high until the liquid begins to tremble, then lower the heat to maintain a simmer. Reduce to 2 tablespoons and set aside.

In a sauté pan, melt half the butter over medium heat. Add the garlic and shallot and sauté until translucent, about 2 minutes. Sprinkle the flour into the pan and stir until it begins to brown, another 2 minutes. Using a whisk, stir in the milk and mix until smooth. Add the hot sauce and lobster reduction. Bring to a simmer and cook until thickened, about 4 minutes. Add the spinach and cook until wilted, about 1 minute. Season with salt and pepper.

In a clean sauté pan, melt the remaining butter and add the artichoke bottoms. Cook until heated through, about 5 minutes. Turn off the heat. Gently portion and rest the lobster meat on the artichoke bottoms; cover to keep warm and set aside.

HOLLANDAISE

3 egg yolks
1 teaspoon water
1 cup (225 g) unsalted butter, cut into tablespoons
2 teaspoons lemon juice

½ vanilla bean, seeds only
Dash cayenne pepper
Sea salt to taste
Tarragon, for garnish

In the bottom of a double boiler, add 1 inch (2.5 cm) water and bring to a simmer over medium heat. Add the egg yolks and water to the top of the double boiler, and whisk until lightened, about 1 minute. Place the mixture over the simmering water and whisk constantly until the mixture coats a spoon, about 4 minutes.

Remove the bowl from the heat and gradually whisk in the butter, 1 tablespoon at a time, until fully incorporated. Return the bowl to the double boiler to help melt the butter, as needed. Finish with the lemon juice, vanilla bean seeds, cayenne pepper, and sea salt. Keep warm.

TO SERVE: Spoon the spinach mixture onto each plate and top with a lobster-filled artichoke bottom. Carefully rest a poached egg onto or next to the lobster filling. Cover with hollandaise. Garnish with tarragon.

CHAPTER ELEVEN

Vegetable Stocks, Broths, and Dishes

E ven though animal-based stocks and broths are fundamental to most chefs' kitchens, plant-based stocks should be used as the seasons provide, and with as much enthusiasm. Flavor, as well as nutrition, is the driver here.

The range of flavors you can extract from vegetables is as vast as their kingdom. An earthy mushroom stock is a great substitute for beef stock; a squash consommé imparts the lightness of chicken stock. Infuse the smoke of applewood into a tomato and apply it to broth—the smoke and fruit suspended in liquid to affect the whole dish. Add seaweed for a boost of minerals and to impart a silky mouthfeel; a satisfying umami emerges from below the vegetal note.

Vegetables are more delicate than bones: Within the first hour of simmering, some vitamins will denature while others will become enhanced (see "On the Criticisms of Bone Broth," page 61). Surprisingly, vegetable stocks can have more calcium than bone broths, and a homemade vegetable stock contains less fat, carbohydrates, and sodium than grocery store alternatives. Locate vegetables from an organic farmer you trust, preferably one that manages an assorted range of crops. More variety on a farm can help enrich the soil and minimize disease in the fields; natural immunity in crops means less need for pesticides and other harmful chemicals. All of these details translate to better health in the stockpot.

The vegetables used in stock are consistent with those in animal-based stocks and broths. Raw onions are sharp; leeks are mild and buttery; carrots are sweet and colorful. Other vegetables, such as fennel and parsnips, impart subtle flavors that add complexity to the base. Vegetables take less time to break down than bones, which means vegetable stocks require considerably less simmering time. The rate of extraction is further influenced by how much vegetable matter is exposed to water: The finer the chop, the less time in the pot.

The recipes in this section follow a repetitive technique while employing varying ingredients. The result is a palette of color and a range of flavor that lends itself to exploration in the kitchen. Don't stop here: Experiment with other vegetables. For instance, corn cobs produce a milky broth with a nutty quality (as seen in the Saffron Emulsion on page 240); yellow beets, roasted and peeled, yield a bright orange broth—both suitable as a foundation upon which to build new dishes.

Vegetable stocks do not contain proteins that bind molecules and thicken the liquid. As such, they lose flavor quickly and should be used or frozen within two days. You can add plant-based thickeners, such as kelp or agar-agar, or a small amount of grass-fed gelatin to stabilize the foundation.

MIXED VEGETABLES

When selecting vegetables for stock, locate a farm that encourages crop diversity on the land. You should be able to find onions, leeks, and carrots—maybe fennel, too—from the same farmer. The vegetables in these stocks are chopped in a food processor to expedite infusion into the liquid. Vegetable stock serves as an all-purpose medium for cooking.

Basic Vegetable Stock

This basic vegetable stock sweats the vegetables in the stockpot before adding the liquid. Processing the vegetables into smaller pieces lessens simmering time and encourages more flavor to be extracted. Vegetable stock is light in body and loses its aroma quickly. Use it within two days, if chilled, or preserve it for up to six months in the freezer.

ACTIVE TIME: ¾ hour | **TOTAL TIME:** 2 hours (including heating, simmering, and initial cooling) | **YIELD:** Makes about 3 quarts (2.8 liters)

½ pound (225 g) white onions, cut into large dice

1 pound (455 g) leeks, dark green parts removed, cut into large dice

¾ pound (340 g) carrots, cut into large dice

1 small fennel bulb, coarsely chopped, fronds removed

3 tablespoons grapeseed oil

½ cup (120 ml) dry white wine, such as Sauvignon Blanc

3 quarts (2.8 L) filtered water, cold

2 sprigs thyme

4 sprigs flat-leaf parsley

2 bay leaves

Sea salt to taste

One at a time, place each vegetable in the bowl of a food processor; pulse until finely chopped. Do not overchop the vegetables. You want small uniform pieces without much liquid. Transfer the vegetables into one large bowl. Reserve.

In a medium stockpot, heat the grapeseed oil over medium heat. When the oil is hot, add the vegetables and cook until softened, 5 to 8 minutes. If the diameter of your stockpot is not large enough to hold the vegetables in one layer, cook the vegetables in two batches. Deglaze with wine while stirring, about 1 minute.

Add the water and herbs to the pot; add more water to cover the vegetables, if necessary. Slowly bring to a gentle boil, then lower the heat to maintain a simmer, skimming the surface as soon as scum appears. Cook for 45 minutes.

Turn off the heat and rest the stock on the stove, about 10 minutes. Line a fine-mesh strainer with cheesecloth and set it on the lid of a container large enough to hold the liquid contents of the pot. Carefully ladle the stock from the pot into the strainer, leaving any cloudy liquid at the bottom of the pot. Discard the solids.

If a more concentrated flavor is desired, return the stock to a clean pot and simmer until reduced. Taste and season with salt. Chill the stock in the refrigerator, stirring occasionally to expedite the cooling process. Refrigerate for up to 2 days or freeze in smaller containers for longer storage.

Roasted Vegetable Stock

This brown vegetable stock incorporates parsnips and garlic into a standard mirepoix. Roasting the vegetables deepens the color and flavor of the stock. Use it to create rich soups or to deglaze vegetables or meat.

ACTIVE TIME: ½ hour | **TOTAL TIME:** 2½ hours (including roasting, heating, simmering, and initial cooling) | **YIELD:** Makes about 3 quarts (2.8 liters)

½ pound (225 g) white onions, cut into small dice
1 pound (455 g) leeks, dark green parts removed, cut into small dice
½ pound (225 g) carrots, cut into small dice
½ pound (225 g) parsnips, cut into small dice
1 small fennel bulb, coarsely chopped, fronds removed

3 cloves garlic, unpeeled
3 tablespoons grapeseed oil
3 quarts (2.8 L) filtered water, cold
2 sprigs thyme
4 sprigs flat-leaf parsley
12 black peppercorns
2 bay leaves
Sea salt to taste

Preheat the oven to 350°F (175°C).

In a large bowl, toss the vegetables with the grapeseed oil. Spread the vegetables in a single layer over two sheet pans. Roast for 1 hour, stirring occasionally.

Transfer the vegetables to a medium stockpot, scraping the pan with a spatula to loosen brown bits. Add the water, herbs, and spices to the pot; add more water to cover the vegetables, if necessary. Slowly bring to a gentle boil, then lower the heat to maintain a simmer, skimming the surface as soon as scum appears. Cook for 1 hour, or until tender.

Turn off the heat and rest the stock on the stove, about 10 minutes. Line a fine-mesh strainer with cheesecloth and set it over a container large enough to hold the liquid contents of the pot. Carefully ladle the stock from the pot into the strainer, leaving any cloudy liquid at the bottom of the pot. Discard the solids.

If a more concentrated flavor is desired, return the stock to a clean pot and simmer until reduced. Taste and season with salt. Chill the stock in the refrigerator, stirring occasionally to expedite the cooling process. Refrigerate for up to 2 days or freeze in smaller containers for longer storage.

Velvety Vegetable Stock

The alginate in kelp, a type of seaweed, is what gives this stock texture. Kelp also flavors the stock with a soft umami. If domestically harvested kelp is unavailable, kombu is a reasonable substitute. Use this stock when you require structure in a dish. If desired, add light soy sauce or tamari to the final stock to intensify the flavor. See "A Word on Vegetable Stocks and Seaweed," page 65, for more information about kelp.

ACTIVE TIME: ¾ hour | **TOTAL TIME:** 2½ hours
(including soaking, heating, and simmering) | **YIELD:** Makes about 3 quarts (2.8 liters)

3 sheets kelp or kombu
3 quarts (2.8 L) filtered water, cold, divided
½ pound (225 g) white onions, cut into large dice
1 pound (455 g) leeks, dark green parts removed, cut into large dice
½ pound (225 g) carrots, cut into large dice
½ pound (225 g) parsnips, cut into large dice
1 small fennel bulb, coarsely chopped, fronds removed
3 tablespoons grapeseed oil
2 sprigs thyme
4 sprigs flat-leaf parsley
2 bay leaves
12 black peppercorns
2 teaspoons light soy sauce or tamari (optional)
Sea salt to taste, if necessary

In a medium stockpot, cover the kelp with 1 quart (960 ml) water. If you have time, soak the kelp for 2 hours to bring out the natural flavor. Turn the heat to medium and slowly bring to a simmer. Skim the liquid as any impurities appear at the surface. As soon as the liquid ripples, turn off the heat and immediately remove the kelp with tongs. Use the kelp for another recipe. Rest the liquid on the stove for 10 minutes. Line a fine-mesh strainer with cheesecloth. Carefully pass the liquid through the strainer into a bowl, leaving any sediment on the bottom of the pot.

Follow the cooking instructions for Basic Vegetable Stock (page 245), adding the kelp liquid with the remaining water after the vegetables are sautéed. Season the final stock with soy sauce or tamari, and adjust with sea salt if necessary.

Wine Grower's Vegetable Terrine with Verjus-Pickled Grapes

Hudson Valley is especially beautiful in the fall—sumac-lined roads that meander across farms and orchards, distilleries, and wineries. Perhaps known more for cider in recent years, the valley actually lays claim to the oldest vineyard in America. Wild grapes are also abundant throughout the region.

If you live in an area where wild grapes adorn walls, harvest vine, fruit, and leaves for this recipe. Alternatively, if you are a friend of a winemaker, double the recipe and offer a terrine in exchange for prime ingredients. Or, better yet, make your own *verjus*—the vinegar from the juice of unripe grapes—and bottle extra for friends and family.

ACTIVE TIME: 1½ hours | **TOTAL TIME:** 10 hours (including heating and chilling) | **YIELD:** Makes 12 servings

TERRINE

6 sticks grapevine, dried, or smoking chips, such as applewood

1 small eggplant, cut on the bias into ¼-inch (.6 cm) slices

2 medium zucchini, cut on the bias into ¼-inch (.6 cm) slices

2 medium crookneck squash, cut on the bias into ¼-inch (.6 cm) slices

2 medium red bell peppers, halved, seeded, and cut into ¼-inch (.6 cm) slices

1 small shallot, minced

½ cup (120 ml) olive oil

Salt and pepper

¾ cup (27 g) fresh green pine needles or rosemary

1 cup (240 ml) Basic Vegetable Stock

2 teaspoons Gelatin Powder or 1 gelatin sheet

½ teaspoon aged sherry or red wine vinegar

8 grape leaves, blanched and drained

½ cup (125 g) ricotta, preferably homemade (see "Whey," page 302)

With a stovetop smoker, heat the grapevine, covered, over medium heat, until smoking, about 10 minutes. Meanwhile, toss all vegetables with the oil in a large bowl. Season with salt and pepper.

Remove the cover from the smoker, scatter the pine needles over the hot wood, and top with a fine grate. If the grate has wide slots, place a sheet of aluminum foil across the grate. Layer vegetables on the grate and replace the cover. Turn the heat to low. Smoke for 15 to 20 minutes. If the vegetables are not fully cooked, finish roasting in a 375°F (190°C) oven until tender. Cool to room temperature.

In a small saucepan, heat the vegetable stock over medium heat until warm. Turn off the heat and soak the gelatin until it melts into the liquid, about 2 minutes. Add the vinegar and set aside to cool. When the vegetables and broth mixture are cool, toss together in a large bowl.

Line a terrine mold with plastic wrap, leaving about 3 inches (7.5 cm) hanging off the side. Line the mold by overlapping blanched grape leaves at an angle, leaving 2 inches (5 cm) hanging off the sides. Layer the eggplant lengthwise into the mold, followed by the zucchini strips. Spread the ricotta on top, then layer the summer squash and end with the bell peppers. Fold the hanging grape leaves over the vegetables, and wrap tightly with the plastic wrap. Place a weight on the terrine (such as full aluminum cans) and refrigerate overnight.

GRAPES

½ pound (225 g) red or black grapes, rinsed and removed from the vine
½ cup (120 ml) apple cider vinegar
¼ cup (50 g) sugar
1 teaspoon mustard seeds

½ teaspoon whole cloves
½ teaspoon black peppercorns
½ teaspoon sea salt
¼ cup (60 ml) verjus

While the terrine is resting, prepare the grapes. Slice the stem end off each grape and discard. Set the trimmed grapes aside in a bowl or layer in canning jars. In a small saucepan, heat the vinegar, sugar, and spices over medium heat until the sugar dissolves. Remove from the heat, stir in the verjus and cool to room temperature. Add the grapes to the cooled brine, wrap the bowl or seal with a lid, and rest in the refrigerator overnight.

TO SERVE: Remove the terrine from the refrigerator, unwrap, and carefully invert onto a cutting board. With a serrated knife, slice into 2-inch (5 cm) pieces and plate with the pickled grapes. Serve with crostini.

Roasted Sesame and Spring Greens Soup

This recipe highlights the significance that kelp can have on a vegetable stock. It adds silken texture and heightens flavor. This spring soup is best when you start with raw sesame seeds—the toasted flavor and texture of homemade tahini blends well into the bright base of the dish. Nevertheless, you can use ready-made tahini in a pinch.

ACTIVE TIME: ¾ hour | **TOTAL TIME:** 1½ hours (including cooling and simmering) | **YIELD:** Makes 4 servings

TAHINI

¼ cup (35 g) hulled sesame seeds

2 tablespoons olive oil

In a clean, dry skillet, heat the sesame seeds over medium-low heat, tossing in the pan to evenly distribute and prevent burning. Toast until lightly browned and fragrant, about 8 minutes. Remove from the heat and cool to room temperature.

Transfer the toasted sesame seeds to a food processor. Pulse until the seeds turn to a paste. While running on low, add the oil in a slow stream until well combined. Transfer to a ramekin and set aside.

SOUP

2 tablespoons unsalted butter
1 tablespoon olive oil
1 medium onion, chopped
2 medium leeks, rinsed and chopped
1 garlic clove, minced
1 large potato, preferably Yukon gold
1 quart (960 ml) Velvety
   Vegetable Stock

2 sprigs thyme
1 small head green lettuce, leaves separated
   (about 4 cups [960 ml])
4 leaves fresh sorrel (optional)
Tahini (above)
1 tablespoon fresh lemon juice
Sea salt and white pepper
Chives, for garnish

In a small stockpot, heat the butter and oil over medium heat. When the oil is hot but not smoking, stir in the onion, leeks, and garlic and cook until softened, about 4 minutes. Add the potato, stock, and thyme, and bring to a simmer. Cook over medium-low heat

until the potato is tender, about 12 minutes. Remove the thyme sprigs. Stir in the lettuce leaves and sorrel and continue simmering, about 8 to 10 minutes.

Carefully transfer the liquid to a blender, working in batches if necessary, and blend until smooth. Add 2 tablespoons of the tahini and blend until combined. Return the soup to the pot, add the lemon juice, and maintain gentle heat. Do not boil or the broth might separate. Season with salt and pepper. Portion into bowls and garnish with chives. Serve immediately.

Creamy Rutabaga Risotto with Stock-Poached Eggs

We see a lot of rutabaga in a Hudson Valley winter. A cross between turnips and cabbage, this root vegetable is less starchy than potatoes and sweeter than turnips, making it a perfect addition to a cold-weather meal. This recipe also illustrates how to poach an egg in stock.

ACTIVE TIME: 1 hour | **TOTAL TIME:** 1¼ hours
(including simmering and poaching) | **YIELD:** Makes 4 servings

RISOTTO

2 tablespoons olive oil
2 tablespoons unsalted butter, divided
1 medium onion, finely chopped
1 medium leek, finely chopped
1 clove garlic, minced
1 medium rutabaga (about 2 pounds [910 g]), cubed

1 cup (200 g) short-grain rice, such as arborio or carnaroli
3 cups (720 ml) Basic Vegetable Stock, warmed
½ cup (50 g) grated fresh Parmesan cheese, plus extra for garnish
½ lemon, zested and juiced
Salt and pepper
Flat-leaf parsley, for garnish

Heat a large saucepan over medium heat. Heat the olive oil and 1 tablespoon of the butter until warm. Stir in the onion, leek, and garlic, and cook until translucent, about 4 minutes. Add the rutabaga and cook until al dente, another 4 minutes. Stir occasionally to prevent the vegetables from sticking to the bottom.

Add the rice to the pan and stir to combine. Toast for 1 minute while stirring. Gradually add the warm stock, stirring after each addition, until absorbed by the rice. Continue to add stock, stirring constantly, until the rice is creamy and al dente, about 30 to 40 minutes.

When the rice is ready, stir in the cheese, lemon zest, and lemon juice. Taste and season with salt and pepper. Rest a lid on edge of the pan to maintain warmth.

POACHING EGGS IN STOCK

Eggs, in their suspended state of incubation, are inherently delicate; they take well to the introduction of flavor. Of an egg poached in chicken stock, Chef Tamar Adler, author of *The Everlasting Meal*, describes it as "delicious if philosophically perplexing." Nevertheless, an egg can be poached in any kind of stock, not just a stock of its own ilk. Better yet, add a clove of garlic or a sprig of thyme to the liquid, and the egg will take on even more flavor.

To poach one or more eggs in stock: In a medium saucepan, bring enough stock to hold the eggs to a rolling boil. If you want to infuse more flavor into the egg, add a peeled garlic clove and/or fresh herbs to the pot. Stir in a glug of vinegar;

this will help set the egg whites. Reduce the heat to medium-low, and carefully slide a cracked egg into the stock, swirling the liquid around the egg with a spoon to prevent it from resting on the bottom. Repeat with any remaining eggs, being careful to not overcrowd the pot. Poach until the whites are firm and the yolks are tender, about 3 to 4 minutes. Using a slotted spoon, carefully remove the eggs one at a time. Serve immediately.

Depending on the recipe, the poaching liquid can be served as broth in the egg dish, or simply passed through a cheesecloth-lined strainer and reserved in cold storage for future use. Using the vinegar-spiked stock to further develop a gastrique is an excellent way to employ the leftover liquid.

EGGS

4 eggs
2 cups (480 ml) Basic Vegetable Stock or water

1 teaspoon apple cider vinegar

Using vegetable stock and apple cider vinegar, poach the eggs according to the instructions in the "Poaching Eggs in Stock" sidebar.

TO SERVE: Portion the risotto into shallow bowls. With a slotted spoon, transfer an egg to each bowl. Grate cheese on top and garnish with parsley. Serve immediately.

Maple Butterscotch Carrots with Carrot Top Chimichurri

My mother had a clever way of getting me to eat vegetables as a child. Her butterscotch carrots—vegetables disguised as candy—was a favorite. This recipe is updated with maple syrup in place of brown sugar and further balanced with herbs and citrus.

Wasting nothing, carrot tops form the base of a chimichurri sauce. Here root and tops come together as a sweet and savory side dish that goes well with grilled meat.

ACTIVE TIME: ½ hour | **TOTAL TIME:** ½ hour | **YIELD:** Makes 4 to 6 servings

CARROTS

2 pounds (910 g) carrots, scrubbed,
   green tops reserved
2 tablespoons olive oil
2 tablespoons unsalted butter
Salt and pepper
¼ cup (60 ml) dry white wine,

such as Sauvignon Blanc
½ cup (120 ml) Roasted Vegetable Stock,
   plus more if needed
2 tablespoons maple syrup
1 tablespoon minced fresh tarragon
1 teaspoon lemon zest

Slice the carrots on the bias into 1-inch (2.5 cm) medallions. In a medium saucepan, heat the oil and butter over medium until hot but not smoking. Add the carrots and stir to coat, about 1 minute. Season with salt and pepper. Pour in the white wine and simmer until reduced, about 2 minutes. Add the vegetable stock and maple syrup; continue to cook, stirring occasionally, until the liquid is reduced and the vegetables are coated and tender. Add more stock or water if the pan becomes dry. Remove from the heat and toss with the tarragon and lemon zest. Serve with the chimichurri.

CHIMICHURRI

1 cup (60 g) carrot greens, coarsely chopped
½ cup (30 g) flat-leaf parsley, coarsely chopped
½ small jalapeño, seeds removed,
   minced
2 cloves garlic, minced

1 teaspoon smoked paprika, preferably sweet
1 teaspoon sea salt
½ teaspoon black pepper
¼ cup (60 ml) red wine vinegar
½ cup (120 ml) olive oil

While the carrots are cooking, combine all ingredients except the oil in a food processor. Pulse until well combined. With the processor running on low, gradually add the oil and blend until emulsified. Transfer to a ramekin and serve with the vegetables.

MUSHROOMS

Mushrooms are a versatile vegetable: There are many varieties—from basic button mushrooms to exotic wild morels—that can be foraged or cultivated, served as an entrée or accompaniment. Mushrooms can be small and delicate, like beech and enoki; medium and layered, like oyster and hen of the woods; or large and beefy, like porcini and king trumpet. Despite the size and texture of a mushroom, all varieties offer an earthy profile that encourages use in comfort-inducing applications—as a base for soup or stew, or enveloped within grains. Mushrooms, and their liquid essence, are an ideal accompaniment to the changing of the seasons, often at their peak in early spring and throughout fall.

Mushroom stock can complement meat or vegetable dishes or be used as a substitute for beef stock. When making stock, grinding fresh, raw mushrooms increases exposure to liquid and therefore decreases simmering time. This was a good discovery for my business: Early in development, we would buy mushroom scraps from cultivators at the end of market days. It served as a way for our suppliers to make a buck on what would otherwise go to waste.

Remember that every mushroom type has a different flavor profile. Consider making stock using a single mushroom variety—such as oyster or lobster mushrooms for a delicate seafood flavor—to achieve a unique base. Mushroom stock will cloud easily if left in the refrigerator overnight. To preserve a clear mushroom stock, use or freeze it immediately.

Basic Mushroom Stock

This white mushroom stock sautés finely chopped button mushrooms with other vegetables to achieve a stock that is light in body and nutty in flavor. Celery root, the sweet vegetable base of celery stalks, imparts another earthy element to the liquid.

ACTIVE TIME: ¾ hour | **TOTAL TIME:** 2 hours (including heating, simmering, and initial cooling) | **YIELD:** Makes about 3 quarts (2.8 liters)

1½ pounds (680 g) button mushrooms, including stems

½ pound (225 g) white onions, cut into large dice

1 pound (455 g) leeks, dark green parts
    removed, cut into large dice
½ pound (225 g) carrots, cut into large dice
1 small celery root, peeled, coarsely chopped
3 tablespoons grapeseed oil
½ cup (120 ml) dry white wine, such as
    Sauvignon Blanc

3 quarts (2.8 L) filtered water, cold
2 sprigs thyme
4 sprigs flat-leaf parsley
12 black peppercorns
2 bay leaves
Sea salt to taste

Follow the cooking instructions for Basic Vegetable Stock (page 245), starting by chopping the mushrooms in a food processor. If a more flavorful stock is desired, gently reduce the liquid after straining until the correct concentration is achieved.

Roasted Mushroom Stock

This brown mushroom stock roasts cremini mushrooms, which are darker than button mushrooms, to color the liquid. Roasted mushrooms have a meaty flavor, making this stock an ideal substitute for an animal stock.

ACTIVE TIME: ½ hour | TOTAL TIME: 2½ hours (including roasting, heating, simmering, and initial cooling) | YIELD: Makes about 3 quarts (2.8 liters)

1½ pounds (680 g) cremini mushrooms,
    including stems
½ pound (225 g) white onions, cut into small dice
1 pound (455 g) leeks, dark green parts
    removed, cut into small dice
½ pound (225 g) carrots, cut into small dice
½ pound (225 g) parsnips, cut into small dice
½ small fennel bulb, coarsely chopped,
    fronds removed

½ head garlic, unpeeled
3 tablespoons grapeseed oil
1 tablespoon dry vermouth (optional)
3 quarts (2.8 L) filtered water, cold
2 sprigs marjoram
4 sprigs flat-leaf parsley
12 black peppercorns
2 bay leaves
Sea salt to taste

Follow the cooking instructions for Roasted Vegetable Stock (page 246), adjusting the oven temperature to 375°F (190°C). If a more flavorful stock is desired, gently reduce the liquid after straining until the correct concentration is achieved.

Dried Mushroom Essence

This essence reconstitutes dried wild mushrooms to develop a woodsy broth. Olive oil is used in place of grapeseed oil to add flavor and increase viscosity. You can also blend in a small amount of white miso at the end for extra umami.

ACTIVE TIME: 1 hour | **TOTAL TIME:** 2 hours (including heating, simmering, and initial cooling) | **YIELD:** Makes about 1 quart (960 ml)

2 ounces (56 g) dried mushrooms, preferably porcini or shiitake

3 tablespoons olive oil

½ pound (225 g) white onions, cut into large dice

½ pound (225 g) leeks, dark green parts removed, cut into large dice

½ pound (225 g) carrots, cut into large dice

½ small fennel bulb, coarsely chopped, fronds removed

1 quart (960 ml) filtered water, cold, plus 1 cup hot water

2 sprigs thyme

4 sprigs flat-leaf parsley

8 black peppercorns

1 bay leaf

1 teaspoon white miso (optional)

Sea salt to taste, if necessary

Place the dried mushrooms in a fine-mesh strainer, and rinse under cold water to remove grit. Transfer the mushrooms to a bowl. Pour 1 cup hot water over the mushrooms and rest until plump, about 7 minutes. Line a strainer with cheesecloth, and pass the liquid through the strainer into a bowl. Reserve both mushrooms and soaking liquid.

While the mushrooms are reconstituting, follow the cooking instructions for Basic Vegetable Stock (page 245), reducing the quantity of water to 1 quart (960 ml) and adding the mushrooms and soaking liquid. Season the final stock with miso, or adjust with sea salt if necessary. After straining, reserve the soaked mushrooms for another use.

Vegetarian French Onion Soup

For vegetarians and carnivores alike, mushroom stock is a great substitute for beef stock. This recipe transforms a basic mushroom stock into the rich foundation necessary for classic French onion soup. Tamari and dry sherry are added to enhance flavor. Take your time when caramelizing the onions! Your patience will be rewarded with a rich, silky soup that satisfies as much as the classic beef version.

ACTIVE TIME: 1 hour | **TOTAL TIME:** 2 hours (including heating and simmering) | **YIELD:** Makes 4 to 6 servings

---

2 tablespoons olive oil
2 tablespoons unsalted butter
4 large onions, thinly sliced
3 cloves garlic, thinly sliced
1 teaspoon brown sugar
½ cup (120 ml) dry white wine, such as
    Sauvignon Blanc
2 tablespoons all-purpose flour
2 tablespoons dry sherry

1½ quarts (1.4 L) Roasted Mushroom Stock
1 teaspoon tamari (optional)
4 sprigs thyme
1 bay leaf
2 cups (60 g) mustard greens
Salt and pepper
1 fresh baguette, sliced on the bias
½ cup (55 g) Gruyère or Emmentaler cheese

In a large Dutch oven or other heavy pot, heat the oil and butter over medium-high heat. When the oil begins to ripple, add the onions and stir to combine. Reduce the heat to medium-low and cook slowly, stirring frequently, until the onions are a light golden brown, about 30 minutes. Temper with a splash of water if the onions stick to the surface, and scrape any brown bits into the mixture. Do not scorch the bottom of the pan.

Stir in the garlic and brown sugar and a splash of white wine. Continue to cook until the onions are a deep golden brown, stirring often, about 20 minutes longer. Add a splash of water to prevent scorching when needed. Deglaze with the remaining wine, scraping the bottom of the pan to incorporate the crust.

Use a sieve to sprinkle the flour over the onion mixture; stir until well combined, about 1 minute. Deglaze with the sherry while stirring. Add the mushroom stock, tamari, thyme, and bay leaf. Simmer until the flavors come together, about 30 minutes. Stir in the mustard greens, and simmer until wilted. Season with salt and pepper.

While the soup is simmering, set the broiler to low. Arrange the bread on a sheet pan in a single layer. Broil until toasted. Set aside.

Portion the soup into deep, wide ramekins or oven-safe bowls. Float one or two slices of bread on the soup, and top with grated cheese. Broil until melted and golden. Serve immediately.

Matsutake-Crusted Roots on Farro Piccolo

Years ago a chef-friend taught me how to sear root vegetables as you would meat in a hot pan. I've since seen adaptations refer to the technique as Osso Buco style, indicating the charred, bone-like appearance the vegetables take on in this dish. When cut into large cylinders and on the bias, the roots will form a gradient of color—golden and crusted on the outside, creamy on the inside.

ACTIVE TIME: ½ hour | **TOTAL TIME:** 1¼ hours | **YIELD:** Makes 4 servings

ROOTS

2 pounds (910 g) mixed white roots, such as parsnips, turnips, burdock, and/or salsify, peeled

2 tablespoons olive oil

2 tablespoons unsalted butter

Salt and pepper

¼ cup (60 ml) dry red wine, such as Pinot Noir

½ cup (120 ml) Basic Mushroom Stock or Dried Mushroom Essence

1 tablespoon pulverized dried mushrooms

½ lemon, juice and zest

Slice the roots into 3-inch (7.5 cm) sections, cutting diagonally on each end. In a large, heavy skillet, melt the oil and butter over medium until hot but not smoking. Add the root vegetables in a single layer and stir to coat. Season with salt and pepper. Cook until browned on all sides, about 4 minutes. Pour in the red wine and simmer until reduced, about 2 minutes. Add the mushroom stock and mushroom powder; continue to cook, stirring occasionally, until the liquid is reduced and the vegetables are crusted. Remove from the heat and toss with the lemon juice and zest. Serve with the farro piccolo.

FARRO

2 cups (480 ml) Basic Mushroom Stock or Dried Mushroom Essence

2 tablespoons dry red wine, such as Pinot Noir

1 cup (200 g) farro piccolo

2 tablespoons unsalted butter

1 pound (455 g) cipollini onions,

blanched and peeled

½ cup (120 ml) heavy cream

¼ cup (56 g) crème fraîche

Dash cayenne pepper

Dash nutmeg

Salt and pepper

In a saucepan, bring the mushroom stock and red wine to a simmer over medium heat. Stir in the farro, cover the pan, and reduce the heat to low. Gently cook until al dente, about 40 minutes.

While the farro is cooking, melt the butter in a wide sauté pan over medium heat. Add the onions and sauté until browned on all sides, about 7 minutes. Pour in the heavy cream, reduce the heat to low, and simmer until thickened, about 10 minutes.

When the farro is done, fold in the creamed onions and stir in the crème fraîche. Season with cayenne pepper, nutmeg, salt, and pepper. Portion into bowls and top with the crusted root vegetables.

French Horn Mushroom "Steak" on Brown Butter Kamut Spaetzle

This recipe highlights the meaty texture of French horn mushrooms. Easily cultivated, this mushroom is also known as king trumpet, king oyster, or my favorite reference, trumpet royale. It is the largest species in the oyster mushroom genus, which makes it perfect for searing like a slab of steak and serving alongside the buttery goodness of spaetzle. If you cannot locate French horn mushrooms, look for a similarly large, dense variety, such as matsutake or porcini.

Spaetzle, dumplings common to southern Germany and Alsace, are formed by pushing a soft egg dough through a slotted cheese grater into simmering liquid until they cook through and float to the top. The spaetzle in this recipe are simmered in mushroom stock, which is then reserved for a sauce, naturally thickened from the gluten of the dough. There is little more comforting than eating a bowl of fresh spaetzle with a glass of Alsatian wine!

ACTIVE TIME: 1 hour | **TOTAL TIME:** 1 hour | **YIELD:** Makes 4 servings

SPAETZLE

¾ cup (180 ml) whole milk

3 eggs

1 teaspoon sea salt

Dash nutmeg

2 cups (240 g) kamut flour, or all-purpose flour

2 cups (480 ml) Roasted Mushroom Stock

½ cup (115 g) unsalted butter

Splash vermouth (optional)

Salt and pepper

2 tablespoons freshly snipped chives

In a blender, pulse the milk, eggs, salt, and nutmeg until combined. Add the flour and blend until smooth. Transfer to a bowl and hold at room temperature.

In a medium stockpot, bring the mushroom stock to a boil. Working in batches, press the batter through a slotted grater into the boiling liquid and simmer until cooked, about 2 minutes per batch. Transfer the cooked spaetzle with a strainer into a bowl; cover to maintain heat. Repeat with the remaining batter. Reserve some of the cooking liquid to coat the spaetzle.

In a large, heavy skillet, cook the butter over medium heat until fragrant and golden brown, about 4 minutes. Add the spaetzle and 2 tablespoons cooking liquid; toss to combine. Deglaze with a splash of vermouth, if desired. Season with salt and pepper. Fold in the snipped chives.

MUSHROOMS

1 pound (455 g) French horn mushrooms, or similarly large mushrooms, such as matsutake or porcini
Salt and pepper
2 tablespoons olive oil

2 small shallots, minced
1 clove garlic, minced
¼ cup (60 ml) Roasted Mushroom Stock
Splash vermouth (optional)

Slice the mushrooms into thick 1-inch (2.5 cm) cross sections, about two or three slices per mushroom. Season with salt and pepper on both sides. Set aside at room temperature while the pan heats.

Heat the olive oil in a heavy skillet until hot but not smoking. Stir in the shallots and garlic and cook until translucent, about 2 minutes. Add the mushrooms in a single layer and sauté until they release their liquid, about 3 minutes. Deglaze the pan with stock and vermouth; simmer until the liquid is reduced and the mushrooms caramelize. Serve immediately with the spaetzle.

SQUASH

Summer squash—simmered in butter with loads of spring onions—was one of my favorite childhood comfort foods. My mother used to make a salty, overcooked version, and I would greedily eat the whole pot when no one was looking. This section offers a refined approach to this adolescent indulgence: Summer squash is developed into a light, brightly flavored stock, and winter squash is dehydrated to coax clear, concentrated sugars into the liquid. Squash stock can be used as a neutral base or in place of chicken stock.

Summer Squash Stock

This stock combines yellow crookneck squash with sautéed onions to develop a sugary, buttery foundation. Vidalia onions, available in the warmer months, are a sweet variety that matches well with summer squash. They have more water than most other onions and take longer to brown in the pan. Spanish onions are an acceptable substitute; with less water content, they cook faster than Vidalia onions. Be certain to stir the onions often and remove before they caramelize in the pan: The goal is to add onions with their flavor, not their color, coaxed out in order to maintain the lemon-yellow hue from the squash.

ACTIVE TIME: ½ hour | **TOTAL TIME:** 1¼ hours (including heating and simmering) | **YIELD:** Makes about 1 quart (960 ml)

---

1 tablespoon olive oil

2 tablespoons unsalted butter

½ pound (225 g) onions, preferably Vidalia, cut into small dice

1 pound (455 g) leeks, dark green parts removed, cut into small dice

2 cloves garlic

1½ pounds (680 g) yellow summer squash, sliced

1 quart (960 ml) filtered water, cold

2 thyme sprigs

1 bay leaf

Sea salt to taste

1 tablespoon fresh lemon juice

In a medium stockpot, heat the olive oil and butter over medium heat. When the oil begins to ripple, add the onions and cook until softened, about 3 minutes. Add the leeks and garlic and continue to sauté while stirring, about 4 minutes longer. Cook until translucent; do not brown the onions.

Add the squash and stir until combined. Pour in the water, adding enough to cover the squash, if necessary, and add the herbs to the pot. Maintain the heat for a gentle simmer, and cook until the squash has melted into the liquid, about 30 minutes.

Turn off the heat and rest the stock on the stove, about 10 minutes. Place a fine-mesh strainer on the lid of a container large enough to hold the liquid contents of the pot. Line the strainer with cheesecloth. Ladle the mixture from the pot into the strainer. Discard the herbs and reserve the solids for another use (for instance, a simple purée). Line the strainer with cheesecloth and repeat the straining process with the liquid.

If a more concentrated flavor is desired, return the stock to a clean pot and simmer until reduced. Taste and season with salt. Finish the stock with lemon juice. Chill the stock in the refrigerator, stirring occasionally to expedite the cooling process. Refrigerate for up to 2 days or freeze in smaller containers for longer storage.

Winter Squash Stock

This stock is made by dehydrating winter squash to intensify sweetness. The drying process makes the squash sturdy, which prevents it from breaking down quickly and helps maintain clarity in the stock.

ACTIVE TIME: 1 hour | **TOTAL TIME:** 10 hours (including dehydrating, heating, and simmering) | **YIELD:** Makes about 2 quarts (1.9 liters)

---

3 pounds (1.4 kg) winter squash,
  such as butternut, delicata, or acorn,
  halved
¼ cup (60 ml) grapeseed oil, divided
½ pound (225 g) white onions, cut into
  small dice
1 pound (455 g) leeks, dark green parts
  removed, cut into small dice
1 pound (455 g) carrots, cut into small dice

½ small fennel bulb, coarsely chopped,
  fronds removed
½ head garlic, unpeeled
2 quarts (1.9 L) filtered water, cold
2 sprigs thyme
8 black peppercorns
1 bay leaf
4 sprigs flat-leaf parsley
Sea salt to taste

Preheat the oven to its lowest temperature setting, preferably 150°F (65°C) and no more than 170°F (75°C).

Carefully slice the squash into 1-inch (2.5 cm) thick half-moons, keeping the seed structure intact. In a large bowl, toss the squash slices with 2 tablespoons grapeseed oil. Place in a single layer on one or two parchment-covered sheet trays. Bake until dry to the touch, about 8 to 10 hours, turning once in the middle of the cooking time. Turn off the oven and cool on the rack.

In a medium stockpot, heat the remaining grapeseed oil over medium heat. When the oil is hot, add the vegetables and cook while stirring, until soft but not brown, about 7 minutes. Add the water, thyme, peppercorns, and bay leaf to the pot; add more water to cover the vegetables, if necessary. Maintain the heat for a gentle simmer, skimming the surface as soon as scum appears. Cook until the liquid is golden and flavorful, about 45 minutes. Add the parsley and simmer for another 5 minutes.

Turn off the heat and rest the stock on the stove, about 10 minutes. Line a fine-mesh strainer with cheesecloth and set it on the lid of a container large enough to hold the liquid contents of the pot. Carefully ladle the stock from the pot into the strainer, leaving any cloudy liquid at the bottom of the pot. Discard the solids.

If a more concentrated flavor is desired, return the stock to a clean pot and simmer until reduced. Taste and season with salt. Chill the stock in the refrigerator, stirring occasionally to expedite the cooling process. Refrigerate for up to 2 days or freeze in smaller containers for longer storage.

Tortilla Española with Txakoli Wine Sauce

Tortilla Española comes with legendary origin. First documented in 1817, this dish was referenced in an anonymous letter to the Navarra court, a complaint that the people of Pamplona were eating a decadent omelet while farmers had nothing to eat. Another tale of its origin is credited to a general during the Carlist wars, when the dish started to spread in popularity.

Whatever its history, Tortilla Española has been adopted around the world. At its base, it is a simple dish akin to a potato omelet, yet some chefs shy from tradition and apply their own interpretation—say, an adjustment in size or the addition of ingredients. This variation starts by blanching sliced potatoes in a stock sweetened with squash, which infuses flavor for the final frying stage. The blanching liquid, naturally thickened from the potato starch, is then reduced to form the base of the sauce, to which an acidic wine is added. Txakoli, a refreshing wine from the Basque Country, is recommended, as the remainder of the bottle is an excellent accompaniment to the tortilla. If you cannot locate Txakoli wine, look for another crisp white varietal from Spain.

ACTIVE TIME: 1 hour | TOTAL TIME: 1¼ hours | YIELD: Makes 6 to 8 servings

TORTILLA

2 cups (480 ml) Summer Squash Stock
4 large russet potatoes, peeled and
    thinly sliced

⅓ cup (80 ml) olive oil
2 medium yellow onions, thinly sliced
4 eggs

In a medium stockpot, bring the squash stock to a boil over medium-high heat. Blanch the potatoes until tender, about 7 minutes. With a slotted spoon, transfer the potatoes to a sheet pan in a single layer. Refrigerate until cold, about 2 hours. Reserve 2 tablespoons potato-squash water for the sauce and use the remainder to thicken soups and stews (see "Thicken as Needed," page 101).

In a large sauté pan, heat the olive oil over medium heat and add the onions, stirring to coat. Cook the onions until translucent, about 5 minutes. Add the potatoes and cook on both sides, gently turning once or twice, to warm through, about 2 minutes. Remove the pan from the heat.

In a separate bowl, beat the eggs until frothy. With a slotted spoon, transfer the potatoes and onions from the pan into the eggs. Hold while the pan heats.

Return the sauté pan to the stove and heat over medium. When hot but not smoking, pour in the egg-and-potato mixture, spreading the potatoes evenly across the pan. Cook until the bottom begins to brown, gently shaking the pan to prevent sticking, about 4 minutes.

Slide a spatula around the edge of the tortilla to ensure that it stays together. When the bottom is set, using oven mitts, place a plate over the pan and quickly turn the pan over so the tortilla falls onto the plate. If the pan is dry, add a small amount of oil. Gently slide the tortilla back into the pan to cook the other side. Cook until the eggs are set, another 3 minutes. Remove from the heat and rest for a few minutes. Transfer to a plate and hold at room temperature until ready to serve.

SAUCE

2 tablespoons olive oil
1 medium shallot, minced
1 clove garlic, minced

1 cup crisp white wine, preferably Txakoli
Zest of 1 lemon
Salt and pepper

In a small saucepan, heat the olive oil over medium heat. Add the shallot and garlic and cook until translucent, about 3 minutes. Add the wine and simmer until reduced by a third. Pour in the reserved 2 tablespoons of the potato-squash water, and continue to simmer until thickened, about 3 minutes. Stir in the lemon zest and season with salt and pepper. Strain the sauce, and serve with wedges of the tortilla.

Tagine of Kabocha Squash and Lemon Confit with Green Couscous

Tagine is a classic Moroccan dish named after its cooking vessel—an earthenware pot with a conical lid that flavors food during a long, slow cook. Tagine is so intrinsic to Moorish culture that seasoned pots are given to newlyweds as a symbol of long-lived unity.

In Morocco, couscous is rolled by hand, but this recipe calls for the store-bought variety that you will rub with herb oil after it is cooked. Look for fine couscous, the type that exhibits small irregular grains, often identified as Moroccan (as opposed to Israeli or Italian). Don't be shy when rubbing the herb oil into the grain! The couscous should reveal a lovely green hue when properly blended by hand.

The lemon confit benefits from being made well in advance; the confit recipe makes more than the tagine calls for. Also known as preserved lemons, the confit holds well when packed and sealed in jars. Alternatively, you can use store-bought preserved lemons if you don't have time to make them at home.

ACTIVE TIME: 1½ hours | **TOTAL TIME:** 5+ days
(including fermentation, simmering, and steaming) | **YIELD:** Makes 4 to 6 servings

CONFIT

3 lemons, scrubbed

3 tablespoons kosher salt, plus more for jar

Trim the ends from each lemon without exposing the flesh. One by one, rest each lemon on a cutting board, cut-side up, and quarter it without cutting through the base. Sprinkle each lemon with 1 tablespoon kosher salt, making certain to reach the interior. One at a time, place each lemon in a mason jar, sprinkle with more salt, and with a wooden spoon, muddle until juice is released. Continue the layering, salting, and muddling process until the lemons reside below the brine, adding salt as necessary. Cover the jar and rest in a dark spot at room temperature, at least 5 days and up to 1 month. Store in the refrigerator to stop the fermentation process, and rinse well before using.

TAGINE

1 cup (220 g) dried chickpeas, soaked overnight
3 tablespoons olive oil
2 medium onions, diced
2 cloves garlic, minced
1 teaspoon ground turmeric
1 teaspoon ground coriander
1 teaspoon ground cumin
½ teaspoon ground cinnamon
½ teaspoon crushed red pepper

2 medium carrots, diced
1 large kabocha squash, peeled and diced
2 cups (480 ml) Winter Squash Stock, divided
½ teaspoon saffron threads, toasted and ground
½ cup (64 g) dried apricots, diced
½ confited lemon, rinsed and minced, from above
¼ cup (15 g) cilantro leaves
Salt and pepper

Place the chickpeas in a saucepan and cover with salted water. Over medium heat, bring the chickpeas to a boil and simmer until tender, about 30 minutes. Drain and set aside.

In a heavy sauté pan, heat the olive oil over medium heat. Add the onions and cook until translucent, about 4 minutes. Stir in the garlic and spices and continue to cook until the onions begin to caramelize, another 6 minutes.

Add the carrots and squash and cook until tender, about 4 minutes.

Dissolve the saffron in the squash stock. Add the stock, apricots, and confited lemon to the pan. Reduce the heat to medium-low, cover, and simmer for 20 minutes. Fold in the chickpeas and warm through, another 10 minutes. Sprinkle with cilantro and season with salt and pepper, to taste.

COUSCOUS

1 tablespoon unsalted butter
1 clove garlic, minced
1 cup (200 g) fine couscous
1¼ cups (300 ml) Winter Squash Stock, divided

Sea salt to taste
½ cup (30 g) flat-leaf parsley leaves
½ cup (30 g) mixed herbs, such as thyme, basil, and chives

In a medium saucepan, melt the butter with the garlic over medium heat. Add the couscous and stir to coat, about 2 minutes. Pour in 1 cup squash stock and enough sea salt to taste; bring to a boil. Cover the pan and turn off the heat. Rest for 10 minutes.

While the couscous is steaming, place the parsley and herbs with the remaining stock in a blender. Blend until smooth. Uncover the steamed couscous and fluff with a fork. With your hands, mix the herb mixture into the couscous until the grain takes on a green hue. Serve with the tagine.

Pasta with Spaghetti Squash, Fried Peppers, and Bread Crumbs

This recipe is adapted from my favorite Southern Italian pasta dish. Traditionally made without stock, the sauce relies on flavorful oil enhanced with dried chilies and anchovies. Stock is used here to enhance the sauce and as a supplement to pasta water.

At the risk of offending the tradition of an Italian grandmother, you can eliminate the pasta entirely to make a side dish with spaghetti squash only. Likewise, you can omit the squash to arrive at a more authentic bowl of pasta. This recipe yields a healthy quantity, great for a family meal.

ACTIVE TIME: 1 hour | **TOTAL TIME:** 2 hours (including roasting and simmering) | **YIELD:** Makes 4 to 6 servings

---

½ small spaghetti squash, seeded
2 tablespoons olive oil
¼ cup (60 ml) olive or avocado oil, divided
1 cup (80 g) day-old crusty bread, cubed and toasted
6 dried mild chilies, such as guajillo or pasilla, stemmed and seeded
1 anchovy, minced

3 cloves garlic, thinly sliced
2 pints (550 g) yellow cherry tomatoes, halved
⅓ cup (80 ml) Winter Squash Stock
1 teaspoon white balsamic vinegar
Salt and pepper
1 pound (455 g) pasta, such as orecchiette or strascinati

Preheat the oven to 400°F (200°C). Rub the squash half with 2 tablespoons olive oil and season with salt. Place the squash on a sheet pan, flesh-side down, and roast until tender, about

45 minutes. Using a fork, gently scrape out the flesh, separating it into long strands. Transfer to a bowl, cover, and set aside.

Place the toasted bread cubes in a food

processor and pulse into coarse crumbs. In a heavy saucepan, combine 2 tablespoons olive oil with the bread crumbs and stir over medium heat until golden, about 7 minutes. Transfer to a bowl.

Wipe the skillet clean with a kitchen towel. Heat the remaining oil and add the chilies, stirring to avoid scorching them. Toast on both sides. Using tongs, transfer the chilies to a bowl. When cool enough to handle, tear into large pieces and reserve.

In the same skillet, smash the anchovy with a wooden spoon. Stir in the garlic slices and cherry tomatoes, tossing in the pan until the tomatoes release their juices, about 7 minutes. Carefully stir in the spaghetti squash. Add the stock and simmer until thickened, about 2 minutes. Add the vinegar and season with salt and pepper.

While the sauce is simmering, make the pasta. Bring a medium stockpot of salted water to a rolling boil. Add the pasta; cook until al dente, about 8 minutes. Using tongs, transfer the pasta to the skillet with the sauce. Add a splash of pasta water to loosen up the sauce if necessary.

Portion the pasta into bowls or serve it family style. Garnish with fried chilies and bread crumbs and serve immediately.

TOMATOES

Though technically a fruit, tomatoes deserve acknowledgment in a book about culinary foundation. Not the tomatoes bred of industrial agriculture—the bland, plastic ones we find in many supermarkets today. Instead, it is the tomato that is truly fresh from vine, perhaps thin of skin and not suitable for long-distance travel. These tomatoes have history innate to their seeds, an undeniable acidity differentiated by variety, and a juiciness that runs down your chin with every greedy bite.

One could argue that stock made from tomatoes is as simple as straining liquid from a pot of blanched tomatoes. By following the process of making a classic stock, however, a sophistication can be achieved: A clear tomato stock is delicate enough to blend into the background of cocktails without overpowering other ingredients, and a fire-roasted tomato stock is bold enough to guide spicy Italian dishes. At the end of the season, when the sun begins to subside and green tomatoes are abundant, you can make a green tomato stock that is light and acidic—ideal for many late-summer soups. Go one step further, and reserve the spent tomatoes from these recipes to make tomato sauce or ketchup.

Basic Tomato Stock

This basic tomato stock serves as a light foundation for any dish or cocktail that would benefit from the color and acidity of the fruit, such as a delicate broth to be accompanied by meat or fish or a classy tomato-based cocktail where clarity of liquid is warranted. It is best made when tomatoes are in season—bright and bulbous, fresh from the vine. Aim to use heirloom tomatoes for this recipe; they have a thin skin that bursts forth with delicious fruit. A small amount of anchovy, though optional, will add umami to the base. For a richer stock, stir in a dash of tomato paste alongside the quartered tomatoes.

ACTIVE TIME: ½ hour | **TOTAL TIME:** 1½ hours (including heating and simmering) | **YIELD:** Makes about 2 quarts (1.9 liters)

2 tablespoons olive oil

½ pound (225 g) white onions, cut into small dice

1 pound (455 g) leeks, dark green parts removed, cut into small dice

½ small fennel bulb, coarsely chopped, fronds removed

½ pound (225 g) carrots, cut into small dice

1 teaspoon oil-packed anchovies (optional)

4 pounds (1.8 kg) tomatoes, quartered

2 quarts (1.9 L) filtered water, cold

½ head garlic, unpeeled

2 sprigs marjoram

4 sprigs flat-leaf parsley

1 bay leaf

12 black peppercorns

Sea salt to taste

In a medium stockpot, heat the olive oil over medium heat. When the oil is hot, add the onions, leeks, and fennel and cook until softened, about 5 minutes. Add the carrots and optional anchovies and continue to cook while stirring, about 4 minutes longer. Stir in the tomato and cook until combined, about 1 minute.

Make an herb sachet by wrapping the herbs and peppercorns in cheesecloth and securing with butcher's twine. Add the sachet, garlic, and filtered water; slowly bring to a gentle boil. Add more water to cover the vegetables, if necessary.

Raise the heat until the water begins to tremble, then lower the heat to maintain a gentle simmer, skimming the surface as soon as scum appears. Gently simmer for 45 minutes. Be careful not to boil, or the tomatoes will become grainy and cloud the liquid.

Turn off the heat and rest the stock on the stove, about 10 minutes. Line a fine-mesh strainer with cheesecloth and set it over a container large enough to hold the liquid contents of the pot. Carefully ladle the stock from the pot into the strainer, leaving any cloudy liquid at the bottom of the pot. Discard the sachet and garlic, and reserve the tomato base for another use.

If a more concentrated flavor is desired, return the stock to a clean pot and simmer until reduced. Taste and season with salt. Chill the stock in the refrigerator, stirring occasionally to expedite the cooling process. Refrigerate for up to 2 days or freeze in smaller containers for longer storage.

Green Tomato Stock

This stock makes use of unripe tomatoes, lending flavor and color that are both green. Roasted garlic introduces a sweetness that counters the immaturity of the fruit. It is a wonderful base for split pea soup with ham.

ACTIVE TIME: ¾ hour | **TOTAL TIME:** 2¼ hours (including roasting, heating, and simmering) | **YIELD:** Makes about 2 quarts (1.9 liters)

---

1 head garlic

2 tablespoons olive oil, divided

2 ounces (58 g) pancetta, cubed (optional)

½ pound (225 g) white onions, cut into small dice

1 pound (455 g) leeks, dark green parts removed, cut into small dice

½ small fennel bulb, coarsely chopped, fronds removed

½ pound (225 g) parsnips, cut into small dice

4 pounds (1.8 kg) green tomatoes, coarsely chopped

2 quarts (1.9 L) filtered water, cold

2 sprigs marjoram

4 sprigs flat-leaf parsley

1 bay leaf

12 black peppercorns

Sea salt to taste

Preheat the oven to 350°F (175°C).

Slice the top off the head of garlic to expose the cloves. Place the garlic head on a sheet of aluminum foil, drizzle with 1 tablespoon olive oil, and seal loosely. Bake in the oven until cloves are tender but not caramelized, about 40 minutes. Remove from the oven and set aside.

Place a medium stockpot over medium heat. When the pot is hot, add the cubed pancetta and cook until rendered, about 2 minutes. Pour in the remaining olive oil and add the onions, leeks, and fennel; cook until softened, about 5 minutes. Add the parsnips and continue to cook while stirring, about 4 minutes longer. Stir in the green tomatoes and cook until warmed through but not browned, about 3 minutes.

Make an herb sachet by wrapping the herbs and peppercorns in cheesecloth and securing with butcher's twine. Add the sachet, garlic, and filtered water; slowly bring to a gentle boil. Add more water to cover the vegetables, if necessary.

Raise the heat until the water begins to tremble, then lower the heat to maintain a gentle simmer, skimming the surface as soon as scum appears. Gently simmer for 45 minutes. Be careful not to boil, or the tomatoes will become grainy and cloud the liquid.

Turn off the heat and rest the stock on the stove, about 10 minutes. Line a fine-mesh strainer with cheesecloth and set it over a container large enough to hold the liquid contents of the pot. Carefully ladle the stock from the pot into the strainer, leaving any cloudy liquid at the bottom of the pot. Discard the sachet and garlic, and reserve the tomato base for another use.

If a more concentrated flavor is desired, return the stock to a clean pot and simmer until reduced. Taste and season with salt. Chill the stock in the refrigerator, stirring occasionally to expedite the cooling process. Refrigerate for up to 2 days or freeze in smaller containers for longer storage.

Fire-Roasted Tomato Stock

The char on the tomatoes deepens color and heightens flavor in this stock recipe. I recommend Roma tomatoes here: They have thick skins that hold their shape and retain juices when roasted. The vegetables are sautéed instead of roasted in order to preserve and highlight the roasted tomato flavor. Use this stock in any dish that would benefit from fire-roasted tomatoes, adding a dash of vinegar should you want to approximate the canned variety, which has a slightly more acidic flavor.

ACTIVE TIME: 1 hour | **TOTAL TIME:** 2 hours
(including roasting, heating, and simmering) | **YIELD:** Makes about 2 quarts (1.9 liters)

---

4 pounds (1.8 kg) whole Roma tomatoes
2 medium white onions, halved with skin on
1 pound (455 g) leeks, dark green parts
    removed, cut into small dice
½ pound (225 g) carrots, cut into small dice
½ small fennel bulb, coarsely chopped,
    fronds removed
½ head garlic, unpeeled
1 teaspoon oil-packed anchovies (optional)

2 quarts (1.9 L) filtered water, cold
2 sprigs marjoram
4 sprigs flat-leaf parsley
12 black peppercorns
1 bay leaf
Sea salt to taste
Special equipment:
    Natural hardwood charcoal, if using an
    outdoor grill

In a charcoal grill, arrange the charcoals in the basin, light, and burn until they are covered with ash. Alternatively, preheat a gas grill with the lid on, or set an indoor broiler to high.

If using a grill, place the whole tomatoes on the grate over the central heat source and the halved onions on the grate over indirect heat. Using tongs, turn the vegetables as they begin to cook. Grill until the tomatoes are blistered on all sides and the onion begins to caramelize. Be careful not to overcook the tomatoes; too much

heat will make them burst, and too much char will discolor the stock. Transfer the tomatoes and onions to a bowl. If using an indoor oven, broil the tomatoes and onions until blistered, about 15 minutes, turning once or twice throughout the cook time.

To complete, follow the cooking instructions for Basic Tomato Stock (page 269), using the roasted tomatoes and onions in place of the uncooked varieties. The stock will be darker with a smoky flavor.

ABOUT TOMATO PASTE

Tomato paste is tomato purée that has been cooked for several hours to produce a thick concentrate. The seeds and skins are removed to render a silky and glossy finish. Many brown stocks call for the addition of tomato paste, which deepens flavor and brightens hue.

Store-bought tomato paste often includes corn syrup or citric acid to increase its shelf life. This recipe offers a healthier homemade alternative, using honey as the sweetener. Packed and sealed in jars, this tomato paste will last indefinitely. If you don't have time to make your own, look for a store-bought variety that lists tomatoes as the only ingredient.

HONEYED TOMATO PASTE

ACTIVE TIME: 1 hour | **TOTAL TIME:** 6 hours (including simmering and baking)
| **YIELD:** Makes about 2 cups (480 ml)

---

8 pounds (3.6 kg) red tomatoes, ripe
2 tablespoons olive oil, plus more
    for packing

⅓ cup (115 g) honey
2 bay leaves
1 tablespoon sea salt

Core and halve the tomatoes. Remove the seeds with your fingers or a spoon. In a medium stockpot, add the tomatoes and the olive oil. Over medium heat, bring the tomatoes to a simmer and cook until softened and juices are released, about 40 minutes. Remove from the heat and cool slightly.

Outfit a food mill with a fine disk and place over a bowl. Pass the tomatoes through the mill. Return the tomatoes to a clean pot; add the honey, bay leaves, and sea salt. Bring to a gentle simmer over medium heat and reduce until thick, stirring often, about 1 hour. If the mixture sputters, place a splatter guard over the pot. Be careful not to scorch the sauce.

Heat the oven to 250°F (120°C). On an oiled baking sheet, spread the tomato purée into a thin, even layer. Bake until the purée becomes thick and tacky, stirring every 20 minutes, about 3 hours total. Remove from the oven and cool to room temperature. Transfer to jars and top with a thin layer of olive oil to prevent discoloration. Keep in the refrigerator, up to 1 month, or for long-term storage process in a water bath canner. Consult the manufacturer's guide of your water bath canner for detailed operating instructions.

Pissaladière Niçoise with Smoked Tomatoes and Dandelion Greens

An old breakfast dish from Nice, *pissaladière* is a savory tart with caramelized onions and anchovies. The origins of the name are Latin—loosely *pissalat* in Niçard, which means "salted fish." This version incorporates smoked grape tomatoes and their respective stock, a pleasant foil to the creamy onions and pungent anchovies.

ACTIVE TIME: 1½ hours | **TOTAL TIME:** 2½ hours (including resting and baking) | **YIELD:** Makes 8 to 12 servings

PASTRY

½ teaspoon sugar
1 teaspoon active dry yeast
¾ cup (180 ml) warm water

2 tablespoons lard, melted, or olive oil
1 teaspoon sea salt
2 cups (240 g) bread flour

In a mixing bowl, sprinkle the sugar and yeast over ½ cup of the warm water. Stir until dissolved. Let stand in a warm place until foamy, about 5 minutes. Add the remaining water, lard, salt, and flour. Mix with a wooden spoon until combined. Transfer to a lightly floured surface. Knead until smooth, about 7 minutes. Split the dough in half and place each half in a lightly oiled bowl. Cover and rest in a warm place until doubled in size, about 1 hour.

TOPPINGS

1 pint (275 g) grape tomatoes
1 cup (90 g) smoking chips, such as applewood, soaked in water
¼ cup (60 ml) olive oil
2 pounds (910 g) yellow onions, thinly sliced
3 cloves garlic, thinly sliced
1 cup (30 g) fresh dandelion greens, trimmed

and coarsely chopped
½ cup (120 ml) Fire-Roasted Tomato Stock
Splash aged sherry vinegar
Salt and pepper
24 Niçoise olives, pitted and halved
12 anchovy fillets
1 tablespoon fresh thyme leaves

While the dough is resting, smoke the tomatoes and prepare the filling. In a stovetop smoker, heat the wood chips, covered, over medium heat, until they start to smoke, about 10 minutes. Reduce the heat to low, place the tomatoes in the smoker, and replace the cover. Smoke for about 15 minutes. Remove the tomatoes and rest at room temperature.

In a heavy skillet, heat the olive oil over medium heat. Add the onions and cook, stirring, until they begin to brown, about 12 minutes. Stir in the garlic and continue to cook, about 5 minutes. When the onions are light brown and creamy, fold in the dandelion greens with the tomato stock. Simmer until the greens are wilted and the liquid is reduced, about 1 minute. Finish with a splash of sherry vinegar and season with salt and pepper.

TO ASSEMBLE: Preheat the oven to 425°F (220°C). Lightly oil two half-sheet pans or round pizza pans. Roll each dough ball to fit each pan. Prick the dough with a fork, cover with plastic wrap, and let rise again, about 30 minutes.

Spread the onion mixture on the dough and arrange the tomatoes, olives, and anchovies in a decorative pattern across the top. Bake the pissaladière until cooked through and the crust is golden brown, about 25 minutes. Garnish with fresh thyme. Season with salt and pepper. Using a pizza cutter, slice into wedges and serve warm or at room temperature.

Chile-Marinated Poached Sturgeon with Herbed Rice Grits

Poaching fish in bouillon is a wonderful way to infuse flavor and maintain moisture. The poaching liquid here is brightened with red wine vinegar, spiced with ancho chilies, and sweetened with tomato and honey. Heavily regulated due to its popularity for both meat and eggs, sturgeon is among the most reliable fish to source.

If you can't locate rice grits—broken rice that comes from milling fragile grains—then make your own. Pulse semi-frozen long-grain rice in a spice mill until coarse, then sift to remove dust. What remains in the sifter can be used in any recipe that calls for rice grits.

ACTIVE TIME: ½ hour | **TOTAL TIME:** 1¼ hours
(including marinating, poaching, and simmering) | **YIELD:** Makes 4 servings

STURGEON

3 tablespoons red wine vinegar, divided
1 tablespoon ancho-chili powder
1 pound (455 g) sturgeon, farm-raised in
    closed tanks, cut into 4 portions
1 cup (240 ml) Basic Tomato Stock

Salt and pepper
1 tablespoon honey
2 tablespoons unsalted butter
1 tablespoon olive oil

In a small bowl, mix 1 tablespoon vinegar with the ancho-chili powder. Sprinkle the portioned sturgeon with the mixture and refrigerate until absorbed, about 20 minutes.

In a medium saucepan, bring the remaining vinegar, tomato stock, and honey to a boil. Season with salt. Reduce the heat, add the sturgeon fillets, and seal with a lid. Poach the fish until nearly cooked through, about 9 minutes. With a slotted spoon, transfer the fish to a plate and tent with aluminum foil. Strain the poaching liquid into a bowl.

In a small saucepan, bring the poaching liquid to a boil, then reduce the heat and maintain a simmer. Reduce to about ¼ cup (60 ml) and mount the butter, 1 tablespoon at a time, into the sauce until silky and smooth. Season with salt and pepper. Cover to keep warm and reserve.

RICE GRITS

1 quart (960 ml) Basic Tomato Stock
3 sprigs fresh thyme, plus more for garnish
1 cup (200 g) rice grits

3 tablespoons unsalted butter
1 tablespoon lemon juice
Salt and pepper

While the sturgeon is marinating, place the stock and thyme in a saucepan. Bring to a boil over medium heat, and stir in the rice grits. Reduce the heat and simmer until al dente, about 15 minutes. Drain the grits in a colander, discard the thyme, and transfer the grits to a bowl. Stir in the butter and lemon juice. Season with salt and pepper.

TO SERVE: Heat the 1 tablespoon olive oil in a heavy skillet. When hot, add the sturgeon fillets and sear on one side until golden brown, about 2 minutes. Portion the grits into bowls, top with the fish, and spoon the sauce over. Garnish with fresh thyme.

Skillet Eggs with Garlicky White Beans in Sofrito Broth

This recipe is a hearty take on *shakshuka*, a popular Israeli breakfast dish of eggs poached in spicy tomato sauce. Here white beans are cooked with garlic and pancetta and enhanced with a sofrito broth—a flavorful foundation made with sautéed vegetables—to form the base for the eggs. I suggest using green tomatoes for the stock, but you can easily substitute red ones instead. Grill some crusty bread and serve on the side for dipping.

ACTIVE TIME: ½ hour | **TOTAL TIME:** 2½ hours
(including simmering and cooking) | **YIELD:** Makes 3 to 6 servings

BEANS

1 cup (220 g) dried cannellini beans,
    soaked overnight
1 quart (960 ml) Green Tomato Stock
1 head garlic, halved

1 slice pancetta (optional)
Sea salt to taste
½ cup (30 g) finely chopped
    flat-leaf parsley

Rinse the soaking liquid from the beans. In a medium stockpot, bring the tomato stock and garlic to a boil. Add the beans, pancetta, if using, and sea salt, and lower the heat to maintain a simmer. Cook, uncovered, until the beans are al dente, about 1½ hours. Slightly cool the beans in their liquid, about 20 minutes. Drain the beans—reserving the liquid and discarding the garlic. Toss with the parsley, and hold in a bowl.

BROTH

2 medium onions, chopped
2 stalks celery, chopped
1 medium carrot, peeled and chopped

⅓ cup (80 ml) olive oil
1 anchovy (optional)
Salt and pepper

While the beans are cooling, make the sofrito. Chop the vegetables, one by one, in a food processor. In a medium stockpot, heat the olive oil until hot but not smoking. Add the vegetables and sauté until translucent, about 7 minutes. Do not brown the vegetables. Stir in the anchovy, if using, and continue to cook, another 3 minutes.

Combine the reserved bean liquid with enough cold water to yield 2 cups (480 ml). Add the broth to the sofrito mixture and continue to heat. When the liquid starts to ripple, before it breaks into a boil, lower the heat to medium and gently simmer until the flavors combine, about 15 minutes. Do not boil the liquid, or the celery will get bitter. Strain the broth into a bowl, discarding the solids, and season the broth with salt and pepper.

EGGS

6 large eggs
Salt and pepper

Parmesan cheese, for grating
Fresh basil, for garnish

In a skillet, add a thick layer of beans and pour enough broth over to create a loose sauce. Heat the beans over medium until warmed through. With the back of a large spoon, make a well in the sauce and crack an egg into the indentation.

Repeat with the remaining eggs. Cook until the whites are set and the yolks remain runny, about 15 minutes. Season with salt and pepper. Grate fresh Parmesan on top and sprinkle with a chiffonade of basil. Serve immediately.

ONIONS

Alliums are a genus of bulbous plants that reside within the lily family. This includes onions, leeks, and ramps; garlic, too, though you'll find a section below that showcases it all on its own. Sauté leeks to develop a light, buttery base, to be used like a white stock; or caramelize onions to make a sweet, dark foundation, to be used like a brown stock. The ramp stock on page 281 is intended as a special-occasion base to brighten spring dishes.

Buttery Leek Stock

This stock makes use of dark green leek tops, the part that is usually reserved for assembling a bouquet garni. It is delicate and sweet; a great match for rabbit or spring vegetables. An optional splash of sherry will round out the flavor to develop a more complex foundation.

ACTIVE TIME: ½ hour | **TOTAL TIME:** 1½ hours (including heating, simmering, and initial cooling) | **YIELD:** Makes about 2 quarts (1.9 liters)

¼ cup (60 ml) olive oil
1 tablespoon unsalted butter
2½ pounds (1.1 kg) leeks, dark green parts only, cut into small dice
1 tablespoon dry sherry (optional)
½ small fennel bulb, coarsely chopped, fronds removed
1 small celery root, peeled, coarsely chopped

1 garlic clove, smashed
¼ cup (60 ml) dry white wine, such as Sauvignon Blanc
2 sprigs marjoram
2 sprigs flat-leaf parsley
1 bay leaf
2 quarts (1.9 L) filtered water, cold
8 black peppercorns
Sea salt to taste

In a large Dutch oven or other heavy pot, heat the oil and butter over medium heat. When the oil is hot but not smoking, add the leeks and cook until translucent, stirring frequently, about 5 minutes.

Add the sherry, if using, and simmer for 30 seconds. Stir in the fennel, celery root, and garlic and cook until softened, about 5 minutes longer. Deglaze the pan with wine and simmer for 1 minute.

Make an herb sachet by wrapping the herbs in cheesecloth and securing with butcher's twine. Add the filtered water, herb sachet, and peppercorns, and slowly bring to a gentle boil. Reduce the heat to medium-low and maintain at a simmer, about 45 minutes.

Turn off the heat and rest the stock on the stove, about 10 minutes. Line a fine-mesh strainer with cheesecloth and set it over a container large enough to hold the liquid contents of the pot. Carefully ladle the stock from the pot into the strainer, leaving any cloudy liquid at the bottom of the pot. Discard the herb sachet and solids. Reserve the leek mixture for soup.

If a more concentrated flavor is desired, return the stock to a clean pot and simmer until reduced. Taste and season the liquid with salt. Chill the stock in the refrigerator, stirring occasionally to expedite the cooling process. Refrigerate for up to 2 days or freeze in smaller containers for longer storage.

Caramelized Onion Stock

Like building a good stock, coaxing sugar from an onion to achieve a syrupy caramel takes time. This stock requires slowly caramelizing the onions before adding liquid. The vinegar, sugar, and spice help balance natural sweetness from the onions.

ACTIVE TIME: ½ hour | **TOTAL TIME:** 2 hours (including heating, simmering, and initial cooling) | **YIELD:** Makes about 2 quarts (1.9 liters)

½ cup (120 ml) olive oil
2½ pounds (1.1 kg) white onions, thinly sliced
1 teaspoon sea salt, plus more to adjust
    seasoning at end
1 teaspoon brown sugar
Dash cayenne pepper
Splash balsamic vinegar
½ small fennel bulb, coarsely chopped,
    fronds removed

½ pound (225 g) parsnips, cut into small dice
1 garlic clove, smashed
½ cup (120 ml) dry white wine, such as
    Sauvignon Blanc
4 sprigs thyme
4 sprigs flat-leaf parsley
1 bay leaf
12 black peppercorns
2 quarts (1.9 L) filtered water, cold

In a large Dutch oven or other heavy pot, heat the oil over medium-high heat. When the oil begins to ripple, add the onions, 1 teaspoon sea salt, brown sugar, and cayenne pepper. Stir to combine. Reduce the heat to medium-low and cook slowly, stirring frequently, until the onions are a light golden brown, about 45 minutes. Temper with a splash of water if the onions stick to the surface, and scrape any brown bits into the mixture. Do not scorch the bottom of the pan.

Add a splash of balsamic vinegar and stir until well combined. Stir in the fennel, parsnips, and garlic, adding a small amount of water if the mixture is too dry. Cook until the vegetables are softened, about 5 minutes. Deglaze the pan with wine and simmer for 1 minute.

Make an herb sachet by wrapping the herbs and peppercorns in cheesecloth and securing with butcher's twine. Add the sachet and filtered water, and slowly bring to a gentle boil. Reduce the heat to medium-low and maintain at a simmer, about 45 minutes.

Turn off the heat and rest the stock on the stove, about 10 minutes. Line a fine-mesh strainer with cheesecloth and set it over a container large enough to hold the liquid contents of the pot. Carefully ladle the stock from the pot into the strainer, leaving any cloudy liquid at the bottom of the pot. Discard the herb sachet and reserve the onion mixture for soup.

If a more concentrated flavor is desired, return the stock to a clean pot and simmer until reduced. Taste and season the liquid with additional salt. Chill the stock in the refrigerator, stirring occasionally to expedite the cooling process. Refrigerate for up to 2 days or freeze in smaller containers for longer storage.

Ramp Stock

Ramps are wild onions found in small patches throughout the northeastern woods in springtime. Their broad leaves and firm bulbs are fragile despite a pungency reminiscent of garlic. This stock is light in body with a bright garlicky flavor, perfect for a lemony risotto. If foraging for ramps, be sure to leave some behind in order to encourage continued growth in the area.

ACTIVE TIME: ¾ hour | **TOTAL TIME:** 2 hours (including heating, simmering, and initial cooling) | **YIELD:** Makes about 1½ quarts (1.4 liters)

1 pound (455 g) ramps, trimmed, green tops
  reserved for another use
2 tablespoons olive oil
½ pound (225 g) leeks, cut into small dice
½ small fennel bulb, coarsely chopped,
  fronds removed
1 small celery root, peeled, coarsely chopped

2 tablespoons dry vermouth
2 sprigs thyme
2 sprigs flat-leaf parsley
1 bay leaf
1½ quarts (1.4 L) filtered water, cold
8 black peppercorns
Sea salt to taste

Rinse the ramp bulbs and pink stems and remove the loose outer skins. Thinly slice the bulbs and stems.

In a medium stockpot, heat the olive oil over medium heat. When the oil is hot, add the ramps, leeks, and fennel and cook until softened, about 5 minutes. Add the celery root and continue to cook, stirring, about 4 minutes longer. Deglaze with vermouth and simmer for 1 minute.

Make an herb sachet by wrapping the herbs and peppercorns in cheesecloth and securing with butcher's twine. Add sachet and filtered water to the pot. Raise the heat until the water begins to tremble, then lower the heat to maintain a gentle simmer, skimming the surface as soon as scum appears. Gently simmer for 45 minutes.

Turn off the heat and rest the stock on the stove, about 10 minutes. Line a fine-mesh strainer with cheesecloth and set it over a container large enough to hold the liquid contents of the pot. Carefully ladle the stock from the pot into the strainer, leaving any cloudy liquid at the bottom of the pot. Discard the herb sachet and reserve the ramp mixture for soup. (Soup is a great destination for the ramp greens, too!)

If a more concentrated flavor is desired, return the stock to a clean pot and simmer until reduced. Taste and season with salt. Chill the stock in the refrigerator, stirring occasionally to expedite the cooling process. Refrigerate for up to 2 days or freeze in smaller containers for longer storage.

Pastured Dairy Onion Dip with Fried Leeks

The key to this onion dip is in the source: Pastured dairy makes all the difference. In addition to being deeply nourishing, pastured dairy has an undeniable flavor—rich, creamy, sometimes nutty—highlighted here in the form of butter, buttermilk, crème fraîche, and whole yogurt.

If you can't locate all four varieties from a good source, I encourage you to adjust amounts in the recipe in favor of those you do procure. Onion dip is a forgiving recipe; aim for a consistency that stands up to a potato chip.

ACTIVE TIME: ½ hour | **TOTAL TIME:** 1½ hours | **YIELD:** Makes 6 servings

LEEKS

Peanut oil (for frying)

2 medium leeks, white and pale green parts only, thinly sliced

Heat the peanut oil in a small saucepan to 350°F (175°C). In small batches, add the leeks and fry until golden brown, about 20 seconds per batch. Remove the leeks with a slotted spoon. Repeat with the remaining leeks. Drain on a kitchen towel and reserve as garnish for the dip. Serve the same day to ensure crispiness.

DIP

1 cup (240 ml) Caramelized Onion Stock
3 tablespoons unsalted butter,
   preferably pastured
2 medium yellow onions, thinly sliced
2 medium shallots, thinly sliced
1 tablespoon fresh thyme leaves
¼ ounce (7 g) dried mushrooms, ground

2 cloves garlic, thinly sliced
Dash aged sherry vinegar
⅓ cup (80 ml) buttermilk, preferably pastured
⅓ cup (85 g) crème fraîche, preferably pastured
⅓ cup (85 g) whole yogurt, preferably pastured
Salt and pepper
2 tablespoons fresh chives, snipped, for garnish

In a saucepan, bring the stock to a boil over medium heat. Lower the heat to medium-low and reduce the liquid to a glaze, approximately 2 tablespoons, about 10 minutes.

In a large skillet, melt the butter over medium heat. Add the onions, shallots, thyme, and mushroom powder. Stir in 1 tablespoon water to prevent sticking. Cook, stirring often, until the onions begin to caramelize, about 30 minutes. Add the garlic and a splash of vinegar and continue to cook while stirring, another 15 minutes. Transfer to a blender and allow to cool.

Add the reduced stock, buttermilk, crème fraîche, and yogurt to the blender. Purée until smooth. Season with salt and pepper. Transfer to a bowl or large ramekin. Garnish with fried leeks and fresh chives.

Caramelized Celery Root and Amaranth Soup

Amaranth is an ancient flower, a perennial cultivated by the Aztecs over eight millennia ago. The Greeks named it *amarantos* for its ability to stay strong after drying. With flowers that produce grain-like buds, amaranth holds remarkable nutrition—high in minerals, easy to digest, and a great source of lysine. It is light in texture and nutty in flavor; often used dry in muesli or moistened to thicken soups and stews.

This recipe simmers amaranth in stock as the base for the soup. Simmering the flower buds in chicken stock builds an exceptional foundation for the introduction of celery root and leek stock. Vegetable stock or water can be used as a substitute for cooking the amaranth.

ACTIVE TIME: ¾ hour | **TOTAL TIME:** 8 hours (including soaking and simmering) | **YIELD:** Makes 4 servings

---

1 cup (200 g) amaranth, uncooked
1 teaspoon apple cider vinegar
4 cups (960 ml) Basic Chicken Stock or Basic Vegetable Stock, divided
2 tablespoons olive oil
1 tablespoon unsalted butter
1 large onion, chopped
1 large leek, sliced
1 large celery root, cubed

½ cup (120 ml) dry white wine, such as Sauvignon Blanc
3 cups (720 ml) Buttery Leek Stock
2 sprigs marjoram
1 tablespoon lemon juice
Sea salt and white pepper
Greek yogurt or crème fraîche, for garnish
Lemon zest, for garnish

Place the amaranth and vinegar in a bowl; cover with water. Soak for at least 6 hours, or overnight. Rinse the grains. In a medium saucepan, bring 2½ cups (600 ml) chicken stock to a boil. Add the amaranth, cover, and reduce the heat to medium-low. Simmer for 25 minutes, or until the liquid has been absorbed. Remove from the heat and keep covered until needed.

In a small stockpot, heat the olive oil and butter over medium until hot but not smoking. Add the onion and leek and cook until translucent, about 4 minutes. Stir in the celery root and continue cooking, another 4 minutes. Deglaze the pan with wine and simmer, about 1 minute. Stir in the remaining chicken stock, leek stock, and marjoram; simmer until the celery root is tender and the liquid is slightly reduced, about 20 minutes.

Carefully transfer the hot soup to a blender in batches; blend until smooth. Return to the pot over low heat. Stir in the lemon juice and season with salt and pepper.

TO SERVE: Spoon the soup into bowls and top with a healthy portion of amaranth. Garnish with yogurt and lemon zest.

Yellow Split Pea Cakes with
Poached Duck Eggs and Ramp Soubise

In addition to being delicious, yellow split peas—hulled and halved field peas—are very good for you. I learned the significance of these tiny legumes during an Ayurvedic cleanse called Panchakarma. Unlike many cleanses, which emphasize an elimination of food, Panchakarma relies on the consumption of restorative foods to help maintain strength. Rich in dietary fiber and protein, yellow split peas play a key role in achieving nutritional balance.

This recipe introduces a dairy-rich soubise—a classic sauce similar to béchamel with puréed onions—and is not suggested for a restorative cleanse. Still, yellow split peas and eggs, especially duck eggs, are a protein powerhouse, making this a wonderful breakfast or brunch dish. Feel free to eliminate the soubise if you desire a healthier meal.

ACTIVE TIME: 1½ hours | **TOTAL TIME:** 2 hours (including chilling and simmering) | **YIELD:** Makes 4 servings

---

YELLOW SPLIT PEA CAKES

1 cup (240 ml) Basic Chicken Stock or
 Parmesan Broth
1 cup (240 ml) Ramp Stock
1 bay leaf
1 cup (225 g) yellow split peas
Dash sea salt
1 duck egg, or 2 chicken eggs

2 medium leeks, white and pale green
 parts only, minced
¼ cup Parmesan, grated
Salt and pepper
1 cup (110 g) panko or dried
 bread crumbs
3 tablespoons olive oil

In a medium saucepan, bring both stocks and the bay leaf to a boil over medium heat. Add the split peas and a dash of sea salt and cook until al dente, about 20 minutes. Strain, reserving the stock. Hold the split peas in a bowl and return the stock to the saucepan. Bring the stock to a simmer and reduce to 2 tablespoons. Toss the reduced stock with the split peas; set aside.

In a medium bowl, whisk the egg until frothy. Fold in the split peas, leeks, and Parmesan until incorporated. Season with salt and pepper. Chill in the refrigerator until firm, about 1 hour.

SOUBISE

2 tablespoons unsalted butter
1 large onion, thinly sliced
1 bunch ramps, tops trimmed and reserved

1 cup (240 ml) raw heavy cream
Salt and pepper
Dash nutmeg

While the split pea mixture is chilling, melt the butter in a medium saucepan over medium heat. Add the onion, ramp bulbs, and 1 tablespoon water; cook until softened, stirring frequently, about 15 minutes. Be careful not to brown the onion mixture. Stir in the heavy cream and continue to simmer until thickened, about 7 minutes. Season with salt, pepper, and a dash of nutmeg.

Transfer the onion mixture to a blender. Pulse until combined, then blend until smooth. For a finer texture, pass through a fine-mesh strainer, or simply transfer to a bowl. Cover and keep warm.

TO FINISH: Remove the split pea mixture from the refrigerator. Form into four cakes and roll in the panko. Heat the olive oil in a heavy skillet over medium until hot but not smoking. Add the split pea cakes, being careful not to crowd the pan, and fry until brown, about 3 minutes on each side. Transfer to a plate and keep warm while poaching the eggs.

EGGS

1 cup (240 ml) Basic Chicken Stock,
    Parmesan Broth, or water
1 tablespoon white wine vinegar

4 duck or chicken eggs
Ramp greens, from above
Smoked paprika, for garnish

Bring the stock and vinegar to a gentle boil in a medium saucepan. Lower the heat to maintain a gentle simmer. One at a time, crack an egg in a bowl, stir the liquid in the pan, and gently slide the egg into the liquid. Repeat with the remaining eggs, stirring to prevent sticking. Cook until the white is opaque and the yolk is still runny, about 5 minutes for duck eggs and 3 minutes for chicken eggs. With a slotted spoon, carefully transfer the eggs to a bowl. While the liquid is still boiling, add the ramp greens and blanch until wilted, about 1 minute. Drain, reserving the stock for another use.

TO SERVE: Spoon the soubise on plates. Place a spoonful of the ramp greens on the sauce, then top with a split pea cake. Gently place an egg on each cake. Season with salt and pepper. Garnish with a dash of smoked paprika.

GARLIC

Despite its natural pungency, garlic has range—from bulb to stalk, young or aged. This section explores garlic in every stage of its life: Scapes are snipped from bulbs early in the season; dried heads are slowly caramelized to achieve a blackened depth. At every step, garlic shows us a unique characteristic; here each stage is imparted to stock. Stocks made with scapes or confit add a soft, savory note to dishes, whereas those made with aged or roasted garlic introduce a pleasant sweetness. Use hardneck varieties, young or cured, to develop a stock when the assertiveness of garlic benefits a dish.

Garlic Scape Stock

Garlic scapes are the stalks that grow from hardneck garlic plants, which are cut off a few weeks before the harvest to encourage last-minute growth. Look for stalks that have closed buds on top; flowering buds tend toward a bitter flavor. Light in body and bright in aroma, this stock is ideal for introducing a clean garlic note to spring dishes.

ACTIVE TIME: ½ hour | **TOTAL TIME:** 1¼ hours (including heating, simmering, and initial cooling) | **YIELD:** Makes about 1 quart (960 ml)

---

1 quart (960 ml) filtered water, cold
24 garlic scapes, green shoots
  coarsely chopped, flower buds reserved
  for another use

2 sprigs thyme
2 bay leaves
8 black peppercorns
Sea salt to taste

Place the water, garlic scapes, herbs, and peppercorns in a small stockpot. Turn the heat to medium and slowly bring to a gentle boil, skimming the surface if any scum appears. Lower the temperature and gently simmer for 45 minutes.

Turn off the heat and rest the stock on the stove, about 10 minutes. Set a fine-mesh strainer over a container large enough to hold the liquid contents of the pot. Line the strainer with cheesecloth. Carefully ladle the stock from the pot into the strainer, leaving any cloudy liquid at the bottom of the pot. Discard the herbs and reserve the garlic scapes for soup.

If a more concentrated flavor is desired, return the stock to a clean pot and simmer until reduced. Taste and season with salt. Chill the stock in the refrigerator, stirring occasionally to expedite the cooling process. Refrigerate for up to 2 days or freeze in smaller containers for longer storage.

Green Garlic Stock

This recipe uses garlic that has been plucked from the ground in early spring. At first, green garlic appears as a spring onion and later develops into a bulb with soft skin. Both can be used here, though the latter is preferable. This stock imparts a mild, sweet flavor to your spring dishes.

If you cannot locate green garlic, or if it is too late in the season to pick from your garden, use cured garlic; this is the type of garlic that is most common in supermarkets. Remove the bitter green germ growing through the center of each clove before chopping the garlic. Crushing garlic releases more flavor into the liquid as well as health-boosting compounds.

ACTIVE TIME: ½ hour | **TOTAL TIME:** 1½ hours (including heating, simmering, and initial cooling) | **YIELD:** Makes about 1½ quarts (1.4 liters)

---

3 heads garlic, preferably young with stalks attached
2 tablespoons grapeseed oil
¼ pound (115 g) white onions, cut into small dice
½ pound (225 g) leeks, cut into small dice, 1 or 2 whole leaves reserved for a bouquet garni
½ small fennel bulb, coarsely chopped, fronds removed

¼ pound (115 g) parsnips, cut into small dice
½ cup (120 ml) dry white wine, such as Sauvignon Blanc
2 sprigs thyme
2 sprigs flat-leaf parsley
1 bay leaf
1½ quarts (1.4 L) filtered water, cold
8 black peppercorns
Sea salt to taste

Remove the loose outer skins from the garlic heads and break into individual cloves. With a mallet, smash the unpeeled cloves, no more than once each, and set aside in a bowl. Coarsely chop the garlic stalks, if using.

In a medium stockpot, heat the oil over

medium heat. When the oil is hot, add the onions, leeks, and fennel, and cook until translucent, about 4 minutes. Add the garlic cloves, optional stalks, and parsnips and continue to cook, stirring, about 4 minutes longer. Deglaze with white wine and simmer for 1 minute. Be careful not to brown the vegetables.

Make a bouquet garni by nestling the herbs in the green exterior of one leek and securing with butcher's twine. Add the water, bouquet garni, and peppercorns to the pot. Raise the heat until the water begins to tremble, then lower to maintain a gentle simmer, skimming the surface as soon as scum appears. Gently simmer for 45 minutes.

Turn off the heat and rest the stock on the stove, about 10 minutes. Line a fine-mesh strainer with cheesecloth and set it on the lid of a container large enough to hold the liquid contents of the pot. Carefully ladle the stock from the pot into the strainer, leaving any cloudy liquid at the bottom of the pot. Discard the solids.

If a more concentrated flavor is desired, return the stock to a clean pot and simmer until reduced. Taste and season with salt. Chill the stock in the refrigerator, stirring occasionally to expedite the cooling process. Refrigerate for up to 2 days or freeze in smaller containers for longer storage.

Aged Garlic Stock

Also known as *black garlic*, aged garlic is the result of a Maillard reaction: Whole heads of garlic are slowly caramelized until the cloves turn black and tacky. Aged garlic is sweet like soft caramel and complex like tamarind. It is said to harness twice the antioxidants of cured garlic. Use this stock to add sweetness to a dish, to develop a marinade for meat, or (reduced) to build a pan sauce.

ACTIVE TIME: ½ hour | **TOTAL TIME:** 2 hours (including roasting, simmering, and initial cooling) | **YIELD:** Makes about 1½ quarts (1.4 liters)

---

3 heads aged garlic
¼ pound (115 g) white onions, cut into
    small dice
½ pound (225 g) leeks, cut into small dice, 1 or
    2 whole leaves reserved for a bouquet garni
¼ pound (115 g) parsnips, cut into small dice
½ small fennel bulb, coarsely chopped,
    fronds removed

3 tablespoons olive oil
2 sprigs thyme
2 sprigs flat-leaf parsley
1 bay leaf
1½ quarts (1.4 L) filtered water, cold
12 black peppercorns
1 teaspoon light soy sauce or tamari
Sea salt to taste

Preheat the oven to 350°F (175°C).

Remove the loose outer skins from the garlic and set aside. Break the heads into individual cloves and reserve with the skins.

In a large bowl, toss the onions, leeks, parsnips, and fennel with the olive oil. Spread the vegetables in a single layer over two sheet pans. Roast for 45 minutes, stirring occasionally.

Transfer the vegetables to a medium stockpot, scraping the pan with a spatula to loosen brown bits. Make a bouquet garni by nestling the herbs in the green exterior of one leek and securing with butcher's twine. Add the water, black garlic, garlic skins, bouquet garni, and peppercorns to the pot; add more water to cover the vegetables, if necessary. Slowly bring to a gentle boil, then lower the heat to maintain a simmer, skimming the surface as soon as scum appears. Cook for 45 minutes.

Turn off the heat and rest the stock on the stove, about 10 minutes. Line a fine-mesh strainer with cheesecloth and set it on the lid of a container large enough to hold the liquid contents of the pot. Carefully ladle the stock from the pot into the strainer, leaving any cloudy liquid at the bottom of the pot. Discard the solids. Reserve the garlic mixture for soup.

If a more concentrated flavor is desired, return the stock to a clean pot and simmer until reduced. Taste and season with soy sauce or tamari; add sea salt to balance, if necessary. Chill the stock in the refrigerator, stirring occasionally to expedite the cooling process. Refrigerate for up to 2 days or freeze in smaller containers for longer storage.

Roasted Garlic Stock

The process of roasting garlic tames its raw pungency and brings out its sweetness. Amber in color, roasted garlic makes a great stock that can be used for fondue pots—broth or cheese—and other dishes where a clean, sweet garlic flavor is beneficial.

ACTIVE TIME: ½ hour | TOTAL TIME: 2 hours (including roasting, heating, simmering, and initial cooling) | YIELD: Makes about 1½ quarts (1.4 liters)

3 heads garlic

3 tablespoons olive oil, divided

¼ pound (115 g) white onions, cut into small dice

½ pound leeks (225 g), cut into small dice, 1 or 2 whole leaves reserved for a bouquet garni

½ small fennel bulb, coarsely chopped, fronds removed

1 small celery root, peeled, coarsely chopped

½ cup (120 ml) fruity red wine, such as Gamay

2 sprigs thyme

2 sprigs flat-leaf parsley

1 bay leaf

1½ quarts (1.4 L) filtered water, cold

12 black peppercorns

Sea salt to taste

Preheat the oven to 350°F (175°C).

Slice the top off the head of garlic to expose the cloves. Place on a sheet of aluminum foil and drizzle with 1 tablespoon olive oil. Wrap in the foil and roast until garlic is tender but not caramelized, about 40 minutes. Remove from the oven and cool. When cool enough to touch, squeeze out the garlic cloves, reserving the papery shells.

In a medium stockpot, heat the remaining olive oil over medium heat. When the oil is hot, add the onions, leeks, and fennel, and cook until translucent, about 4 minutes. Add the celery root and continue to cook while stirring, about 4 minutes longer. Deglaze with red wine and simmer for 1 minute.

Make a bouquet garni by nestling the herbs in the green exterior of one leek and securing with butcher's twine. Add the water, roasted garlic cloves and skins, bouquet garni, and peppercorns to the pot. Raise the heat until the water begins to tremble, then lower to maintain a gentle simmer, skimming the surface as soon as scum appears. Gently simmer for 45 minutes.

Turn off the heat and rest the stock on the stove, about 10 minutes. Line a fine-mesh strainer with cheesecloth and set it over a container large enough to hold the liquid contents of the pot. Carefully ladle the stock from the pot into the strainer, leaving any cloudy liquid at the bottom of the pot. Discard the solids. Reserve the garlic mixture for soup.

If a more concentrated flavor is desired, return the stock to a clean pot and simmer until reduced. Taste and season with salt. Chill the stock in the refrigerator, stirring occasionally to expedite the cooling process. Refrigerate for up to 2 days or freeze in smaller containers for longer storage.

Garlic Confit Broth

This recipe makes use of bulk, peeled garlic cloves. A slow confit tempers the sharp bite of fresh garlic without introducing too much sugar. This broth is rich, golden, clean, and clear: ideal for a soup base or a hot pot brimming with fresh vegetables.

ACTIVE TIME: 1 hour | **TOTAL TIME:** 2½ hours (including heating, simmering, and initial cooling) | **YIELD:** Makes about 1½ quarts (1.4 liters)

1½ cups (360 ml) olive oil
48 cloves garlic
¼ pound (115 g) white onions, cut into small dice
½ pound (225 g) leeks, cut into small dice

½ small fennel bulb, coarsely chopped, fronds removed
1 small celery root, peeled, coarsely chopped
1½ quarts (1.4 L) filtered water, cold

½ cup (120 ml) dry white wine, such as
    Sauvignon Blanc
2 sprigs thyme
2 sprigs flat-leaf parsley

1 bay leaf
12 black peppercorns
Sea salt to taste

In a small saucepan, add the olive oil and garlic cloves. Heat on medium-low—just below a simmer, with bubbles coming to the surface but not breaking—until the cloves are soft but not browned, about 1 hour. Turn off the heat and cool. Carefully strain the garlic cloves from the oil; hold the cloves in the strainer while preparing the vegetables. Reserve the oil for another use.

Follow the cooking instructions for Green Garlic Stock (page 288), using the garlic confit in place of the raw garlic cloves. After straining, reserve the garlic confit for another use.

Garlic Scape Skordalia and Brown Butter Beet Greens on Rye Toast

Skordalia is a Greek potato and garlic dip often served with beets. This adaptation introduces garlic scapes to the spread and features beet greens in the final presentation. I recommend serving roasted beets—sliced and simply dressed with rich olive oil—alongside the spread. You can assemble the ingredients as a tartine or serve in ramekins on a platter.

ACTIVE TIME: ¾ hour | **TOTAL TIME:** 1 hour (including simmering and chilling) | **YIELD:** Makes 4 to 6 servings

SKORDALIA

1 pound (455 g) Yukon gold potatoes, peeled
    and halved
2 cups (480 ml) Garlic Scape Stock
2 garlic scapes, chopped

1 cup (115 g) walnuts, toasted
½ cup (120 ml) olive oil
1 lemon, juiced and zested
Salt and pepper

Place the potatoes in a saucepan and cover with garlic stock. Over medium heat, slowly bring the liquid to a boil, reduce to maintain a simmer, and cook until the potatoes are tender, about 15 minutes. Turn off the heat, cover, and hold until the potatoes are soft enough to be milled but not mushy. Strain; reserve the poaching liquid. With a food mill, or in the bowl of a standing mixer, mix the potatoes until smooth. Transfer to a large bowl and keep warm.

In a food processor, pulse 1 cup poaching liquid with the garlic scapes until a paste forms. Add the walnuts and pulse until combined. Fold the nut mixture into the warm potatoes. With a wooden spoon, stir the potato mixture while gradually adding the olive oil in a slow stream until the oil is fully incorporated. Add the lemon juice and zest. Season with salt and pepper. Cover and chill until ready to serve.

GREENS

2 tablespoons unsalted butter
1 tablespoon coconut oil
1 cup (38 g) beet greens, stems and leaves
    separated and chopped individually

1 clove garlic, minced
½ cup (120 ml) garlic-potato broth, reserved
    from above

In a small skillet, melt the butter with the coconut oil over medium heat until hot but not smoking. Add the chopped beet green stems and cook until al dente, about 1 minute. Stir in the chopped leaves and garlic with the reserved garlic-potato broth; cook until reduced and thickened, about 2 minutes longer. Season with salt and pepper. Cover and keep warm.

TOASTS

1 clove garlic, halved
½ loaf dense rye bread, thinly sliced

2 tablespoons unsalted butter, melted

Set your broiler to high. With your hands, lightly swipe an exposed garlic clove across each slice of bread. Brush melted butter on both sides of the bread. Broil until brown and toasted, about 1 minute each side.

TO SERVE: Slather a generous scoop of skordalia on each slice of warm toast and top with wilted greens. Alternatively, serve the skordalia and beet greens in individual ramekins with toasts on the side.

Broth-Steamed Spring Artichokes
with Black Garlic Sauce

Spring arrives late in the Hudson Valley. A short-lived perennial, artichokes require the hands of a farmer who knows how to protect this thistly plant from intense cold. Luckily, the valley has very dedicated farmers, and artichokes sometimes make a local appearance.

Do your best to locate young, delicate artichokes and rich, aged garlic for this recipe. The bright yellow-green of the artichokes offers a striking contrast to the black-caramel garlic cloves, both vegetal and sweet on the palate. If you have time, make your own preserved lemons. See Tagine of Kabocha Squash and Lemon Confit, page 265, for instructions on preserving lemons.

ACTIVE TIME: ½ hour | **TOTAL TIME:** ¾ hour (including heating and simmering) | **YIELD:** Makes 4 to 6 servings

ARTICHOKES

2 cups (480 ml) Roasted Chicken Stock
1 cup (240 ml) Aged Garlic Stock
½ cup (120 ml) dry white wine, such as
    Sauvignon Blanc
2 tablespoons olive oil

2 lemons, halved
2 bay leaves
1 teaspoon lemon juice or apple cider vinegar
12 spring artichokes
Salt and pepper

Place the stocks, wine, oil, lemons, and bay leaves in a large stockpot. Set over medium heat and bring to a gentle boil.

While the broth is heating, prepare the artichokes. Add the vinegar to a large bowl of water. Cut the artichoke stems on the bias, about 1 inch (2.5 cm) from the base. Remove any tough petals from the surface of each artichoke. Hold the prepared artichokes in the vinegar-water until the stock comes to a boil.

Add the artichokes to the boiling stock, then reduce the heat to maintain a simmer. Cook until the artichokes are tender, about 30 minutes. With a slotted spoon, transfer the artichokes to a bowl, cover, and keep warm. Reduce the poaching liquid to ½ cup (120 ml), and reserve for the sauce.

SAUCE

12 cloves black garlic
2 tablespoons preserved lemon, rind only,
 chopped

Reduced poaching liquid, from above
2 tablespoons unsalted butter,
 room temperature

Place the black garlic cloves and preserved lemon into a blender; pulse until combined. Gradually add the warm poaching liquid and blend until smooth. Transfer the warm sauce to a bowl. Mount with butter, stirring until melted, and whisk until frothy.

TO SERVE: Season the artichokes with salt and pepper. Serve the sauce on the side for dipping.

SEAWEED

Kelp—the largest subgroup of seaweed—forms vast forests within ocean waters and serves as nursery and feeding ground for many sea creatures. Easily cultivated, edible kelp has long been used as a food source in Japan, Korea, and China; only recently has it gained popularity in America. Also known as *kombu*, kelp is known to be dense with nutrients and effective for reducing blood cholesterol and hypertension.

The key to making stock with kelp is to gently coax natural glutamates into water. No heat is applied to a basic kelp stock, and only a short, gentle heat is used to further develop dashi. Both stocks are full in body, slightly sweet, and pleasantly salty. With the introduction of bonito flakes, dashi has a stronger taste of the sea than kelp on its own. You can use dashi to feed bone stocks, especially pork or lamb, enhancing the depth of flavor. Kelp also contains an enzyme that makes beans more digestible; kelp stock is an ideal foundation for cooking beans.

If possible, locate edible kelp from a local and/or domestic source, such as those found in Maine. If unavailable, look for high-quality imported kelp, preferably *ma-kombu* or *rishiri-kombu*, in the Asian section of your supermarket. These varieties have thick, wide leaves and possess a subtle sweet and salty characteristic. To ensure a rich, clear stock, seek out yellowish brown kelp instead of dark brown or black kelp; the latter tend toward a slippery texture and inky hue when simmered in water.

Kelp Stock

This stock can be used on its own for soups and stews or as the foundation for dashi. It is mildly salty and pleasantly sweet. Reserve the kelp for a secondary extraction or slice for use in other dishes.

ACTIVE TIME: ½ hour | **TOTAL TIME:** 8 hours (including soaking) | **YIELD:** Makes about 2 quarts (1.9 liters)

---

1 ounce (28 g) dried kelp sheets (*ma-kombu* or *rishiri-kombu*)

2 quarts (1.9 L) filtered water, cold

Gently wipe the kelp sheets with a moist, clean kitchen towel to remove surface impurities. Do not remove the white residue—it is dense with minerals and flavor! Using scissors, cut the kelp into smaller pieces. Place the water and kelp in a medium stockpot. Cover the pot and place it in the refrigerator overnight.

The next morning, line a fine-mesh strainer with cheesecloth and set it over a container large enough to hold the liquid contents of the pot. Carefully pour the stock from the pot into the strainer, leaving any cloudy liquid at the bottom of the pot. Reserve the kelp for a secondary batch of dashi or julienne for a rice dish.

Refrigerate for up to 3 days or freeze in smaller containers for longer storage.

Dashi

Dashi is an essential stock used in Japanese cooking. It is simply kelp stock enhanced with bonito flakes, which produces a liquid that speaks of the sea. Briny and viscous, dashi is the building block for miso soup and can be used to poach fish or glaze vegetables. Combine dashi with pork or seafood stocks to deepen the flavor of the foundation.

ACTIVE TIME: ½ hour | **TOTAL TIME:** ¾ hour (including simmering) | **YIELD:** Makes about 2 quarts (1.9 liters)

1 batch (2 quarts [1.9 L]) Kelp Stock, from above

¼ cup (3 g) high-quality bonito flakes (*katsuobushi*)

In a medium stockpot, slowly heat the Kelp Stock over medium heat until the liquid begins to tremble. Add the bonito flakes and swirl the liquid to distribute the flakes without force. When the stock simmers, turn off the heat and rest the liquid, about 10 minutes.

Line a fine-mesh strainer with cheesecloth and set it over a container large enough to hold the liquid contents of the pot. Carefully ladle the stock from the pot into the strainer, leaving any cloudy liquid at the bottom of the pot. Reserve the bonito flakes for a secondary batch of dashi.

Chill the stock in the refrigerator, stirring occasionally to expedite the cooling process. Refrigerate for up to 3 days or freeze in smaller containers for longer storage.

Korean Seaweed Soup

Known as *miyeokguk* in Korea, this seaweed soup is commonly made with wakame, a dried kelp known to be high in magnesium, potassium, and dietary fiber. This soup is both celebratory and cleansing in Korean culture, often consumed on birthdays and by women who are recovering from childbirth.

ACTIVE TIME: ¼ hour | **TOTAL TIME:** 1 hour (including simmering) | **YIELD:** Makes 4 servings

---

¼ cup (5 g) dried wakame
2 cups (480 ml) filtered water, cold
2 cups (480 ml) Kelp Stock
2 tablespoons toasted sesame oil, divided
12 fresh shiitake, thinly sliced

1 small jalapeño, thinly sliced (optional)
2 cloves garlic, thinly sliced
2 teaspoons tamari
1 teaspoon high-quality fish sauce
2 cups (340 g) cooked brown rice
Salt and pepper

Soak the dried wakame in 2 cups water until reconstituted, about 30 minutes. Strain, reserving the seaweed water. Slice the wakame and set aside.

In a medium saucepan, heat 1 tablespoon sesame oil until hot but not smoking. Add the shiitake and cook while stirring, until the mushrooms release their liquid, about 3 minutes. Add the jalapeño, if desired, and sauté another 2 minutes. Stir in the garlic and cook, about 1 minute longer.

Add the reserved seaweed water and Kelp Stock. Bring to a boil and maintain on medium-high heat for 5 minutes. Season the broth with tamari and fish sauce. Add the wakame to the pot, reduce the heat, and simmer another 15 minutes.

Spoon the brown rice into serving bowls. Top with shiitake-seaweed broth and drizzle with the remaining sesame oil. Season with salt and pepper. Serve hot.

Shabu Shabu with Sesame Milk Dashi

Shabu shabu is a Japanese dish named after the swishing sound the broth makes when meat is stirred in the cooking pot. Similar to *sukiyaki* in flavor, but not in style, shabu shabu is delivered to the table in pieces: A ceramic hot pot, called *donabe*, of dashi is accompanied by thinly sliced meat and a selection of dipping sauces.

Don't forget to participate in the customary end to the meal, called *shime*! When all the meat is consumed, add any remaining rice to the hot pot; the beef-enriched broth will soak up the grains and offer a delicious finale. The sesame milk is also exceptional on its own or as part of a tonic, as illustrated in Chicken Sesame Milk Sipping Broth (page 328).

ACTIVE TIME: 1 hour | **TOTAL TIME:** 8 hours (including soaking and simmering) | **YIELD:** Makes 4 to 6 servings

SESAME MILK

½ cup (71 g) hulled white sesame seeds

2 cups (480 ml) filtered water, cold

Soak the sesame seeds in water for at least 1 hour or overnight. Drain and transfer the seeds to a blender. Add the water and blend until emulsified. Strain, reserving both the liquid and the solids. The sesame milk keeps in the refrigerator for about 1 week; freeze the solids and use in other recipes (such as baked goods).

SESAME MILK DASHI

1 quart (960 ml) Dashi
2 tablespoons sake
8 fresh shiitake, thinly sliced
8 leaves napa cabbage

4 scallions, sliced on the bias
1 cup (240 ml) Sesame Milk, from above
2 tablespoons white miso

In a medium Dutch oven, gently heat the Dashi and sake over medium heat until the liquid trembles. Add the shiitake, napa cabbage, and scallions; simmer for 10 minutes. Stir in the sesame milk and gently heat through, another 5 minutes. Dissolve the miso into the broth. Cover to keep warm. The liquid should be hot enough to cook the beef but not so hot that the broth separates.

DIPPING SAUCE

1 tablespoon white miso
2 teaspoons brown sugar
1 tablespoon light soy sauce

2 teaspoons rice vinegar
2 tablespoons water
Toasted sesame seeds

Combine all ingredients except the sesame seeds in a small bowl. Whisk until combined.

Serve in one or more small bowls with the sesame seeds on top.

TOPPINGS

½ pound (225 g) sirloin beef, preferably grass-fed
½ cup (30 g) chrysanthemum leaves, blanched (optional)

1 block (455 g) silken tofu, cubed
3 cups (510 g) cooked sticky white rice

Place the sirloin in a covered container and chill in the freezer, about 30 minutes, or while making the broth. This step will allow for easier slicing of the beef.

Remove the sirloin from the freezer and slice into thin strips. Place the strips between two sheets of plastic wrap and pound with a meat hammer.

Arrange the sirloin in a decorative manner on a platter. Top with the chrysanthemum leaves.

Spoon the rice and tofu into serving bowls. Place the sirloin platter and dipping sauce on the table. Bring the Dutch oven to the center of the table, remove the cover, and instruct your guests to dip the sirloin in the hot broth to cook.

CHAPTER TWELVE

Dairy Bases and Dishes

In most kitchens, it's a stretch to refer to bases made with dairy as stock. Classic French technique typically reserves milk and cream for sauces. Nevertheless, I believe dairy has a place as a foundation: When stripped of its solids, milk turns into whey, a slightly cloudy, protein-rich liquid that blends well with poultry, seafood, legumes, and vegetables. Whey also works well as a structural cooking component when combined with other stocks, such as pork, chicken, fish, and vegetable. Extracting the delicate, nutty flavor from cheese rinds also produces a delicious base. This section examines how to make the most from cooking with dairy—using whey and cheese as a mechanism for extending ingredients and enhancing dishes in your kitchen.

The careful approach with which you select meat, fish, and produce should also be applied to sourcing quality dairy products. Most milk is pasteurized as a means to destroy bacteria and prevent separation; advocates of pasteurization claim that this process does not reduce its nutritional value. Raw milk, by contrast, is bottled at the farm, often from pastured animals, contains no additives, and boasts a richer, sweeter flavor profile. Due to its lack of processing and fears about the spread of bacteria, it is illegal to sell in some areas and heavily regulated elsewhere—in some states, you can only purchase it straight from the farm. There are a few studies that point to health benefits of drinking raw milk, and the claims, as with bone broths, are striking—from curing asthma to autism. Some people who are lactose-intolerant claim they can drink raw milk without reaction. Nevertheless, more research is required and encouraged to support these hypotheses; after all, raw milk is delicious and often comes from happy animals. Regardless of treatment process, seek out milk that is produced within your region and from animals that are raised on grass and without added hormones.

Cheese, too, should be purchased with care. When seeking out cheese made in Italy, such as Parmesan, look for the *Denominazione di Origine Protetta* label. This label translates to "Protected Designation of Origin," and applies to special products that abide by Italian standards of production. Many cheeses that are made in the United States and labeled as Parmesan are false imitations. They often contain additives, such as potassium sorbate and cheese cultures, that are not found in authentic Parmesan. In recent history, some commercially available shredded versions of the cheese have been identified as containing wood pulp—labeled as cellulose powder—used to prevent clumping in the package and to reduce manufacturing costs. In addition to containing additives, cheese that is grated for purchase quickly loses its aroma, flavor, and freshness. As a general rule, it is better to buy cheese in block form and to grate it by hand before use.

WHEY

Whey, the liquid that remains when solids are removed from milk, is not technically stock, yet its composition is more than suitable as a foundation. Whey is traditionally used as a culture starter for lacto-fermentation and as a thickener in cultured dairy. You may know it as the liquid that rises above your yogurt, for example. Whey is also often fed to pigs on small farms. Nevertheless, the physical structure of whey, with its high protein content, makes it excellent as a base—to be matched with fish fumet in a seafood stew or as a rich component in vegetarian dishes.

The whey recipes in this book employ cow's milk in various formats—pasteurized and raw, as well as cultured. You can also make whey with other types of milk, such as sheep's or goat's milk. I encourage you to experiment with these types of whey in your cooking, too. In addition to producing whey, all of these recipes yield cheese curds. You can make ricotta simply by adding a dash of salt to the curds or paneer by weighting it in the refrigerator overnight.

Basic Whey

This whey is separated from curd by introducing lemon juice to warm cow's milk. You can use pasteurized milk, preferably organic, or from a trusted source. Do not use ultra-high-temperature (UHT) pasteurized milk, as the process interferes with the protein structure of the milk and prevents separation. The curds can be used to make ricotta.

ACTIVE TIME: ½ hour | **TOTAL TIME:** 1 hour (including simmering and draining) | **YIELD:** Makes about 2 cups (480 ml)

---

2 quarts (1.9 L) organic whole cow's milk, not ultra-high-temperature pasteurized

⅓ cup (80 ml) fresh lemon juice
Sea salt to taste

Clip an instant-read thermometer to a medium stockpot. Add the milk and turn the heat to medium. Slowly warm the milk until it reaches a temperature of 190°F (85°C). If the milk foams and starts to rise, remove the pot from the heat to prevent the milk from boiling.

When the temperature reaches 190°F (85°C), turn off the heat and stir in the lemon juice and salt. Rest the milk for a few minutes to allow the curds to separate from the whey.

Line a fine-mesh strainer with cheesecloth and set it over a container large enough to hold the liquid contents of the pot. Carefully ladle the curds and liquid from the pot into the strainer. Tie the cheesecloth to hold the curds, letting the whey drain into the pot for half an hour, or until it stops dripping. Reserve the curds for another use, such as ricotta.

Taste and season with salt. Chill the whey in the refrigerator, stirring occasionally to expedite the cooling process. Refrigerate for up to 3 days or freeze in smaller containers for longer storage.

Buttermilk Whey

This whey employs cultured buttermilk to encourage separation. Include the cream if you want a richer, thicker whey. Avoid ultra-high-temperature pasteurized milk.

ACTIVE TIME: ½ hour | **TOTAL TIME:** 1 hour (including simmering and draining) | **YIELD:** Makes about 2 cups (480 ml)

1½ quarts (1.4 L) organic whole cow's milk
1½ cups (360 ml) organic cultured buttermilk
½ cup (120 ml) organic whole cream (optional)
Sea salt to taste

Follow the cooking instructions for Basic Whey (above), replacing the lemon juice with cultured buttermilk and adding the whole cream.

Raw Milk Whey

A high-quality source is key when acquiring fresh raw milk. In the Hudson Valley, we buy raw milk directly from the farm. Some farmers store their milk in small chillers and allow residents to retrieve it on an honor system. It makes delicious whey that can be used for fermentation, and the curds can be weighted to make paneer (see Adzuki Bean Stew with Homemade Paneer and Whey Flatbread, page 307).

ACTIVE TIME: ½ hour | **TOTAL TIME:** 2 to 3 days
(including clabbering and draining) | **YIELD:** Makes about 2 cups (480 ml)

2 quarts (1.9 L) organic raw cow's milk,
preferably with cream on top

Sea salt to taste

Pour the raw milk into a clean glass container with a lid, such as a widemouthed mason jar. Screw the lid on loosely. Rest the jar, undisturbed, at room temperature for 2 to 3 days. Do not stir or shake the contents. The milk should separate into whey and curds due to the ambient temperature.

Check daily to monitor separation. If curds do not develop within 3 days, place the jar on a heat pad on its lowest setting to help aid the souring process.

Line a fine-mesh strainer with cheesecloth and set it over a container large enough to hold the liquid contents of the jar. Carefully pour the curds and liquid from the jar into the strainer. Tie the cheesecloth to hold the curds, letting it drain into the pot for half an hour, or until it stops dripping. Reserve the curds for another use, such as paneer.

Taste and season with salt. Chill the whey in the refrigerator, stirring occasionally to expedite the cooling process. Refrigerate for up to 3 days or freeze in smaller containers for longer storage.

Yogurt Whey

This probiotic whey is great to use for lacto-fermentation projects. Look for full-fat yogurt containing acidophilus, and without thickeners or stabilizers, to ensure separation.

ACTIVE TIME: ½ hour | **TOTAL TIME:** 2 to 3 days
(including clabbering and draining) | **YIELD:** Makes about 2 cups (480 ml)

---

2 quarts (1.8 kg) full-fat yogurt, not Greek-style
Sea salt to taste

Follow the cooking instructions for Raw Milk Whey, replacing the raw milk with full-fat yogurt.

Razor Clam Chowder

Jimmy's No. 43 is a legendary bar in the East Village, with a beer selection from all over the world—tulip glass often hand-delivered (with a kiss!) by Jimmy Carbone himself. Loved by the food community for his warmth and generosity, Jimmy is a boisterous advocate for farmers and activists. Many plans for an improved food system have hatched in his space.

Jimmy also hosts amateur food competitions—a long-held tradition to celebrate classic dishes, including cassoulet, brisket, and chowder. This is an adaptation of my chowder recipe—it won Judge's Choice in the 2012 chowder cook-off.

ACTIVE TIME: 1 hour | **TOTAL TIME:** 2 hours (including heating and simmering) |
YIELD: Makes 8 to 10 servings

SEAFOOD STOCK

3 cups (720 ml) filtered water, cold
2 pounds (910 g) razor clams

1 cup (240 ml) Basic Fish Fumet or
    Shellfish Stock
Salt and pepper

In a medium stockpot, bring the filtered water to a boil. Add the clams, cover, and steam until they open, about 3 minutes. Using tongs, transfer the clams to a bowl as they open. When all the clams have opened, reduce the heat to achieve a simmer and reduce the liquid by one-third. You should have 2 cups (480 ml) of clam stock.

Line a fine-mesh strainer with cheesecloth and place over a container. Strain the liquid into the container. Stir in the fish fumet. Season with salt and pepper.

CREAM BASE

2 cups (480 ml) Buttermilk Whey
½ cup (115 g) crème fraîche

1 cup (240 ml) heavy cream

In a saucepan, gently heat the whey over medium heat until the liquid trembles. Stir in the crème fraîche until fully incorporated. Remove from the heat and stir in the heavy cream.

CHOWDER

½ cup (115 g) cubed thick-cut bacon
2 medium onions, chopped
3 medium leeks, sliced
5 cloves garlic, minced
½ pound (225 g) sunchokes, cubed
½ pound (225 g) fingerling potatoes, cubed
1 pound (455 g) winter squash, preferably
    kabocha, cubed
¼ cup (56 g) unsalted butter

¼ cup (30 g) all-purpose flour
1 bay leaf
½ pound (225 g) monkfish, cubed
1 pound (455 g) scallops, side muscles
    removed, sliced on the bias
Pinch nutmeg
Pinch cayenne pepper
Salt and pepper

When the clam shells are cool enough to touch, remove the meat, chop, and reserve in a bowl. Discard the shells.

Heat a Dutch oven over medium until hot but not smoking. Add the bacon and sauté until rendered and golden, about 4 minutes.

Remove the bacon with a slotted spoon and reserve in a bowl.

Add the onions to the pan and sauté until translucent, about 4 minutes. Stir in the leeks and garlic and sauté another 3 minutes. Add the sunchokes to the pan and cook, stirring frequently, about 3 minutes. Stir in the potatoes and squash and continue cooking until al dente, another 4 minutes. Transfer the vegetable mixture to a bowl and set aside.

In the same pan, melt the butter and slowly sprinkle the flour on top while stirring. Continue stirring until the roux darkens slightly, about 2 minutes. With a whisk, gradually add the clam stock until smooth. Add the bay leaf to the pot. Return the vegetables to the pan and simmer until tender, about 10 minutes.

With a wooden spoon, slowly stir in the cream base, then add the monkfish and scallops. Lightly simmer until the seafood is cooked through and the soup thickens slightly, another 10 minutes. Stir in the chopped clams. Season with nutmeg, cayenne pepper, salt, and pepper. Garnish with bacon and serve immediately.

Adzuki Bean Stew with Homemade Paneer and Whey Flatbread

This recipe illustrates how to create cheese, bread, and stew from one primary ingredient: a quart of milk. The cheese is made by separating curds from whey, and the whey is used in place of water in the flatbread and as you would stock in the stew. Whey is also used to soak the adzuki beans, a legume that is rich in flavor and meaty in texture.

Originating from Northeast Asia, adzuki beans are also a significant source of magnesium, potassium, iron, and B vitamins. This recipe suggests soaking the adzuki beans a full day before beginning the stew—a step that encourages the legumes to begin germination, which eases digestion and enhances the bioavailability of nutrients. To gain the correct consistency, however, the beans are heated for a long time, which destroys some of the nutrients brought to the surface during the soaking period. For this reason, it is unnecessary to soak the beans until they fully sprout (see "Soaking versus Sprouting," page 160).

ACTIVE TIME: 2 hours | **TOTAL TIME:** 1 day
(including pressing, soaking, and simmering) | **YIELD:** Makes 4 to 6 servings

PANEER

1 quart (960 ml) whole cow's milk

2 tablespoons fresh lemon juice

In a large stockpot, carefully heat the milk over medium until it trembles. When the milk comes to a gentle boil, stir in the lemon juice and lower the heat to prevent scalding. Continue to stir until the curds separate from the whey.

Line a fine-mesh strainer with cheesecloth and set over a bowl large enough to hold the whey. Remove the pot from the heat and pour the contents into the strainer. Lift the cheesecloth and twist to squeeze any remaining whey from the curds into the strainer. Hold in the strainer and let drain, about 10 minutes. Reserve the whey.

Squeeze the curds in the cheesecloth into the shape of a block. Set on a plate and top with a weight or another plate. Chill until firm, at least 1 hour or overnight.

THE BEANS

1 cup (180 g) dried adzuki beans
¼ cup (60 ml) whey, from above
1 tablespoon maple syrup

1 bay leaf
1 dried chili pepper
Sea salt to taste

The day before, place the dried beans with ¼ cup whey in a bowl. Fill with water and loosely cover with a kitchen towel. Let the beans soak in a warm area for 24 hours. Drain and rinse.

Place the soaked beans in a medium stockpot with enough filtered water to cover. Add the maple syrup, bay leaf, dried chili, and some sea salt. Bring to a boil over medium heat, reduce to maintain a simmer, and cook until al dente, about 90 minutes. Skim the surface occasionally. Drain and rinse under cold water. Reserve.

FLATBREAD

2 cups (240 g) all-purpose flour
1 teaspoon baking soda
1 teaspoon sugar
½ teaspoon sea salt

¾ cup (180 ml) whey,
    from above
1 teaspoon apple cider vinegar
½ cup (120 ml) olive oil, divided

In a large bowl, combine the flour, baking soda, sugar, and salt. In a small bowl, whisk the whey and vinegar with 2 tablespoons olive oil and fold into the flour mixture. Stir until combined. Transfer the dough to a lightly floured surface and knead until smooth, about 5 minutes. Divide the dough into six balls and cover with a towel. Rest for 20 minutes.

On a lightly floured surface, roll each ball of dough into a long oval. Heat the remaining oil in a heavy skillet and fry the flatbreads until golden brown and cooked through, about 3 minutes on both sides. Keep warm.

STEW

3 tablespoons coconut oil
Paneer, from above
2 large shallots, minced
4 cloves garlic, minced
2 tablespoons minced ginger
1 teaspoon coriander, toasted and ground
1 teaspoon fennel seeds, toasted and ground
1 tablespoon cardamom seeds, toasted and ground

½ teaspoon ground turmeric
¼ teaspoon cayenne pepper
2 cups (400 g) chopped tomatoes
1 cup (240 ml) Basic Whey, from above, divided
½ cup (120 ml) coconut milk
1 bunch Swiss chard, ribs removed, chopped
Salt and pepper

In a large skillet, melt the coconut oil over medium heat. Cube the paneer and add to the hot skillet, searing until golden brown on all sides. With a slotted spoon, transfer the paneer to a bowl. Cover and reserve.

In the same skillet, add the shallots, garlic, and ginger and sauté until caramelized, about 3 minutes. Stir in the spices and continue to cook until toasted, another 3 minutes. Stir in the tomatoes, whey, and coconut milk, stirring until combined, and simmer until slightly reduced, about 15 minutes. A few minutes before serving, stir in the Swiss chard and cook until wilted, another 3 minutes. Top with the cubed paneer. Season with salt and pepper. Serve with flatbread.

AGED CHEESE

In the efficiency of an Italian kitchen, where minimal ingredients show off their quality in a composite dish, it is not uncommon to see cheese rinds floating in a pot of simmering soup. The heat of the stock slowly melts the cheese and melds into the liquid, creating a rich, silky broth. In addition to a soup base, the broth is great for making pasta sauce and simmering grains. You can also add it to cheese-laden dishes where more liquid is required, or to a dish that would benefit from enhanced umami.

Parmesan Broth

This recipe makes a clear, nutty broth that offers the essence of cheese without overwhelming your palate. Parmesan is the most common cheese suggested for a broth made with rind, but other aged types can be used, such as Pecorino, Asiago, or most other mild, hard cheese varieties. You can hoard rinds in the freezer until you have enough to make a batch.

ACTIVE TIME: ½ hour | **TOTAL TIME:** 2½ hours
(including heating and simmering) | **YIELD:** Makes about 1 quart (960 ml)

---

2 tablespoons olive oil
¼ pound (115 g) white onions, cut into
    small dice
1 head garlic, halved
½ small celery root, peeled, coarsely chopped
½ cup (120 ml) dry white wine, such as
    Pinot Grigio

2 quarts (1.9 L) filtered water, cold
1 pound (455 g) Parmesan rinds
2 sprigs thyme
2 sprigs flat-leaf parsley
1 bay leaf
12 black peppercorns
Sea salt to taste

In a medium stockpot, heat the olive oil over medium heat. When the oil is hot, add the onions and garlic. Sauté until the onions are translucent, about 5 minutes. Add the celery root and continue to cook while stirring, about 4 minutes longer. Deglaze with wine and simmer for 1 minute.

Add the water, Parmesan rinds, herbs and peppercorns to the pot. Raise the heat until the water begins to tremble, then lower to maintain a gentle simmer, skimming the surface as soon as scum appears. Stir occasionally to prevent the Parmesan from sticking to the bottom of the pot. Simmer for 2 hours, enough time for the Parmesan rinds to melt into the liquid.

Turn off the heat and rest the stock on the stove, about 10 minutes. Line a fine-mesh strainer with cheesecloth and set it over a container large enough to hold the liquid contents of the pot. Carefully ladle the stock from the pot into the strainer, leaving any cloudy liquid at the bottom of the pot. Discard the solids.

Return the stock to a clean pot and return it to a simmer. Reduce the liquid by half. Taste and season with salt. Chill the stock in the refrigerator, stirring occasionally to expedite the cooling process. Refrigerate for up to 2 days or freeze in smaller containers for longer storage.

Whole Asparagus Parmesan Soup

A version of this asparagus soup was my introduction, some twenty years ago, to using the all-of-everything in a recipe. I recall thinking how genius the idea was: Blending the woody, inedible asparagus stalks to extract flavor, and passing through a sieve to refine texture. Certainly this is learned in culinary school, and yet for me, it was the start of an education (and obsession) about culinary efficiency.

ACTIVE TIME: ½ hour | **TOTAL TIME:** 1¼ hours (including heating and simmering) |
YIELD: Makes 6 to 8 servings

2 pounds (910 g) asparagus
3 tablespoons unsalted butter
2 medium onions, sliced
1 clove garlic, minced
½ cup (120 ml) dry white wine, such as
    Pinot Grigio

3 cups (720 ml) Basic Chicken Stock
2 cups (480 ml) Parmesan Broth
4 sprigs thyme
2 tablespoons fresh lemon juice, zest reserved
    for garnish
Salt and pepper

Slice the tips from the asparagus. Using a mandolin, shave the asparagus tips by running them lengthwise across the blade. Set aside in a bowl of ice water. Coarsely chop the remaining asparagus parts, including the woody bottoms. Reserve.

In a medium stockpot, heat the butter over medium heat until melted. Add the onions and garlic and cook until translucent, about 5 minutes. Stir in the chopped asparagus, then add the wine and cook until the liquid is reduced, another

3 minutes. Add the chicken stock, Parmesan Broth, and thyme. Bring to a boil then reduce the heat to maintain a simmer, about 30 minutes.

Working in batches, carefully transfer the hot soup to a blender and purée until smooth. Place a fine-mesh strainer over the stockpot and pass the soup through to achieve a silky texture. Heat the soup on medium heat until hot; do not boil. Stir in the lemon juice and season with salt and pepper. Serve the soup in small cups garnished with shaved asparagus tips and lemon zest.

Sprouted Minestrone Soup with Prosciutto Crisps

This hearty soup is best (and better for you) when you sprout the beans. You can use any selection of beans and legumes you like, such as cannellini, mung, garbanzo, and any variety of lentils. Depending on humidity, sprouting from seed can take two to three days. When seeds are germinated, their nutrients become more available to you. The benefits are significant, including high levels of dietary fiber, antioxidants, digestive enzymes, and vitamin C.

Sprouted beans cook faster than soaked beans. Keep in mind that cooking them at high temperatures can harm the nutrients. This recipe introduces the sprouted beans as the final step, gently simmering until warmed through. If the result is too raw for your liking, you can simmer until the flavors come together.

ACTIVE TIME: 1 hour | **TOTAL TIME:** 3 days (including soaking and simmering) | **YIELD:** Makes 4 to 6 servings

CRISPS

½ cup (115 g) prosciutto, sliced

1 tablespoon olive oil

Preheat the oven to 375°F (190°C). In a small bowl, toss the sliced prosciutto with olive oil. Place the slices in a single layer on a baking sheet. Bake until the edges begin to curl, about 12 minutes. Remove from the oven and cool to achieve crispness.

SOUP

1 cup (230 g) mixed dried beans, for sprouting
3 tablespoons olive oil
½ cup (115 g) cubed pancetta or guanciale
1 medium onion, chopped
1 teaspoon cumin, toasted and ground
½ teaspoon smoked paprika
½ teaspoon ground turmeric
½ teaspoon red pepper flakes
3 cloves garlic, minced
1 medium carrot, peeled and chopped
1 medium parsnip, peeled and chopped

3 medium tomatoes, preferably fire-roasted, chopped
1 tablespoon maple syrup
2 cups (480 ml) Basic Pork Stock or Roasted Vegetable Stock
2 cups (480 ml) Parmesan Broth
1 cup (75 g) dried pasta, such as bow ties or fusilli
1 cup (160 g) thinly sliced savoy cabbage
2 tablespoons oregano, chopped
Salt and pepper
Parmesan, for garnish

Starting 3 days before you intend to eat, follow the guidelines outlined in "Soaking versus Sprouting," page 160, to sprout the dried beans. Store between kitchen towels in the refrigerator until ready to use.

In a medium stockpot, heat the oil until hot but not smoking. Add the pancetta and sauté until crisp, about 2 minutes. Stir in the onion, cumin, smoked paprika, turmeric, and red pepper flakes and cook until the onion is soft, about 4 minutes. Add the garlic, carrot, and parsnip and continue to cook, stirring, another

3 minutes. Stir in the tomatoes and maple syrup until combined, about 1 minute longer. Pour in the stock and Parmesan Broth and simmer over medium heat, about 20 minutes.

When the soup has thickened a little and become flavorful, add the dried pasta and cabbage. Continue to simmer until the pasta is al dente, another 10 minutes. Add the sprouted beans and simmer until warmed through. Stir in the oregano and season with salt and pepper. Garnish with grated Parmesan and prosciutto crisps.

CHAPTER THIRTEEN

More Cooking
with Stocks and Broths

When you have fundamental knowledge about preparing stocks and broths, your kitchen becomes a laboratory for limitless creations—from complex dishes to homemade gelatin powder. If you're anything like me, you sometimes find your home freezer stocked with more than one stock type and begin to craft ways to diminish your reserve in hopes of freeing space. Should this resonate with the state of your kitchen, this chapter will help you devise ways to use more than one stock type at a time and for more than only savory cooking.

This chapter begins with a review of classic dishes that combine multiple stock types to develop compound flavors—paella with its combination of meat and seafood, ramen with its umami-intense seaweed, mushroom, and pork profile. Desserts are included, too—broths made with fruit, confections made with grass-fed gelatin, and pastry made with animal fats, an homage to using the all-of-everything. A section on beverages introduces healthy broth-based tonics and concludes with hedonistic classic cocktails. Bouillon in its preserved form—gelatin, cubes, powder, even gummy candies—is also covered.

MIXED BROTH RECIPES

Multiple stocks are commonly combined to develop complex flavors within a unified dish. A splash of veal stock is often added to other animal stocks—its neutrality blends into the background while heightening depth of flavor. Some dishes, like paella and ramen, rely on combining stocks to acquire a signature foundation. Review the Razor Clam Chowder recipe (page 305) for an example of how to combine seafood stocks with a dairy base.

If your cooking plans involve the preparation of multiple stock types, consider how you will store them first. You can use fresh stock from the refrigerator up to a few days, or you can store it in the freezer for many months. Be sure to make time for defrosting your frozen stocks before you embark on the cooking process. See "Guidelines for Making Stocks and Broths," page 88, for storage and defrosting tips.

Grand Seafood Paella

Paella, the national dish of Spain, is a glistening rice dish that illustrates how stocks from different sources can blend to create the sublime. The origins of paella are in Valencia—where Romans introduced irrigation and Arabs brought rice—and the dish traditionally involved rabbit and snails. Today, many variations exist, such as this one, which includes clams, mussels, and scallops. The name of the dish refers to the cooking pan itself: A flat bottom, large diameter, and dimpled surface all promote even cooking, ideal for setting the *patélla* over fire.

The key to good paella is patience: Don't stir the rice after you add the stock. Your reward will be *soccarat*, a golden crust that caramelizes at the bottom of the pan, topped with moist saffron rice that has absorbed the flavors of land and sea. If you cannot find short-grain Spanish rice, such as Bomba (also known as Valencia), you can use arborio or carnaroli rice instead.

ACTIVE TIME: 1 hour | **TOTAL TIME:** 1¼ hours | **YIELD:** Makes 8 to 10 servings

4 tablespoons olive oil, divided

2 medium onions, finely chopped

4 cloves garlic, minced

2 medium tomatoes, grated

1 teaspoon smoked paprika, preferably sweet, divided

½ teaspoon red pepper flakes

Salt and pepper

¼ teaspoon saffron threads

1 cup (240 ml) dry white wine, such as Albariño

2 cups (400 g) short-grain Spanish rice, such as Bomba

2 cups (480 ml) Basic Fish Fumet

1 cup (240 ml) Lobster Stock or Shellfish Stock

1 cup (240 ml) Basic Chicken Stock

2 pounds (910 g) clams, scrubbed

1 pound (455 g) mussels, scrubbed and debearded

12 sea scallops, side muscles removed

1 cup (225 g) shelled English peas

½ cup (30 g) finely chopped flat-leaf parsley

2 lemons, cut into wedges

In a large, flat pan, heat 2 tablespoons olive oil over medium-high heat. Add the onion and cook until it begins to caramelize, about 7 minutes. Stir in the garlic and sauté for 2 minutes longer. Add the tomatoes, smoked paprika, and red pepper flakes; season with salt and pepper. Cook until reduced, stirring occasionally, about 15 minutes.

While the tomato mixture is simmering, toast the saffron threads in a small, dry pan. Cool and combine with the white wine in a small bowl. Reserve.

Add the rice to the pan and stir to combine. Toast, stirring, about 1 minute. Deglaze with the saffron-wine mixture. Pour the fish fumet and lobster and chicken stocks over the rice, making sure the liquid covers the rice. Add water to cover, if necessary. Simmer *without* stirring until half of the liquid is absorbed, about 20 minutes or until al dente. Gently shake or rotate the pan as needed to ensure even cooking of the rice. If the rice becomes dry before it is finished, add more water, but be careful to not add too much.

The goal is for the liquid to evaporate so that the top layer of rice becomes al dente while the bottom layer forms a crust.

When the rice has almost finished cooking, nestle the clams and mussels in the mixture, deep enough for the ambient heat to coax the shellfish open, about 10 minutes. Meanwhile, sear the scallops in a hot pan with the remaining oil, about 1 minute per side. Cover and reserve the scallops.

During the last few minutes of cooking, toss the peas on top of the paella to steam, and scatter the scallops across the top.

To test for the soccarat, dip the tip of a wooden spoon into the rice in a few areas. You will feel a crust forming on the bottom of the pan. If the bottom layer of rice is loose, increase the heat and continue to cook, while rotating the pan, another minute or so. Be careful not to burn the rice.

Remove paella from the heat and rest for a few minutes before serving. Garnish with parsley and lemon wedges.

Tonkotsu Ramen

My experience with making ramen has been a slow process—more of an eater's education. Chef John McCarthy, a Hudson Valley favorite, features a different type of ramen every week at his restaurant The Crimson Sparrow, serving those lucky few who arrive before the broth runs out. With wry humor, he always asks my opinion of the broth, knowing full well the lesson is mine.

Chef McCarthy uses the word *hammer* to describe the long, rapid boil of his ramen broth. This method differs from most of the stock recipes in this book—the French favor a smile to a boil. Here the difference is a cultural preference: clarifying for structure versus emulsifying for flavor. If you've ever had a perfect bowl of steaming ramen, then you know that flavor reigns supreme in this application.

ACTIVE TIME: ¾ hour | **TOTAL TIME:** 4 hours (including braising and simmering) | **YIELD:** Makes 8 servings

PORK

¼ cup (34 g) kosher salt
¼ cup (50 g) sugar

1 pound (455 g) pork belly

In a small bowl, mix the salt and sugar until combined. Nestle the pork belly in the mixture, making sure it is coated on both sides. Cover the bowl and refrigerate, about 8 hours or overnight.

Preheat the oven to 325°F (165°C). Remove the pork belly from the cure and shake off the excess salt and sugar. Place skin-side up on a baking sheet. Roast until tender, about 2½ hours.

Raise the heat to 400°F (200°C) and roast until the skin is crisp, about 15 minutes. Remove from the oven and rest before cutting, about 10 minutes. Slice the pork belly into ½-inch (1.25 cm) slices. If you intend to eat immediately, cover and reserve at room temperature. Alternatively, refrigerate the pork, covered, up to 2 days. Gently reheat the pork in the oven before serving.

BROTH

2 cups (480 ml) Kelp Stock
2 cups (480 ml) Basic Mushroom Stock
2 cups (480 ml) Basic Chicken Stock
2 cups (480 ml) Smoked Pork Stock
1 quart (960 ml) Basic Pork Stock
12 shiitake, fresh or dried

1 head garlic, halved
1 3-inch (7.5-cm) piece ginger, sliced on the bias
¼ cup (60 ml) mirin
¼ cup (60 ml) sake
½ cup (120 ml) light soy sauce
1 tablespoon brown sugar

In a large stockpot, combine all five stocks with the shiitake, garlic, and ginger. Over medium heat, slowly bring the broth to a boil and hold at a hard simmer to infuse the flavors, about 15 minutes. Strain, reserving the mushrooms. Julienne the ginger for garnish. Discard the garlic.

In a small bowl whisk the mirin, sake, light soy sauce, and brown sugar until combined. Taste the broth and season sparingly with the mirin mixture. You will have more mirin mixture than you need. Cover the broth to maintain warmth.

TO SERVE

1 pound (455 g) fresh ramen noodles
1 bunch tatsoi, leaves separated
1 cup (120 g) sliced bamboo shoots
12 shiitake, from broth step above, thinly sliced

1 bunch scallions, thinly sliced on the bias
8 eggs, poached
8 sheets nori

Bring a pot of water to a boil. Add the noodles and cook until al dente, about 4 minutes. Drain.

With tongs, divide the noodles among eight serving bowls. Pour enough broth into the bowls to cover the noodles. Arrange the tatsoi, bamboo, shiitake, and scallions around the edges of each bowl. Add pork belly slices to the side. Top each with a poached egg and a sheet of nori. Serve hot.

DESSERTS

A cookbook isn't complete without a section devoted to dessert. You can infuse liquid with fruit and spices to develop a sweet broth in the same way we use vegetables to create distinctive broths. This section also employs lard to make pastry dough and chocolate cake and gelatin powder to make marshmallows. I encourage you to wash and use the fat remaining from pork stock for the lard listed in these recipes (see chapter 14).

Sweet Ginger Broth with Dark Chocolate Mousse and Maple Cashew Meringue

This recipe is an open-minded take on *ile flottante*, or "floating island," where gently poached meringue floats on crème anglaise. Offering similar textures to the original, this version features a crisp meringue set atop dark chocolate mousse, an island resting in ginger-sweetened broth.

ACTIVE TIME: 1 hour | **TOTAL TIME:** 6+ hours (including chilling and resting) | **YIELD:** Makes 4 to 6 servings

---

BROTH

½ pound (225 g) fresh ginger, grated
2 cups (480 ml) filtered water, cold

¼ cup (75 ml) maple syrup
¼ teaspoon smoked sea salt, preferably Maldon

In a medium saucepan, bring the ginger and water to a boil over medium heat. Maintain a boil for about 3 minutes. Turn off the heat and infuse the ginger, about 20 minutes.

Line a fine-mesh strainer with cheesecloth and strain the liquid into a bowl. Stir in the maple syrup and smoked sea salt until dissolved. Chill in the refrigerator.

MOUSSE

4 ounces (115 g) dark chocolate
¼ cup (56 g) unsalted butter
2 pastured eggs, separated

2 tablespoons maple syrup
1 tablespoon dark rum
Pinch sea salt

In the top of a double boiler, combine the chocolate and butter and set over hot water, stirring until melted and smooth. Remove from the heat and cool until tepid.

Bring the water in the bottom of the double boiler to a simmer. Place the egg yolks, maple syrup, and rum in a separate heatproof bowl, and place the bowl over the simmering water. The bottom of the bowl should not touch the water. Whisk the yolk mixture until it thickens and ribbons form as the whisk is lifted, about 3 minutes. Remove from the heat and continue to whisk until slightly cooled. Fold into the chocolate mixture.

In a clean bowl, whisk the egg whites with a pinch of salt until frothy. Continue to whisk until thick and shiny, about 3 minutes. Spoon a couple of dollops onto the chocolate mixture and fold until the whites are just combined and the chocolate mixture is lightened. Carefully fold the remaining egg whites into the mixture; in order to maintain volume, do not overmix. Chill in the refrigerator until set, at least 4 hours.

MERINGUES

2 egg whites
½ cup (155 ml) maple syrup

¼ cup (30 g) cashews, ground

Heat the oven to 200°F (95°C). In the top of a double boiler, combine the egg whites and maple syrup. Set over simmering water and whisk until glossy peaks form, about 4 minutes. Remove from the heat. Carefully fold in the ground cashews; do not overmix. Transfer the meringue to a pastry bag fitted with a wide star tip. Holding the pastry bag perpendicular to a parchment-lined baking sheet, pipe kisses by squeezing and releasing with even pressure, spacing the kisses about 1 inch (2.5 cm) apart. Bake for 2 hours, rotating the sheets once during baking. Turn off the heat, open the oven door, and leave the meringues to cool, at least 1 hour and up to overnight. The meringues will become crunchy as they cool.

TO SERVE: Pour some ginger broth in a shallow bowl. Using two spoons, shape a quenelle of mousse and center it on the plate. Top with a few meringues.

Cider Apple Pie with Lard Whey Crust

Steve Wood of Farnum Hill Ciders is a master cider maker—an influencer in the revival of cider apple varieties in the Northeast—and the gentleman who introduced me to my favorite apple: Ashmead's Kernel, important for traditional hard cider, delicious on its own or baked in a pie. You can't go wrong with this variety. Luckily, cider apples are abundant in the Hudson Valley, so I'm never too far from a bushel.

This classic pie concentrates apple cider as you would a stock to intensify flavor. If you can't locate Ashmead's Kernel apples, select a type with firm flesh and a sweet-tart profile. Do your best to avoid the wax-coated apples commonly found at supermarkets.

ACTIVE TIME: 1 hour | **TOTAL TIME:** 3 hours (including chilling and baking) | **YIELD:** Makes 8 to 12 servings

CRUST

2½ cups (300 g) all-purpose flour
1 tablespoon sugar
½ teaspoon sea salt
½ cup (115 g) unsalted butter, chilled

½ cup (115 g) lard, chilled
1 teaspoon apple cider vinegar, chilled
5 tablespoons Yogurt Whey, cold

In the bowl of a food processor, combine the flour, sugar, and salt. Pulse until combined. Cut the butter and lard into small pieces and scatter across the flour mixture. Pulse until coarse crumbs form.

In a separate bowl, whisk the vinegar and whey together. Sprinkle on top and pulse until the mixture forms a ball. Transfer to a lightly floured surface and knead lightly until smooth. Wrap and rest in the refrigerator, at least 1 hour.

PIE

2 cups (480 ml) apple cider
3 pounds (1.4 kg) cider apples, such as
    Ashmead's Kernel
1 tablespoon lemon juice
½ cup (115 g) packed light brown sugar

1 teaspoon ground cinnamon
¼ teaspoon freshly grated nutmeg
2 tablespoons all-purpose flour
1 tablespoon heavy cream, for baking

In a saucepan, bring the apple cider to a boil and reduce by half. Remove from the heat and cool to room temperature.

Peel, core, and thinly slice the apples; sprinkle with lemon juice. In a large bowl, toss the brown sugar, cinnamon, nutmeg, and flour together. Add the apples and stir until combined. Stir in the reduced cider. Cover and reserve.

TO ASSEMBLE: Preheat the oven to 425°F (220°C). Remove the pastry dough from the refrigerator 30 minutes before rolling. Cut in two equal pieces. On a lightly floured surface, roll out one piece of the dough to fit the bottom of a 9-inch (23 cm) pie pan. Lay the dough in the pan, leaving a 1-inch (2.5 cm) overhang. Spoon the filling into the crust. Roll out the second piece of pastry and fit on top of the filling. Lift the excess dough from the bottom to meet the top, and use your fingers to crimp the edges.

Brush the pastry with the heavy cream. Bake until golden and apples are tender, about 1 hour. If the top starts browning before the apples are done, tent a piece of aluminum foil over the pie. Remove from the oven and cool slightly before serving.

Chocolate Lard Bourbon Cake

Always a raucous time, Grrls Meat Camp is an annual gathering of female farmers, butchers, and chefs: Every year a different location, it's an endeavor that gives voice to women in a male-dominated industry. Kathy Skutecki, a pastry chef by trade and a meat grrl by heart, offered this decadent cake during a recent gathering. For the lard in this recipe, you can reserve and wash the fat from pork stock (see chapter 8, "Pork," page 151). See the instructions for washing fat in chapter 14, "Using Animal Fats," page 339.

ACTIVE TIME: 1½ hours | **TOTAL TIME:** 2½ hours (including baking and cooling) |
YIELD: Makes 12 servings

CAKE

1¾ cups (210 g) unbleached
    all-purpose flour
¾ cup (63 g) Dutch process cocoa powder
1½ teaspoons baking powder
1½ teaspoons baking soda
1 teaspoon kosher salt

2 cups (400 g) sugar
2 large eggs
1 cup (240 ml) whole milk
1 tablespoon bourbon
½ cup (110 g) lard, melted but not hot
1 cup (240 ml) boiling water

Preheat the oven to 375°F (190°C) and place a rack in the bottom third of the oven. Spray a 1-inch (2.5 cm) high rimmed half-sheet pan or jelly roll pan with cooking spray and line the bottom with a piece of parchment trimmed to fit.

In a large bowl, whisk together the flour, cocoa, baking powder, baking soda, salt, and sugar until combined. Whisk in the eggs, milk, and bourbon until well blended. The mixture will be thick. Whisk in the melted lard in a thin, steady stream until well combined. Add the boiling water, carefully mixing until well combined. The batter will be liquid.

Pour the batter into the prepared pan and carefully transfer to the preheated oven. Bake for 15 minutes until the top is firm, with a bit of a spring, and a toothpick inserted just off-center comes out clean with moist crumbs. Cool completely on a wire rack.

GANACHE

1½ pounds (680 g) bittersweet chocolate,
    finely chopped

4 cups (910 g) sour cream, room temperature
1 tablespoon bourbon

Melt the chocolate over a double boiler until smooth. Cool slightly. Add the sour cream (at room temperature—cold sour cream will make the chocolate seize) and stir with a spatula until smooth. Stir in the bourbon and set aside.

TO ASSEMBLE: With a sharp knife, cut the cake away from the pan sides if necessary and slide the cake, parchment-side down, onto a work surface. Cut the cake, width-wise, through the parchment into three even pieces about 5½ inches (14 cm) wide. Use a ruler to make sure your slices are even, if necessary.

On a large platter, place a dab of ganache to hold the cake in place and top with one slice of the cake, parchment-side up. Remove the sheet of parchment and top with a little less than a third of the ganache. Smooth the ganache into an even layer.

Top with the next slice of cake, parchment-side

up. Remove the parchment and smooth a little less than a third of the ganache on top. Top with the final piece of cake, parchment-side up, and remove the parchment. Use the remaining ganache to evenly coat the top and sides. A boning knife works quite well in making nice, tight corners and edges. If you have leftover ganache, transfer to a piping bag and place decorative dots or swirls along the edges.

The cake is best served at room temperature and keeps very well for several days if tightly wrapped.

Strawberry Cream Marshmallow Bars

This recipe illustrates how to make a healthier version of marshmallows at home. Arrowroot is used in place of cornstarch; honey or maple syrup is used in place of corn syrup. And the powdered gelatin can be made from grass-fed cows—either in your kitchen or from a mindful manufacturer. Strawberries are a highlight of early spring and late summer in the Hudson Valley.

ACTIVE TIME: 1 hour | **TOTAL TIME:** 7 hours (including chilling) |
YIELD: Makes 8 to 10 servings

CRUST

1½ cups (140 g) raw almonds
¼ cup (56 g) unsalted butter, melted

1 tablespoon honey or maple syrup
Pinch sea salt

Place the almonds in the bowl of a food processor. Pulse until a crumbly meal forms. Transfer the nuts to a bowl and mix with the remaining ingredients. Press into an oblong baking dish. Set aside.

MARSHMALLOWS

1 teaspoon grapeseed oil, for greasing the pan
1 tablespoon arrowroot powder, for dusting the pan
1 cup (240 ml) filtered water, cold, divided
½ cup (85 g) Gelatin Powder

1 cup (340 g) honey, or 1 cup (310 g) maple syrup
½ vanilla bean, scraped to remove seeds, seeds reserved
Pinch sea salt

Oil an 8-inch (20 cm) square pan and line with parchment paper, leaving an overhang on two sides. Lightly oil the paper and sprinkle with arrowroot powder. Set aside.

Place ½ cup of the water in the bowl of a mixer, and sprinkle the gelatin over the water. Gently whisk the mixture and rest for 5 minutes, until the gelatin blooms.

In a small saucepan, mix the remaining water with the honey or maple syrup. Whisk in the vanilla bean pod and seeds and sea salt. Place a candy thermometer in the pan. Bring the mixture to a boil over medium heat. If the mixture foams up, remove the pan from the heat until it settles, then return it to a slightly lower setting. Boil until the mixture reaches the soft ball stage (240°F to 242°F [115°C]), about 12 to 15 minutes. Keep an eye on the mixture as it gets closer to the correct temperature.

With the whisk attachment, turn the mixer on medium and slowly pour the syrup in a thin stream over the softened gelatin until incorporated. Turn the mixer to high and whip until the mixture triples in volume and gentle peaks form, about 10 to 15 minutes. Pour the marshmallow into the prepared pan and smooth with a spatula. Cool to room temperature.

CREAM

Marshmallow, from above
½ cup (120 ml) whole milk
1 cup (240 ml) heavy whipping cream

1 pint (330 g) fresh strawberries, rinsed and sliced
½ cup (57 g) slivered almonds, toasted

Scoop half of the cooled marshmallow mixture into a small saucepan. (The remaining marshmallows can be cut when firm and tossed with arrowroot powder for classic marshmallows.) Add the milk. Gently melt the marshmallow and stir to combine. Transfer to a bowl and set aside to cool.

Meanwhile, whip the heavy cream until stiff peaks form. Fold into the cooled marshmallow mixture until incorporated. Spread half of the cream mixture over the almond base, top with the sliced strawberries, and spread the remaining marshmallow cream over the berries. Sprinkle with almonds. Chill in the refrigerator until set, about 6 hours or overnight.

BEVERAGES

As mentioned early on, I live my life by the rule of responsible hedonism. In my world, a healthy diet is tempered with the occasional adult beverage, a reminder about the merits of balance. Herbal tonics and broth-spiked cocktails have been used for centuries to restore and invigorate the body, each in their own way. Here we introduce sipping broths for that purpose—savory tonics, sweet teas, and one lacto-fermented soda—followed by a collection of classic and contemporary cocktails to help you find balance.

Tonics

An old South American proverb says, "Good broth will resurrect the dead." Intended for sipping as you would tea, these broth-based tonics were developed with this holistic intention in mind.

Classic Beef Tea

ACTIVE TIME: 20 minutes | **TOTAL TIME:** ½ hour (including roasting) | **YIELD:** Makes 2 servings

½ pound (225 g) lean beef, such as top round
   or rump roast
½ cup (120 ml) warm water

Sea salt to taste
1 long strip lemon zest (optional)

Turn the broiler on low. Trim any fat and skin from the beef. Place on a sheet pan and broil until meat juices begin to emerge, about 2 minutes on each side. Remove from the oven and transfer to a cutting board. Cut the beef into small pieces and wrap in a thin layer of cheesecloth.

In a small saucepan, squeeze the beef to release juices into the warm water. (At this point, you can use the beef for another dish.) Lightly season with sea salt. Heat on medium-low until tea is warm and soothing. Do not boil. Pour into a mug and garnish with lemon zest, if desired. Drink immediately.

Maple Ginger Beef Brew

ACTIVE TIME: ¼ hour | **TOTAL TIME:** ¼ hour | **YIELD:** Makes 4 to 6 servings

1 quart (960 ml) Beef Bone Broth
½ pound (225 g) fresh ginger
¼ cup (75 g) maple syrup

Dash cayenne pepper
Pinch sea salt, preferably
    smoked Maldon

In a medium stockpot, gently heat the stock over medium-low heat until warm. Juice or grate the ginger and add it to the pot. Stir in the maple syrup. Season with cayenne pepper and sea salt. Serve hot.

Chicken Sesame Milk Sipping Broth

ACTIVE TIME: ¼ hour | **TOTAL TIME:** ¼ hour | **YIELD:** Makes 4 to 6 servings

1 quart (960 ml) Chicken Bone Broth
1 cup (240 ml) Sesame Milk

2 tablespoons honey
Pinch cayenne pepper

In a medium stockpot, gently heat the stock over medium-low heat until warm. Whisk in the Sesame Milk and honey until dissolved. Season with cayenne pepper. Serve hot.

Turmeric Molasses Chicken Tonic

ACTIVE TIME: ¼ hour | **TOTAL TIME:** ½ hour | **YIELD:** Makes 4 to 6 servings

1 quart (960 ml) Chicken Bone Broth
2 tablespoons blackstrap molasses
1 tablespoon coconut oil

1½ teaspoons ground turmeric
½ teaspoon ground cinnamon
¼ teaspoon ground ginger

Pinch sea salt
Pinch black pepper

Pinch cayenne pepper
Pinch ground nutmeg

In a medium stockpot, gently heat the stock over medium-low heat until warm. Stir in the molasses and coconut oil until dissolved. Whisk in the remaining spices until incorporated. Steep for 10 minutes. Serve warm.

Turkey Broth with Grapefruit and Fennel

ACTIVE TIME: ¼ hour | **TOTAL TIME:** ½ hour | **YIELD:** Makes 4 to 6 servings

1 quart (960 ml) Turkey Bone Broth
1 tablespoon fennel seeds
2 tablespoons grapefruit juice

2 tablespoons honey
Strips of grapefruit zest for garnish

In a medium stockpot, gently heat the stock with the fennel seeds over medium-low heat until warm. Whisk in the grapefruit juice and honey until dissolved. Steep 10 minutes; do not boil or the tonic will become bitter. Pour through a fine-mesh strainer. Serve hot with a grapefruit twist.

Barley Miso Tahini Vegetable Sipper

ACTIVE TIME: ¼ hour | **TOTAL TIME:** ½ hour | **YIELD:** Makes 4 to 6 servings

1 quart (960 ml) Velvety Vegetable Stock
2 tablespoons barley miso

1 tablespoon tahini
2 teaspoons maple syrup

In a medium stockpot, gently heat the stock over medium-low heat until warm. Whisk in the barley miso, and then the tahini and maple syrup. Infuse for 10 minutes; do not boil or the miso will separate. Pour through a fine-mesh strainer. Serve hot.

Medicinal Sipping Broth

ACTIVE TIME: ¼ hour | **TOTAL TIME:** 2¼ hours (including simmering) |
YIELD: Makes 8 servings

---

2 quarts (1.9 L) filtered water, cold,
    plus more as needed
2 ounces (56 g) dried reishi mushrooms, sliced

4 slices ginger
2 tablespoons honey

In a medium stockpot, slowly bring the water to a boil, then reduce the heat to maintain a simmer. Add the mushrooms, ginger, and honey. Simmer for 2 hours, adding water to prevent concentration, if necessary. Carefully strain the liquid into a heatproof container. The first extraction will be bitter. You can repeat the process to yield a less bitter secondary extraction. Divide into ½-cup (120 ml) portions—more might cause a stomachache—or store in the refrigerator, up to 3 days.

Honey Sumac Whey Tonic

ACTIVE TIME: ½ hour | **TOTAL TIME:** 3+ days
(including steeping and fermentation) | **YIELD:** Makes 6 to 8 servings

---

6 dried sumac buds
1 quart (960 ml) filtered water,
    warm

½ cup (120 ml) Raw Milk Whey
⅓ cup (115 g) local honey
1 cinnamon stick

Place the sumac buds and warm water in a 1½-quart (1.4-liter) or slightly larger container. Steep at room temperature for a few hours or overnight. Use a fine-mesh strainer to strain the tea; discard the solids. Place the tea in a clean mason jar. Add the whey, honey, and cinnamon. Seal tightly and shake to blend. Loosen the lid to allow for carbonation to develop. Rest at room temperature, 2 to 3 days, or until fermented and bubbly. Drink when carbonated, or keep in the refrigerator, up to a week.

Coconut Matcha Tea

ACTIVE TIME: ¼ hour | **TOTAL TIME:** ½ hour | **YIELD:** Makes 2 to 4 servings

2 cups (480 ml) Raw Milk Whey
¼ cup (60 ml) coconut milk
1 teaspoon coconut oil

1 tablespoon maple syrup
1 teaspoon green matcha tea powder

In a medium stockpot, gently heat the whey, coconut milk, coconut oil, and maple syrup until warm. Whisk in the green matcha tea and infuse for 10 minutes. Do not boil or the whey will separate. Pour through a fine-mesh strainer. Serve hot.

Cocktails

It might take a minute to warm up to the idea of sipping a cocktail that features broth as an ingredient. The concept has been around for a while, however; once taken up by celebrities in the 1950s, when the Bullshot was introduced in Detroit's Caucus Club. Animal-based stocks add umami to a drink, a savory note that coats the mouth in a pleasing way.

Warm Sherry Aperitif

PREP TIME: 10 minutes | **YIELD:** Makes 1 serving

1 ounce (30 ml) hot water
1 ounce (30 ml) Basic Veal Stock
1 ounce (35 g) honey

1 ounce (30 ml) dry sherry
1 dash Angostura bitters
1 lemon twist

Pour the hot water into a mug; whisk the veal stock and honey into the liquid until dissolved. Add the sherry and a dash of bitters. Twist the lemon above the drink, then drop the twist into the mug. Serve warm.

Fundamental Martini

PREP TIME: 5 minutes | **YIELD:** Makes 1 serving

Splash dry vermouth, such as Dolin
3 ounces (90 ml) top-shelf gin, such as Plymouth

1 ounce (30 ml) Basic Veal Stock
Green olives, such as Cerignola d'Bella

Splash a martini glass with dry vermouth; roll the spirit around in the glass and dump it out. Fill the glass with ice and set aside while making the drink. In a mixing glass, add enough ice to nearly fill the glass. Pour the gin and veal stock over the ice. With a bar spoon, stir in a circular motion until the glass is very cold. Toss out the ice in the martini glass; strain the liquid into the chilled glass. Garnish with green olives.

Warm Cassia Bourbon Punch

ACTIVE TIME: 10 minutes | **TOTAL TIME:** ½ hour | **YIELD:** Makes 6 servings

2 cups (480 ml) apple cider
½ cup (120 ml) Basic Chicken Stock or
   Chicken Bone Broth
6 orange slices

1 teaspoon cassia berries, or 1 stick cinnamon
¾ cup (180 ml) bourbon
4 dashes orange bitters

In a medium saucepan, gently heat the apple cider, chicken stock, orange slices, and cassia over medium-low until heated through. Infuse for 20 minutes. Transfer the hot liquid to a punch bowl. Stir in the bourbon and bitters. Ladle into small cups and serve immediately.

MORE COOKING WITH STOCKS AND BROTHS

The Happy Bullshot

PREP TIME: 10 minutes | YIELD: Makes 1 serving

Celery salt, for rim
1 lemon wedge, for rim
1½ ounces (45 ml) vodka
2 ounces (60 ml) Basic Beef Stock or
  Beef Bone Broth

2 teaspoons fresh lemon juice
2 dashes tamari
2 dashes hot sauce
1 lemon twist

On a small plate, place a mound of celery salt. Swipe the rim of an old-fashioned glass with the lemon wedge, then dip the glass into the celery salt and twist to coat. Fill the glass with ice; reserve.

Fill a shaker with ice. Add the vodka, beef stock, lemon juice, tamari, and hot sauce. Shake until chilled. Strain into the glass. Garnish with the lemon twist.

Bloody Bouillon

ACTIVE TIME: ¼ hour | TOTAL TIME: 1¼ hours (including chilling) |
YIELD: Makes 3 servings

¾ cup (180 ml) Basic Tomato Stock
¾ cup (180 ml) Basic Beef Stock or
  Beef Bone Broth
¾ cup (180 ml) tomato juice
4 ounces (120 ml) gin
3 tablespoons grated fresh
  horseradish
3 tablespoons maple syrup
1 tablespoon apple cider vinegar
1 tablespoon hot sauce
1½ teaspoons tamari

1 lemon, juiced and zested
1½ teaspoons black pepper
¼ teaspoon mustard powder
¼ teaspoon garlic powder
¼ teaspoon smoked paprika
¾ teaspoon celery seed
¾ teaspoon sea salt
Pinch cayenne pepper
2 lemon wedges, for rim
Coarse sea salt, for rim
Pickled vegetables, for garnish

Line a fine-mesh strainer with cheesecloth. Strain the tomato stock into a clean container; do not force solids through the strainer. The goal is a clear tomato water.

In a mixing glass, combine the tomato water with all remaining ingredients, except the lemon wedges, coarse sea salt, and pickled vegetables. Stir until well incorporated. Refrigerate until chilled, a minimum of 1 hour.

Run the lemon wedges across the rims of three Collins glasses. Place some coarse sea salt on a small plate. Dip the rim of each glass into the salt and twist to coat. Fill the glasses with ice.

Remove the beverage from the refrigerator and stir to loosen the mixture. If you prefer a thicker consistency, pour directly into the glasses; or strain for a thinner consistency. Garnish with pickled vegetables.

Bloody Caesar

ACTIVE TIME: ¼ hour | **TOTAL TIME:** 1¼ hours (including chilling) | **YIELD:** Makes 2 servings

1 tablespoon fennel seeds, toasted and ground
1 tablespoon black pepper
2 tablespoons coarse sea salt
4 ounces (120 ml) vodka
½ cup (120 ml) Clam Liquor
2 ounces (60 ml) tomato juice

2 teaspoons tamari
2 teaspoons hot sauce
2 teaspoons black pepper
½ cup (120 ml) lime juice
Lime wedges, for rim
Celery hearts, for garnish

In a small bowl, mix the ground fennel, black pepper, and sea salt. Place some on a shallow plate. Reserve.

In a mixing glass, combine all the remaining ingredients except the rim and garnish ingredients. Stir until well incorporated. Refrigerate until chilled, a minimum of 1 hour.

Run the lime wedge across the rim of two Collins glasses. Dip the rim of each glass into the reserved fennel salt and twist to coat. Fill the glasses with ice.

Stir the chilled mix and pour into the prepared glasses. Garnish with lime wedges and celery hearts.

PRESERVING YOUR BOUILLON

Due to its high protein content, concentrated bouillon made from animal-based stocks can be preserved for later use. The simplest method is reducing animal stock or bone broth until it holds its shape, or you can go further by dehydrating stock or broth to produce a powder. If you are short on time or materials, substitute store-bought gelatin, preferably grass-fed, in recipes that call for powder.

Soup Cubes

This recipe is the modern-day equivalent of portable soup—it provides a fast, convenient way to make soup when time is limited. The broths from veal, beef, pork, and poultry make an especially rich cube. The process of reducing broth to an even more gelatinous state concentrates flavors; there is no need to add sea salt at the end. If you don't have much freezer space for quarts of stock, soup cubes are an excellent way to keep a concentrated stock on hand without taking up too much room.

ACTIVE TIME: ½ hour | **TOTAL TIME:** 12 hours (including simmering and chilling) | **YIELD:** Makes 16 cubes

---

4 quarts (3.8 L) animal stock or bone broth, fat removed

1 tablespoon Gelatin Powder

Place the stock or broth in a large pot. Bring the stock to a boil over medium heat. When the liquid begins to tremble, lower the heat to maintain a simmer and slowly reduce to 2 cups. As the liquid thickens, small bubbles will rise to the surface. Depending on the size of your pot, this should take a few hours.

When the liquid is reduced, ladle it through a strainer lined with cheesecloth into a measuring cup. Stir in the gelatin until dissolved. The liquid should be thick and silky.

Pour the reduced stock into silicon ice cube trays. Refrigerate until set, about 8 hours or overnight. Reserve the cubes in the refrigerator for up to 2 weeks, or transfer to a sealed container and freeze for many months. To use, dissolve a cube into 1 cup hot water, stir, and use immediately.

Gelatin Powder

This recipe produces a versatile powder that can be used as a thickening agent. When made with grass-fed bones, your powder will be superior to most commercial varieties. Use it to make Soup Cubes and Gelatin Gummies. If you prefer to reserve your stock or broth for cooking, you can use the gelatin rendered from a batch of spent beef, pork, or lamb bones (see chapter 8).

ACTIVE TIME: ½ hour | **TOTAL TIME:** 3 days
(including simmering and dehydrating) | **YIELD:** Makes ½ cup

---

4 quarts (3.8 L) animal stock or bone broth,
fat removed

Special equipment:
Dehydrator, non-stick sheets

Follow the instructions for Soup Cubes (above) to reduce the stock to 2 cups. The reduction should be thick and silky. Remove from the heat and cool slightly.

On a dehydrator's non-stick drying sheet, pour the reduced stock onto the surface and spread into a thin layer across the sheet using an offset spatula. Dehydrate on high until brittle, checking each day, about 2½ to 3 days total. Cool completely.

Transfer to a powerful blender, such as a Vitamix, and blend until pulverized. One teaspoon is the equivalent of 1 cup (240 ml) of broth. Store in a glass jar at room temperature.

Gelatin Gummies

These gummies make a delicious after-school snack. You can experiment with other juices and eliminate the dairy as needed.

ACTIVE TIME: ¼ hour | **TOTAL TIME:** 1¼ hours (including chilling) |
YIELD: Makes 24 gummies

---

1 tablespoon lime juice
1 cup (240 ml) tart cherry juice
3 tablespoons maple syrup

¼ cup (43 g) Gelatin Powder
⅓ cup (76 g) Greek yogurt
Dash sea salt

Place the lime juice, cherry juice, and maple syrup in a small saucepan. Turn the heat to medium-low and slowly warm the mixture, stirring until the maple syrup is incorporated. Sprinkle the gelatin on the liquid and whisk until dissolved. Remove from the heat and cool to room temperature. Whisk the yogurt and salt into mixture until silky and smooth.

Transfer to a measuring cup and pour into silicon molds or a small glass dish. Chill until set, about 1 hour. Remove the gummies from the mold or cut into small squares. Store in refrigerator, up to 2 weeks.

Dehydrated Bouillon Cubes

This recipe is a much better alternative to store-bought bouillon cubes. It is ideal for the home cook who has limited freezer space, or hikers who need a restorative beverage on the trail. For a delicious compound butter, whip a crushed cube into room-temperature unsalted butter, and slather it on seared meat.

ACTIVE TIME: ½ hour | **TOTAL TIME:** 10½ hours (including dehydrating) |
YIELD: Makes 8 cubes

1 teaspoon dried parsley
1 teaspoon dried onion
1 teaspoon dried garlic
1 teaspoon dried carrot
¼ teaspoon fennel seed, toasted

¼ teaspoon black peppercorns
¼ teaspoon honey granules (optional)
1 tablespoon nutritional yeast
1½ tablespoons sea salt
1 cup (240 ml) Liquid Gelatin (page 353)

In a mortar and pestle, combine the parsley, onion, garlic, carrot, fennel seed, and peppercorns. Grind to a powder. Transfer the mixture to a small bowl. Grind the honey granules, if using, and nutritional yeast; add to the spice mixture. Stir in the sea salt until well combined. Set aside.

In a small saucepan, heat the gelatin over low heat until melted. Pour the gelatin over the spice mixture and stir until a paste forms. Rest until the spices are absorbed into the liquid, about 20 minutes. The mixture should be firm enough to hold its shape when molded with your hands. If the mixture is still loose, add more dried herbs until the mixture comes together. Maintain the ratio of salt to herbs and spices.

With your hands, scoop about 2 tablespoons of the mixture and form into a cube. Place on a dehydrator sheet. Repeat with the remaining mixture. Dehydrate on medium heat until completely dry, about 10 hours. The inside should be as dry as the outside to ensure shelf stability. Store in a closed container at room temperature.

CHAPTER FOURTEEN

Working with Animal Fat and Spent Bones

One of the benefits of using high-quality bones is the elongated life of the bones themselves—both the rendered fat and the spent bones can be used after the lengthy simmering process. This chapter illustrates how to use tallow, lard, and schmaltz in a variety of cooking, cosmetic, and preservation applications. Spent bones—despite appearing limp and soggy from the stockpot—maintain certain integrity, a by-product that can be turned into gelatin, dog food, fertilizer, and charcoal. Truly ashes to ashes! This is the final lesson in using all-of-everything when it comes to culinary stocks.

USING ANIMAL FATS

These recipes show you how to use washed animal fats for making food and cosmetics, even a suet feeder for birds. When chilled, the fat from animal stocks will rise to the top and harden for easy removal.

You will need to wash the fat before using in recipes. Here's how: Place the fat with some water—about 1 cup water (240 ml) for every 4 cups fat (820 g)—in a medium stockpot. Gently heat the mixture on low until the fat melts. The fat and water will separate, leaving the fat on top. When the mixture is fully separated, pour through a strainer into a large container. Refrigerate until firm. Remove the top layer of fat; discard the water. For a purer fat, repeat the process.

Washed and dried fats keep for many weeks in the refrigerator and indefinitely in the freezer. You can also pack and seal washed fats in jars to store in your pantry.

For Eating

The following recipes make use of tallow, lard, and schmaltz. Stocks made from beef and pork bones will yield more fat than stocks made from poultry bones.

Scots Cock-a-Leekie Pie

Originating in Scotland, this savory pie dates back to the sixteenth century when poultry, leeks, and prunes were simmered to create a hearty stew. The crust is made with lard.

ACTIVE TIME: 1 hour | **TOTAL TIME:** 2½ hours (including braising and baking) | **YIELD:** Makes 8 to 12 servings

---

1 whole chicken (about 4 to 6 pounds [1.8 to 2.7 kg]), preferably pastured, skin on, cut into 8 parts
Salt and pepper to taste
½ teaspoon smoked paprika, preferably sweet
¼ cup (56 g) unsalted butter, divided
½ cup (115 g) pancetta, cubed
3 cups (720 ml) Basic Chicken Broth, divided

4 medium leeks, white and pale green parts only, sliced
1 tablespoon dry sherry
2 tablespoons all-purpose flour
½ cup (65 g) pitted and chopped prunes
2 tablespoons thyme leaves
1 batch lard pastry (page 132)
1 egg, beaten

Season the chicken with salt, pepper, and paprika. Hold at room temperature while cooking the pancetta.

In a Dutch oven, melt 1 tablespoon butter over medium heat. Add the pancetta and cook, stirring, until lightly browned, about 2 minutes. With a slotted spoon, transfer the pancetta to a plate.

In the same Dutch oven, melt 1 tablespoon butter until hot but not smoking. Add the chicken pieces in batches, being careful not to crowd the pan, and cook until brown, about 3 minutes per side. Transfer to a plate and repeat with any remaining chicken pieces. Pour 2 cups of broth into the pan, scraping the brown bits with a wooden spoon, and return the chicken to the pan. Reduce the heat to medium-low. Braise, covered, until cooked through, about 20 minutes.

Transfer the chicken to a plate to cool. Strain the braising liquid into a small saucepan. Heat over medium heat and reduce by half. Whisk in the remaining broth; set aside.

In a medium skillet, melt the remaining butter over medium heat. Add the leeks and cook, stirring, until softened, about 3 minutes. Deglaze with sherry and continue cooking until the leeks are silky, another 3 minutes. Sprinkle the flour over the leek mixture and stir until incorporated, about 2 minutes. Gradually whisk in the braising liquid until smooth. Simmer until thickened, about 4 minutes. Season with salt and pepper.

In a large bowl, shred the chicken; reserve the bones for another recipe. Mix in the leek mixture, pancetta, chopped prunes, and thyme. Season with salt and pepper. Set aside.

Preheat the oven to 375°F (190°C).

On a lightly floured surface, roll out half of the lard dough to fit a deep pie dish. Transfer the dough to the dish, leaving a 1-inch (2.5 cm) overhang. Spoon the filling into the dish. Roll out the second half of the dough to fit the top of the dish. Place on top of the filling and turn the excess dough to cover the top, forming a decorative edge. With a sharp knife, slice a few vents in the top dough. Brush with the beaten egg.

Bake until the filling is cooked through and the pastry is golden brown, about 1 hour. Serve warm.

Schmaltz Knishes

In the early 1900s, Jewish immigrants introduced knishes—flaky pastry wrapped around starchy filling—to New York City. The pastry is traditionally made with schmaltz, or rendered chicken fat, considered liquid gold in Jewish cookery.

ACTIVE TIME: 1 hour | **TOTAL TIME:** 3 hours (including chilling and baking) | **YIELD:** Makes 8 servings

DOUGH

2 cups (240 g) all-purpose flour
1 teaspoon baking powder
½ teaspoon sea salt
2 eggs, divided

½ cup (115 g) schmaltz, melted
1 teaspoon apple cider vinegar
3 tablespoons Basic Chicken Stock, warm

In a medium bowl, stir the flour, baking powder, and salt together. In a small bowl, whisk one egg with the schmaltz and vinegar until smooth. Fold the wet ingredients into the dry mixture until combined. Add the warm chicken stock 1 tablespoon at a time and stir until the mixture comes together. Transfer the dough to a lightly floured surface and knead until smooth, about 2 minutes. Wrap in plastic wrap and chill, at least 2 hours and up to 2 days.

FILLING

6 medium russet potatoes
Salt and pepper
3 tablespoons olive oil
2 medium onions, thinly sliced
1 bunch Swiss chard, ribs removed,
coarsely chopped
1 tablespoon thyme leaves
1 egg
Pinch nutmeg
Pinch cayenne pepper

Place the potatoes in a large pot and cover with salted water. Turn the heat to high and bring to a boil. Reduce the heat to medium and cook until the potatoes are tender but not mushy, about 20 minutes. Drain, reserving the potato water for other uses, and transfer the potatoes to a bowl. With a potato masher, mash the potatoes until relatively smooth, adding potato water as necessary. The mashed potatoes should be thick enough to hold their shape. Season with salt and pepper. Set aside.

In a medium skillet, heat the olive oil over medium heat. Add the onions and cook, stirring often, until they begin to caramelize, about 20 minutes. Stir in the Swiss chard and cook until wilted, about 2 minutes. Add the fresh thyme. Season with salt and pepper. Transfer to a bowl and cool.

In a small bowl, whisk the egg with the nutmeg and cayenne pepper. Mix half of the egg mixture into the potatoes and the other half into the onion-chard mixture. Reserve while preparing the dough.

TO ASSEMBLE: Remove the dough from the refrigerator and bring to room temperature. Preheat the oven to 375°F (190°C).

Divide the dough in half. On a floured surface, place one piece of dough in the center and roll into a large rectangle. Spread half of the potato filling across one-third of the dough, leaving a 1-inch (2.5 cm) border. Layer the Swiss chard mixture on top of the potatoes. Roll the dough around the filling.

Carefully slice to make 3-inch (7.5 cm) wide knishes. With your fingers, pinch the ends shut on each knish. Place flat-side down on a parchment-lined baking sheet, leaving space in between. Repeat with the second dough half.

Whisk the remaining egg with a little water to create a wash for the dough. Brush the tops of the knishes with egg wash. Bake for 25 minutes, or until golden brown. Serve warm or at room temperature.

Baked Sweet Potato Fries with Duck Salt

This recipe is a great way to make use of excess duck fat and skin—the fat helps crisp sweet potatoes in the oven, and the skin is dehydrated and blended with spices to make a delicious seasoning. The duck salt is an interpretation of chicken salt, a popular Australian spice for fish-and-chips. You can wash, dry, and use the fat from a batch of duck stock, or you can start by rendering duck skin to produce both fat and cracklings.

ACTIVE TIME: 1 hour | **TOTAL TIME:** 4 hours
(including rendering, simmering, and dehydrating) | **YIELD:** Makes 6 to 8 servings

SALT

½ cup (115 g) duck skin,
  trimmed
½ cup (68 g) kosher salt

1 tablespoon brown sugar
½ tablespoon smoked paprika
1 teaspoon black pepper

Preheat the oven to 350°F (175°C). On a sheet pan, arrange the duck skin in a single layer. Roast for 20 minutes. Remove from the oven and strain any rendered duck fat into a heat-proof container. With tongs, turn the duck skin over. Return the tray to the oven and continue to roast until golden, about another 10 minutes. Strain again; reserve the duck fat for the fries.

Set the oven temperature to its lowest setting, no higher than 190°F (85°C).

Return the skin to the sheet pan and dehydrate in the oven until dry to the touch, about 3 hours. Cool.

Place the duck skin and kosher salt in the bowl of a food processor. Pulse until fine. Transfer to a bowl and toss with the remaining ingredients. Store in an airtight container.

FRIES

½ cup (115 g) duck fat, reserved
  from above

⅓ cup (80 ml) Basic Duck Stock
3 medium sweet potatoes, peeled

In a small stockpot, bring the reserved duck fat and duck stock to a simmer, and slowly cook until reduced by half, about 20 minutes.

Preheat the oven to 450°F (230°C). With a sharp knife, cut the sweet potatoes into ¼-inch (.6 cm) strips. Place the strips in a bowl and toss with the reduced sauce. On a sheet pan, spread the sweet potato strips in a single layer. Bake until golden brown, turning as needed, about 20 minutes. Remove from the oven and cool until crisp, about 5 minutes. Toss with some of the duck salt and serve immediately.

Mincemeat

Similar to plum pudding, mincemeat was developed as a way of preserving meat in animal fat and sugar. Suet is melted to coat and seal sweetened fruit; hearty enough to hold for months in the refrigerator or indefinitely in pressurized jars. Mincemeat, used as a pie filling or served alongside cooked meats, originated in England and remains a holiday tradition to this day.

ACTIVE TIME: ½ hour | **TOTAL TIME:** 2+ weeks
(including macerating and maturing) | **YIELD:** Makes 3 pints

---

1½ cup (225 g) yellow raisins
2½ cups (355 g) dried black currants
¼ cup (115 g) chopped citron or other
    candied citrus peel
¼ cup (37 g) chopped dried figs
¼ cup (60 ml) brandy
1 large apple, quartered, cored, and diced
½ cup (115 g) suet, or rendered beef fat,
    chilled and grated

¾ cup (165 g) muscovado sugar
1 orange, juice and zest
1 lemon, juice and zest
½ teaspoon ground cinnamon
½ teaspoon ground nutmeg
½ teaspoon ground allspice
½ teaspoon ground cloves
¼ teaspoon sea salt

Toss the raisins, currants, citron, and figs in a bowl. Cover with the brandy and soak at room temperature until the fruit is plump, about 1 hour. In a small saucepan, gently heat the remaining ingredients until the suet melts.

Combine the macerated fruit, any brandy in the bowl, and the melted mixture; stir until incorporated. Pack into sterilized jars and wait for the flavors to come together, at least 2 weeks. Refrigerate up to 6 months.

Plum Pudding

The Christmas pudding of Great Britain dates back to the early 1400s, when animals were harvested in autumn and preserved in quantity for winter. Standing pies were first made of meat or fish, held together with flour, preserved with animal fat, and sweetened with dried fruits. Prepared alongside the harvest, these pies were ready before the holidays, originally eaten as a fasting meal in advance of the festivities. Over time, the pudding was enhanced in texture with eggs and flavor with spirits and evolved into a customary holiday dessert.

ACTIVE TIME: 2 hours | **TOTAL TIME:** 1+ months (including macerating, soaking, steaming, and maturing) | **YIELD:** Makes 12 to 14 servings

PUDDING

2 cups (300 g) yellow raisins

2½ cups (355 g) dried black currants

1 cup (150 g) dried mulberries, whole, or chopped dried figs

½ pound (225 g) citron, finely diced

1 cup (130 g) nuts, such as walnuts or hazelnuts, toasted

1 tablespoon grated lemon zest

1 teaspoon ground cinnamon

½ teaspoon ground nutmeg

½ teaspoon ground mace

¼ teaspoon ground allspice

¼ teaspoon ground cloves

¼ teaspoon ground black pepper

1 pound (455 g) suet, or rendered beef fat, chilled and grated

1¾ cups (420 ml) Armagnac, divided

8 eggs

1 cup (200 g) sugar

1 cup (240 ml) buttermilk

½ cup (170 g) blackstrap molasses

5 cups (200 g) fresh bread crumbs

½ cup (100 g) hulled millet (optional)

1 teaspoon sea salt

In a large bowl, toss the dried fruits, nuts, zest, and spices together. Fold in the grated suet until well combined. Stir in 1 cup (240 ml) Armagnac. Cover and refrigerate for a week.

After the mixture has matured for a week, place the eggs and sugar in the bowl of a mixer with the whisk attachment. Whisk on the medium setting until doubled in volume, about 6 minutes. Gradually beat in the buttermilk and molasses until incorporated. With a spatula, fold in the bread crumbs, millet, and sea salt. Transfer to the refrigerator and chill until the bread crumbs are evenly moist, about 1 hour.

Preheat the oven to 275°F (135°C). Fill a roasting pan with 2 inches (5 cm) boiling water. Reserve in the oven.

Butter a 3-quart (3-liter) mold. Fold the macerated fruit, including any Armagnac left in the bowl, into the chilled egg mixture. Turn into the mold, leaving a couple of inches on top, and tap on the counter to settle the mixture. Wrap the mold with foil and secure the foil with butcher's twine. Place the mold in the roasting pan; make sure that the water is not high enough to get into the mold. Steam for 4 to 5 hours, adding water to the pan as necessary. Remove the mold from the oven and rest on a wire rack, about 10 minutes. Tap the mold and carefully invert the pudding to unmold it. Drizzle ½ cup (120 ml) Armagnac over the top and cool completely.

When cool, wrap the pudding in cheese-cloth, then double wrap in plastic. Store in a cool place for a minimum of a few weeks, and ideally a year.

HARD SAUCE

⅓ cup (76 g) unsalted butter,
    room temperature
2 tablespoons lard, room temperature

1½ cups (170 g) powdered sugar, sifted
½ vanilla bean
2 tablespoons Armagnac

Place the butter and lard in the bowl of a mixer with the paddle attachment. Beat until light and fluffy, about 3 minutes. While beating on low, gradually sift in the powdered sugar until incorporated. With a paring knife, split the vanilla bean lengthwise, and scrape the seeds; reserve the pod for another use. Add the Armagnac and vanilla bean seeds and beat until the mixture is smooth. Use immediately or store in the refrigerator. Serve at room temperature.

TO SERVE: Using the steaming method above, return the pudding to the mold and steam for 2 hours. Unmold the pudding onto a platter. At the table, drizzle the remaining ¼ cup (60 ml) Armagnac over the pudding and carefully ignite to flame the pudding. Cut into small portions and serve with hard sauce.

For the Body

It might seem odd to find a section on cosmetics in a book about stocks and broths. In the spirit of using all-of-everything, however, soap and lotion are a great way to make use of excess animal fats. The most technical of these recipes is the body soap, which is made by combining tallow with lye. Wear gloves and goggles when working with caustic agents. All other instructions rely on the careful emulsification of animal fats and essential oils.

Body Soap

ACTIVE TIME: 1 hour | **TOTAL TIME:** 1½ days (including soaking and resting) | **YIELD:** Makes 8 to 10 bars

---

2½ cups (600 ml) filtered water, cold
7 ounces (200 ml) lye
4 cups (910 g) tallow

1.5 ounces (45 g) cocoa butter
2 cups (480 ml) olive oil

Select a mold for the soap: Wood or silicone molds are preferable; avoid glass or metal. Wood molds are structured as long rectangles for making bars; silicon molds offer unique shapes and are easy to clean. Soap requires more drying time in silicon molds. If using a wooden mold, soak in water for an hour, then line it with a clean, damp cheesecloth, leaving a 2-inch (5 cm) overhang. Place the mold inside a larger pan that can be covered with a kitchen towel.

Select a large nonreactive container that is not aluminum. Add the water. Put on gloves and goggles before handling the lye. Carefully pour the lye into the water, stirring until dissolved. Cool to 80 to 85°F (25 to 30°C).

In a saucepan, melt the tallow and cocoa butter over low heat. Stir in the olive oil. Remove from the heat and cool, stirring occasionally, until the mixture starts to congeal. The temperature of the fats should be 100 to 110°F (35 to 40°C).

Confirm that both the lye mixture and the fat mixture are within correct temperature ranges. In a thin, steady stream, slowly pour the lye solution into the fat while stirring. It is important to add the solution gradually; this helps avoid separation. Stir until the liquid begins to thicken, about 15 to 20 minutes.

Pour the mixture into the lined wooden box or silicon mold. Cover the outer pan with a kitchen towel. Rest the soap until it hardens, about 24 hours in a wooden mold and up to 4 days in silicon. Use the cheesecloth to lift the soap from the wooden pan and transfer it to a cutting board. Slice into bars with a sharp knife or fine wire. For silicon molds, simply bend and flex the mold to release the soap.

Face Lotion

ACTIVE TIME: ¼ hour | TOTAL TIME: ¼ hour | YIELD: Makes 1½ cups

1 cup (225 g) tallow, room temperature
1 tablespoon castor oil

10 drops bergamot oil
10 drops geranium oil

In the bowl of a mixer, using the balloon attachment, cream the tallow on medium speed until fluffy, about 2 minutes. Scrape the sides and continue to whip until doubled in volume, another 4 minutes. Whip in the castor oil and essential oils until smooth. Transfer to a sealed cosmetic container. Keep at room temperature.

To use, scoop out a small amount with clean hands and gently rub on your face. Steam with a hot, damp washcloth. Gently wipe the excess lotion from your face. Pat dry with a clean towel. This lotion is best for balanced skin.

Hand Cream

ACTIVE TIME: ½ hour | TOTAL TIME: ¾ hour (including cooling and emulsifying) | YIELD: Makes 3½ cups

¾ cup (170 g) lard
¼ cup (56 g) shea butter
¼ pound (115 g) beeswax
½ cup (120 ml) sweet almond oil
½ cup (120 ml) apricot kernel oil

1 tablespoon vitamin E oil
20 drops myrrh essential oil (optional)
20 drops cedarwood essential oil (optional)
1 cup (240 ml) warm water

Place the first five ingredients in the top of a double boiler, and gently melt the fats over barely simmering water. Remove from the heat and set aside at room temperature to cool slightly. When tepid, transfer to the bowl of a mixer and add the vitamin E and essential oils. Using the balloon attachment, whisk on medium speed until combined, then gradually add the warm water while mixing, until emulsified, about 10 minutes.

Spoon into a sterilized jar and store in the refrigerator. If the mixture separates, repeat the whipping process. To use, scoop a small amount with your fingers and rub into your hands and wrists until smooth and absorbed.

Body Butter

ACTIVE TIME: ½ hour | TOTAL TIME: 1½ hours (including cooling) |
YIELD: Makes 2 cups

½ cup (110 g) lard
¼ cup (56 g) cocoa butter
¼ cup (56 g) shea butter
½ cup (120 ml) coconut oil

½ cup (120 ml) almond oil
20 drops rose essential oil (optional)
20 drops frankincense essential oil
(optional)

Place the first five ingredients in the top of a double boiler, and gently melt the fats over barely simmering water. Remove from the heat and set aside at room temperature until set, about 1 hour.

Transfer the fats to the bowl of a mixer. Add the essential oils. Using the balloon attachment, whip until light and fluffy, about 5 minutes. Spoon into a sealed cosmetic container. Keep at room temperature.

To use, scoop a small amount with your fingers and gently rub onto your skin in a circular motion. This formula is good for your arms, legs, hands, feet, chest, and torso.

Anti-Fungal Foot Salve

ACTIVE TIME: ½ hour | TOTAL TIME: 8 hours (including infusing) |
YIELD: Makes 1½ cups

¼ cup (60 ml) olive oil
2 tablespoons lavender buds
2 tablespoons calendula leaves

1 cup (225 g) tallow, room temperature
1 teaspoon vitamin E oil
5 drops tea tree oil

In a small saucepan, combine the olive oil with the lavender buds and calendula leaves. Gently heat over medium heat until warm, then reduce the temperature to low. Infuse for 1 hour. Turn off the heat and steep overnight. Strain into a bowl.

Place the tallow in the top of a double boiler, and gently melt over barely simmering water. Stir in the infused olive oil, vitamin E oil, and tea tree oil until fully incorporated. Remove from the heat and pack into sterilized jars. Rest at room temperature until set.

This salve is best used at bedtime. Scoop a small amount with your fingers and rub into the base and top of your feet and in between your toes. Wear socks to seal the moisture in overnight.

Baby's Butt Balm

ACTIVE TIME: ½ hour | **TOTAL TIME:** ¾ hour (including cooling) | **YIELD:** Makes 1 cup

¼ cup (56 g) tallow
¼ cup (56 g) shea butter
¼ cup (60 ml) coconut oil

2 tablespoons cod liver oil
2 tablespoons arrowroot powder

Place the first three ingredients in the top of a double boiler, and gently melt the fats over barely simmering water. Remove from the heat and set aside at room temperature until tepid, about 15 minutes. Stir in the cod liver oil. Sift the arrowroot powder evenly over the mixture while whisking to incorporate. Continue to whisk until smooth.

Transfer the mixture to a sterilized jar and store in the refrigerator. To use, scoop a small amount with your fingers and slather onto your baby's bottom to help relieve diaper rash.

Lip Balm

ACTIVE TIME: ¼ hour | **TOTAL TIME:** 4 hours (including cooling) | **YIELD:** Makes 1½ cups

1 cup (225 g) lard
5 ounces (140 g) beeswax pastilles

½ teaspoon food-grade essential oil, such as lemon or peppermint

Place the lard and beeswax in the top of a double boiler, and gently melt over barely simmering water. Remove from the heat and stir in the essential oil. Immediately pour into lip balm containers or a small jar. Stand containers on end and rest at room temperature until solid. To use, rub on your lips and smack them together until absorbed.

For the Birds

Making bird feeders with leftover fat and grain was popularized in the early 1900s. It remains a wonderful home craft.

Bird Feeder

ACTIVE TIME: ½ hour | **TOTAL TIME:** 2½ hours (including cooling and setting) | **YIELD:** Makes 4½ cups

---

3 cups (675 g) tallow, washed
½ cup (55 g) dried bread crumbs
¼ cup (50 g) hulled millet
¼ cup (35 g) sunflower seeds

1 tablespoon poppy seeds
¼ cup (20 g) chopped dried apples
¼ cup (36 g) dried black currants

In a small saucepan, melt the tallow over low heat. Remove from the heat and cool until tepid. Toss the remaining ingredients in a large bowl until combined. Stir in the slightly thickened tallow and mix until the fruit and seeds are interspersed throughout. Pack into molds, such as a parchment-lined tray or a silicone container, or feeders. Refrigerate or freeze until hardened. Remove from the molds and place outside during the warm months.

RECIPES USING SPENT BONES

The evolution of Brooklyn Bouillon is told through the farmers it supports and the ingredients they have to offer. When we started, many bones didn't make it past the processor—there was simply not enough consumer demand to merit the carting of heavy bones back to the farm or to markets. Demand is so significant now that quality bones sell out at farms and markets in record time.

For the company to survive, we needed to look beyond stocks to determine how best to succeed in our zero-waste mission. As it turns out, the life of bones extends well beyond the primary stock and its secondary remouillage, ending as compostable bone char. Here I share some ideas about how you can make use of spent bones in a home kitchen.

Deviled Bones

As soon as the term *deviled* emerged in the late 1700s, so did references to deviled bones. The descriptor has evolved over the years—first it was a reference to highly seasoned fried or broiled dishes, and then it was simplified as a way to describe food with demonic levels of spice.

This technique works well with any meaty bones that are left over from the cooking process. Rib bones are ideal, but other types, such as shank bones, can also be used—provided they have not been picked clean. The meaty bones left over from beef, pork, or lamb stock should yield enough quantity for one batch.

ACTIVE TIME: ½ hour | **TOTAL TIME:** 1 hour (including simmering and roasting) | **YIELD:** Makes 6 servings

BONES

2 cups (480 ml) animal stock, to match bone type
¼ cup (56 g) unsalted butter, or marrow butter (page 118), melted
2 teaspoons red wine vinegar

3 tablespoons all-purpose flour
Salt and pepper
5 pounds (2.3 kg) meaty bones (beef, pork, or lamb), cooked
1 cup (40 g) fresh bread crumbs

In a small saucepan, reduce the stock to a glaze, about 3 tablespoons. Transfer 1 tablespoon to a small bowl and stir in the melted butter and vinegar. Reserve the remaining 2 tablespoons for the sauce.

Preheat the broiler. In a separate bowl, toss the flour with salt and pepper. Dredge the beef bones in the flour mixture and set aside. Place the bread crumbs in another bowl. Dip the ribs in the butter mixture, and then coat with bread crumbs.

Arrange the ribs on a sheet pan and place in the middle rack of the oven. Broil, turning often, until crisp and golden, about 15 minutes.

SAUCE

1 tablespoon unsalted butter
1 medium shallot, minced
⅓ cup (80 ml) dry red wine, such as
   Cabernet Sauvignon

Reduced stock, from above
2 teaspoons Dijon mustard
Pinch cayenne pepper
Salt and pepper

In a small saucepan, melt the butter over medium heat. Add the shallot and sauté until translucent, about 2 minutes. Stir in the red wine and simmer until reduced by half, about 4 minutes.

Whisk in the reduced stock and mustard until well combined. Stir in the cayenne pepper. Simmer until the sauce thickens slightly, another 3 minutes. Taste before seasoning with salt and pepper.

Serve the bones with the sauce on the side, alongside crusty bread and marrow butter, should you have it on hand.

Liquid Gelatin

Liquid gelatin can be used as a neutral thickening agent in cooking, or you can go one step further and dehydrate it to make Gelatin Powder (page 336). This gelatin is best made with bones from large animals, such as beef, pork, or lamb bones. It will hold in the refrigerator for a few days, or in the freezer indefinitely.

ACTIVE TIME: ½ hour | TOTAL TIME: 8+ hours (including simmering) |
YIELD: Makes about 2 quarts (1.9 liters)

10 pounds (4.5 kg) spent bones (beef, pork, or lamb)

Place the spent bones in a large stockpot and cover with cold water. Over medium heat, slowly bring the water to a boil, then lower the heat to maintain a soft simmer. Render the bones until the liquid reduces and thickens, about 8 hours.

Set a China cap over a large container and pass the bones and liquid through the cap. Line a fine-mesh strainer with cheesecloth. Strain the liquid into a clean stockpot. Bring to a gentle boil and reduce by half. Transfer the reduced liquid to a clean container, and chill until solidified. If your bones are still strong after simmering, you can repeat the process to render more gelatin. Store in the refrigerator or freezer.

Bone Meal

Bone meal is a common industrial by-product used to make fertilizer and animal feed. The process of crushing bones into meal makes their nutrients more available to the soil and easier for animals to digest.

In a home kitchen, bone meal is best made from the bones of small animals, such as poultry and fish. Bone meal made from larger animal bones, such as cows, pigs, and sheep, requires industrial grinding equipment. Use this bone meal to make Bone Meal Fertilizer (the next recipe) or Dog Food (page 356).

ACTIVE TIME: 2½ hours | **TOTAL TIME:** 10+ hours
(including simmering and drying) | **YIELD:** Makes about 1 quart (960 ml)

**10 pounds (4.5 kg) spent bones,
   from small animals only
Vinegar, for sterilizing surface**

**Special equipment:
   Safety glasses, heavy mallet, high-wattage
   electric meat and bone grinder**

Place the bones in one or two large stockpots. Cover with water and bring to a boil over medium-high heat. Boil until the fat, gristle, and marrow have rendered from the bones. This can take many hours. With tongs, transfer the bones to a cutting board and pat dry with a kitchen towel. Discard the liquid.

Preheat the oven to 275°F (135°C). Arrange the bones on two to three sheet trays and bake until very dry, about 4 hours. Remove from the oven and cool until dry and brittle.

Select a hard surface that can take a pounding, such as an outside table. Scrub with hot water and soap. With a towel, wipe the surface with vinegar.

Place a few bones at a time in the center of the surface. Wearing safety glasses, pound the bones with a heavy mallet to break into smaller chunks.

Using a high-wattage electric meat and bone grinder, grind the bones in batches to achieve a fine powder. Run the bone powder through the grinder a second time if needed. Store in a closed container at room temperature.

Bone Meal Fertilizer

This fertilizer adds calcium and phosphorous to acidic soil. It is good for perennials and shrubs. Use sparingly in alkaline soil.

ACTIVE TIME: 1 hour | **TOTAL TIME:** 1¼ days (including resting) |
YIELD: Makes 12 quarts (11.5 liters)

---

1 cup (230 g) Bone Meal (above), made from fish bones
¼ cup (25 g) wet kelp, from Kelp Stock

1 cup (240 ml) Liquid Gelatin, made from beef bones
Special equipment:
  Soil test kit or commercial soil thermometer

Using a soil test kit or a commercial soil thermometer, test your soil to determine its pH and nutrient composition. If your soil is acidic, this fertilizer will work well for your soil. Use sparingly on alkaline soil.

In a large stockpot, mix the Bone Meal with 8 quarts (7.5 L) water. Gently heat over medium heat, stirring often, until the water is warm. Turn off the heat and rest at room temperature for 24 hours. Stir occasionally.

Place the wet kelp in a blender and pulse until a paste forms. In a separate container, mix the kelp with 4 quarts (3.8 L) water. Rest for 24 hours.

The next day, line a fine-mesh strainer with cheesecloth and set over a large container. Strain the bone meal liquid into the container. Into the same container, strain the kelp water. Discard both solids.

In a small saucepan, melt the Liquid Gelatin over low heat. Stir into the liquid mixture until incorporated. Your fertilizer is ready to use.

To test on soil, use 2 cups for perennials and 3 cups for shrubs. After 72 hours, test the soil again to monitor any shifts in nutrient content. Continue to monitor over time for a response. Adjust the fertilizer amount based on calcium and phosphorous levels in your soil.

Dog Food

This recipe incorporates bone meal and wet kelp, both by-products from stock recipes, with meat, offal, vegetables, eggs, and oil—a combination that is generally healthy for dogs. You can add ground multivitamin tablets for additional supplemental value.

Check with your veterinarian to see if this recipe is good for your dog. Never feed a dog spent bones directly from the pot—they are brittle and pose a digestive risk.

ACTIVE TIME: ½ hour | **TOTAL TIME:** ½ hour |
YIELD: Makes about 1 quart (910 g)

2 cups (455 g) cooked bulgur wheat
¾ cup (170 g) cooked meat, shredded
2 tablespoons cooked liver, beef, chicken,
   or pork, chopped
1 large carrot, finely chopped

1 tablespoon Bone Meal
½ teaspoon wet kelp, from Kelp Stock,
   minced
1 egg, preferably pastured
2 teaspoons fish oil

In a large bowl, mix the bulgur wheat, shredded meat, liver, carrot, Bone Meal, and kelp until thoroughly combined. Crack the egg over the mixture and top with fish oil. Stir until the mixture comes together. Serve immediately or portion and freeze in vacuum-sealed packs.

Bone Charcoal

A resourceful idea, bone charcoal is a middle point between spent bones and bone char compost. It was popularized by Chef Dan Barber and his team at Blue Hill when they endeavored to carbonize spent bones as a heat source several years ago. Now their bone char is making an appearance as ash on cheese—a collaboration with Vermont Creamery and Murray's Cheese Shop.

To make your own bone charcoal, you need a vented grill that allows for control of oxygen supply and heat control. The goal is to heat your grill as high as it will go, and then leave the bones to smolder as the heat slowly subsides.

WORKING WITH ANIMAL FAT AND SPENT BONES

ACTIVE TIME: 1 hour | **TOTAL TIME:** 8+ hours (including heating and charring) |
YIELD: Makes about 5 pounds (2.3 kilograms)

---

10 pounds (4.5 kg) spent bones, from large animals, such as veal, cow, pig, or sheep, or hollow shellfish, such as oysters or clams

Lay aluminum foil on the base of a charcoal grill. Starting at the center of the base, stack a large amount of charcoal in a pyramidal shape. Light some kindling and/or newspaper. With one hand, start the charcoal with the kindling while fanning with the other hand. Avoid the use of lighter fluid. Allow flames to develop and fan with your hands to catch all of the charcoal. Place a grate above the charcoal.

Keep the bottom vents closed to reduce the oxygen supply and the top vents open to release heat. The goal is to achieve a very high heat, upward of 700°F (370°C).

Let the flames subside before placing bones or shells on the grate.

While the grill is heating, remove any meat and fat from the bones or tough muscles from the shells. Place the bones or shells on the grate in a single layer, directly above the charcoal. When the smoke turns grayish blue and the charcoal turns white, close the lid to create an airtight seal. Char the bones or shells until the heat subsides; this will take several hours. The bones and shells should be carbonized and look like charcoal.

Using tongs, transfer the bone charcoal to a heatproof container and cool completely. If the pieces are too large, you can use a hammer or wood chipper to break them into pieces. Use bone charcoal as you would regular charcoal. If it does not light easily, supplement with natural hardwood charcoal and use bone charcoal as an additional seasoning agent in the grill.

Bulk Recipes and Simplified Methods

If you work in a commercial kitchen, producing stock in large batches is a realistic notion. One day of stock making can streamline production and create a frozen stockpile of stocks always at the ready.

In a home kitchen, however, space and time are often limitations. Instead of a bulk supply, there is benefit to using slow-cooking appliances that work when you are not present. This chapter reviews how to make large batches in a commercial setting and small batches using hands-free cookers at home.

MAKING LARGE BATCHES

The standard ratio for making a quality stock is 2 parts bones to 3 parts water. You will see slight variations throughout this text, sometimes more bones or more water, depending on the intended concentration of the final stock. Using eyesight alone, the general guideline for water amount is to use enough to cover solids in a stockpot. This method works well for a home cook but can throw a commercial batch into an unbalanced state: All the ingredients are delivered in bulk, and adjusting a stock in large quantities requires a quantity of source material that is relative to the size of the equipment used. For a large batch of stock, whether in a large stockpot or in a commercial kettle, we recommend weighing your ingredients to achieve the correct ratio.

Before you begin making stocks in bulk, consider your cold storage: You need to plan for rapid cooling and short- or long-term storage. For large batches, I recommend an ice paddle or a blast chiller to rapidly cool the stock. Alternatively, you can cool stocks quickly by filling stainless steel pans with ice water and placing stock-filled containers in the ice bath. To further expedite cooling, store the containers in the ice bath in the refrigerator, if room permits.

For storage, ask yourself: Will you be holding stocks in the refrigerator and using them within a couple of days? Or portioning in quart containers and storing in a walk-in freezer? Make certain you have enough room in your kitchen to manage the yield. If you miscalculate space, simply reduce the liquid into a more concentrated stock, store in smaller containers, and reconstitute with filtered water upon cooking.

Bulk Beef Stock

ACTIVE TIME: 3 hours | **TOTAL TIME:** 10 hours (including roasting, heating, simmering, and initial cooling) | **YIELD:** Makes about 15 to 18 quarts (14 to 17 liters)

---

40 pounds (18 kg) meaty beef bones, from the neck or leg, preferably grass-fed or pastured

3 calf's feet, preferably grass-fed or pastured (optional)

1 cup (240 ml) grapeseed oil, divided

45 quarts (42 L) filtered water, cold, plus water for rinsing

7 pounds (3 kg) white onions, 4 onions halved, the rest cut into large dice

5 pounds (2.25 kg) leeks, dark green parts removed, cut into large dice

5 pounds (2.25 kg) carrots, cut into large dice

6 heads garlic, split in half, broken into pieces

½ pound (225 g) flat-leaf parsley

1 ounce (28 g) thyme

½ ounce (14 g) bay leaves

1½ ounces (42 g) black peppercorns

Sea salt to taste

Using a 20-gallon stockpot, commercial kettle, or braiser, follow the directions for Roasted Beef Stock (page 125). When the stock is ready to strain, make sure you have buckets large enough to hold the liquid. After straining, if a more concentrated broth is desired, return the stock to a clean pot and simmer until reduced. Be sure to adjust the seasoning at the end of the cooking time. Cool the stock with an ice paddle, in a blast chiller, or in an ice bath. Refrigerate for up to 2 days or freeze in smaller containers for longer storage.

Bulk Chicken Stock

ACTIVE TIME: 3 hours | **TOTAL TIME:** 5 to 6+ hours (including heating, blanching, simmering, and initial cooling) | **YIELD:** Makes about 18 to 20 quarts (17 to 19 liters)

---

30 pounds (13.5 kg) chicken bones, necks and backs

5 pounds (2.25 kg) chicken feet

20 quarts (19 L) filtered water, cold, plus water for rinsing and/or blanching

15 pounds (7 kg) ice cubes, if making white stock, or 10 quarts (9.5 L) water if making brown stock

2½ pounds (1.1 kg) carrots, cut into large dice

2½ pounds (1.1 kg) white onions, cut into large dice

5 pounds (2.25 kg) leeks, dark green parts removed, cut into large dice

½ ounce (14 g) bay leaves

Sea salt to taste

Using a 20-gallon stockpot, commercial kettle, or braiser, follow the directions for Basic Chicken Stock (page 166, for a white stock) or Roasted Chicken Stock (page 168, for a brown stock). If making a brown stock, replace the ice cubes with equal parts water, since the chicken fat was rendered during the roasting process.

When the stock is ready to strain, make sure you have buckets large enough to hold the liquid. After straining, if a more concentrated broth is desired, return the stock to a clean pot and simmer until reduced. If a more viscous broth is preferred, repeat the simmering process with additional chicken feet until the gelatin is extracted from the joints, about 4 hours. The feet will ensure that the stock achieves a gelatinous state. Be sure to adjust the seasoning at the end of the cooking time. Cool the stock with an ice paddle, in a blast chiller, or in an ice bath. Refrigerate for up to 2 days or freeze in smaller containers for longer storage.

Bulk Fish Fumet

ACTIVE TIME: 3 hours | **TOTAL TIME:** 9+ hours (including soaking, heating, simmering, and initial cooling) | **YIELD:** Makes about 25 quarts (23.5 liters)

---

25 pounds (11.5 kg) fish bones, tails, skin, and fins removed

4 pounds (1.8 kg) ice cubes

¾ cup (180 ml) grapeseed oil, divided

3 pounds (1.4 kg) carrots, cut into large dice

2½ pounds (1.1 kg) white onions, cut into large dice

5 pounds (2.25 kg) leeks, dark green parts removed, cut into large dice

2½ pounds (1.1 kg) fennel, coarsely chopped, fronds removed

1 bottle (750 ml) dry white wine, such as Sauvignon Blanc

1 ounce (28 g) thyme

½ pound (225 g) flat-leaf parsley

½ ounce (14 g) bay leaves

1 ounce (28 g) black peppercorns

30 quarts (28 L) filtered water, cold, plus water for soaking

Sea salt to taste

Using a 20-gallon stockpot, commercial kettle, or braiser, follow the directions for Basic Fish Fumet (page 213). When the stock is ready to strain, make sure you have buckets large enough to hold the liquid. After straining, if a more concentrated broth is desired, return the stock to a clean pot and simmer until reduced. Be sure to adjust the seasoning at the end of the cooking time. Cool the stock with an ice paddle, in a blast chiller, or in an ice bath. Refrigerate for up to 2 days or freeze in smaller containers for longer storage.

Bulk Vegetable Stock

ACTIVE TIME: 1½ hours | **TOTAL TIME:** 2½ hours (including heating, simmering, and initial cooling) | **YIELD:** Makes about 15 to 18 quarts (14 to 17 liters)

6 pounds (2.7 kg) leeks, dark green parts removed, cut into large dice

3 pounds (1.4 kg) white onions, cut into large dice

4 pounds (1.8 kg) carrots, cut into large dice

4 pounds (1.8 kg) fennel, coarsely chopped, fronds removed

1 cup (240 ml) grapeseed oil

½ pound (225 g) flat-leaf parsley

1 ounce (28 g) thyme

½ ounce (14 g) bay leaves

18 quarts (17 L) filtered water, cold, plus water for rinsing and/or blanching

Sea salt to taste

½ bottle (375 ml) dry white wine

Using a 20-gallon stockpot, commercial kettle, or braiser, follow the directions for Basic Vegetable Stock (page 245). When the stock is ready to strain, make sure you have buckets large enough to hold the liquid. After straining, if a more concentrated broth is desired, return the stock to a clean pot and simmer until reduced. Be sure to adjust the seasoning at the end of the cooking time. Cool the stock with an ice paddle, in a blast chiller, or in an ice bath. Refrigerate for up to 2 days or freeze in smaller containers for longer storage.

SIMPLIFIED METHODS

Despite my proclivity toward slow cooking, there are days when convenience dictates what happens (or what doesn't happen) in my kitchen. These times call for one-pot, and preferably hands-free, cooking. It is in these rare moments when cooking does not dominate my thoughts that I reach for tools intended to simplify.

For those of you short on time, or when you need homemade stock within an hour or two, a pressure cooker will create a base with concentrated flavor, rich mouthfeel, and decent clarity. A pressure cooker works by building heat and trapping steam inside the chamber, which increases the temperature without agitating the contents. This means that collagen in bones converts to gelatin more rapidly in a pressurized environment. Likewise, flavor is extracted from vegetables in about a third of the time it takes to make vegetable-based stock on the stove. Nevertheless, the high heat also means some vitamins will be denatured during the cooking process.

In addition to making a flavorful stock, a pressure cooker is a handy tool to have in the kitchen, especially if you are keen on preserving. Look around yard sales for old pressure cookers—they last for years! If you find one, have it tested through your local cooperative extension service before use. This step is especially important for old pressure cookers: They can be dangerous if defective or improperly handled. In all cases, read the manufacturer's instructions before use.

For those of you short on patience, or when you are unable to tend the pot, a slow cooker will produce a stock that is light in flavor and body, and clearer than most. The slow cooker approach still takes time—a minimum of eight hours—but the benefit is that you can throw the ingredients in the cooker, walk away for some, or all, of the cook time, and return to a finished stock. This method yields less gelatin and more vitamins.

Another benefit to using a pressure or slow cooker is the savings in energy. Both methods require less gas or electricity than their long-simmering counterparts. Stocks made in a pressure or slow cooker will also experience less evaporation and therefore yield more quantity. If necessary, you can reduce a strained stock on the stove to achieve your desired concentration.

Pressure Cooker Method

ACTIVE TIME: 1 hour | TOTAL TIME: 8+ hours (including heating, simmering, and cooling) | YIELD: Makes about 2 quarts (1.9 liters)

Select a stock or broth recipe in this book and use half the ingredients. Place all the ingredients except the water and salt into a 7-quart (6-liter) pressure cooker. Pour water into the cooker to cover the ingredients; do not fill past the "maximum fill" line. Cover and lock the lid.

Set the pressure cooker over high heat until fully pressurized. Reduce the heat to low and maintain until done. Vegetable stocks will cook in 15 minutes; fish stocks in 30 minutes; poultry stocks in 40 minutes; and beef, pork, and lamb stocks in 50 minutes.

Turn the heat off and rest the cooker until fully depressurized. Allow the entire pressure cooker to cool before opening. *Do not remove the lid before the cooker is cool; improper handling can cause severe burns.* When the display shows 0, carefully unlock the pressure cooker and remove the lid with your face held away from the steam.

Line a fine-mesh strainer with cheesecloth and set it over a container large enough to hold the liquid contents of the pot. Carefully ladle the stock from the cooker into the strainer, leaving any cloudy liquid at the bottom. Reserve the solids for another use. Taste the stock and season with sea salt.

Chill the stock until the fat solidifies, at least 4 hours or overnight. Remove the fat; reserve for another use. Refrigerate for up to 2 days or freeze in smaller containers for longer storage.

Slow Cooker Method

ACTIVE TIME: 1 hour | **TOTAL TIME:** ½ to 1 day (including heating, simmering, and cooling) | **YIELD:** Makes about 2 quarts (1.9 liters)

Select a stock or broth recipe in this book and use half the ingredients. Place all the ingredients except the water and salt into a 6-quart (6.5-liter) slow cooker. Pour water into the cooker to cover the ingredients; do not fill past the "maximum fill" line. Cover.

Turn the slow cooker on; set to the low setting. Cook vegetable stocks for 5 hours; fish stocks for 6 hours; poultry stocks for 8 to 10 hours; beef, pork, and lamb stocks for 10 to 16 hours, depending on how concentrated you want the stock or broth. Periodically remove the lid and skim the surface to remove impurities. When the stock reaches your desired consistency, turn off the heat and rest the stock, about 15 minutes. Carefully remove the lid.

Line a fine-mesh strainer with cheesecloth and set it over a container large enough to hold the liquid contents of the pot. Gently ladle the stock from the cooker into the strainer, leaving any cloudy liquid at the bottom. Reserve the solids for another use. Taste the stock and season with sea salt.

Chill the stock until the fat solidifies, at least 4 hours or overnight. Remove the fat; reserve for another use. Refrigerate for up to 2 days or freeze in smaller containers for longer storage.

A Convivial Finish

In the Southwest of France, there is an old Occitanian custom: To the end of a warm soup bowl, one adds a generous splash of red wine, swirls to blend, and with elbows firmly rooted on table, brings bowl to lips and gulps the enhanced broth as a signature to a satisfying meal. This convivial conclusion is called *faire le chabrot*, loosely meaning "to drink like a goat." At some tables, this old custom might be seen as uncouth, and yet broth has had the undeniable mark of providing comfort and initiating camaraderie throughout the ages.

Trends come and go, fleeting moments that celebrate ingredients and producers, a time and place where people gather around an idea or concept. Stocks and broths, in this way, are a curious thing. They stand the test of time—sometimes in the limelight, as with the recent popularity of bone broths, and yet most often residing in the background. Stocks, after all, are the foundation of good cooking, and broths are pure comfort in the bowl. A certain inherent confidence guides their purpose—to showcase other ingredients—as if the backbone of a family. Perhaps this is why we remember our grandmothers upon walking into a warm kitchen.

Chefs and cooks will remind us, collectively, that taking the time to start from scratch is well worth the effort. And in these moments, despite a world in constant flux and an industrial food system that confounds, we come together to celebrate slow cookery. Take a day, or as the passionate cooks around me often do, an entire weekend, to live in the process—a trip to the farmers market and a chat with your farmer, followed by the meditative process of cleaning, chopping, simmering, and waiting patiently until meal time. With your elbows firmly rooted on the table, I encourage you to tip a bowl back to those who came before us and to continue the tradition with your loved ones.

Sourcing Guidelines

This section provides high-level guidelines about how to source materials for making stocks and broths. For meat and poultry, farming practices of land animals are listed by life span—from birth to harvest—and reflect a consolidation of methods. For fish and seafood, a review of current population status and best fishing practices for each species was conducted for this book.

Keep in mind that farmers in your area and fishermen in your region might operate with different breeds or species and by different mechanisms. Some farmers manage their business without certifications, and yet uphold highly regarded standards of operation. Global water systems are constantly changing, as is the stock quality of fish and seafood; it is important to review up-to-date information when making purchasing decisions.

These guidelines adhere to parameters set by governing bodies in the United States. They are not exhaustive. Get to know the hardworking people who grow and harvest your food; they will be your best source for information about the food available in your area.

TABLE A.1. Sourcing Guidelines for Meat

Animal	Example Breeds	Farming Practices	Labels to Look For	Bone Types
Young Cattle	Dairy cattle, such as: • Pedigree Holstein *Note:* Bull (male) calves only. The females are raised for dairy production.	**Birth:** Start with mothers **Land:** Pastured paddock early in life; rotational pastures in summer, and high-quality hay in winter **Feed:** Fed milk directly from cattle every day; no hormones or antibiotics **Life span:** Raised until 22 to 54 weeks **Harvest:** Processed in a reduced-stress environment	Rose Veal Pastured Veal Free-Raised Veal Animal Welfare Approved certification	Knuckle Neck Back Marrow Breast
Adult Cattle	Beef cattle, such as: • Angus • Hereford • Shorthorn Or rarer breeds, including: • Devon • Dexter • American Low-Line	**Birth:** Start with mothers **Land:** Pastured paddock early in life; rotational pastures in summer and high-quality hay in winter **Feed:** Fed milk directly from cattle every day until weaned to pasture; no hormones or antibiotics **Finish:** On grass (grass-fed only) or quality grain (pastured or grain-finished), 90 to 160 days before slaughter **Life span:** Raised until 18 to 24 months **Harvest:** Processed in a reduced-stress environment	Grass-Fed Beef Pastured Beef Grain-Finished Beef Animal Welfare Approved certification	Knuckle Marrow Neck
Pig	Heritage breeds, such as: • Berkshire • Hereford Or rare breeds, including: • Tamworth • Gloucestershire Old Spot • Large Black • Ossabaw Island • Red Wattle	**Birth:** Born at the farm, preferably in spring; properly weaned at 6 to 8 weeks; inoculated against cholera and wormed early **Land:** Live continuously on rotational pasture, fields, and woods; free to roam and forage; comfortable structures for rooting and nesting in winter **Feed:** Farmer-grown grass, grains, vegetables, fruits, and plants; bugs in the soil; sometimes fortified with whey and acorns; no hormones, antibiotics, or growth enhancers **Life span:** Processed 5 to 6 months, typically when a certain weight (around 225 pounds [100 kg] or so) is achieved **Harvest:** Certified humane environment, either farm or processor, depending on quantity	Heritage Breed Pig Rare Breed Pig Animal Welfare Approved certification	Neck Shoulder Leg Trotter
Lamb	Breeds that are suited for pasture, such as: • Dorset • Hampshire • Katahdin • Southdown • Suffolk Or more common breeds from a reliable source: • Dorper • White Dorper	**Birth:** Born in spring **Land:** Live continuously on rotational pasture; shade in summer and shelter in winter **Feed:** Dense pasture with legumes and balanced pH level; mineral supplements; constant water supply **Life span:** Processed 6 to 8 weeks for "young lamb" or under 1 year; classified as mutton after teething occurs **Harvest:** Certified humane environment, either farm or processor, depending on quantity	Grass-Fed Sheep Pastured Sheep Animal Welfare Approved certification	Neck Shank Breast

TABLE A.2. Sourcing Guidelines for Poultry

Animal	Example Breeds	Farming Practices	Labels to Look For	Bone Types
Chicken	Slow-growing meat or egg breeds selected for climate, geography, and temperament. For example, breeds that are well adapted to the Hudson Valley include: • Dominique • Plymouth Rock • Rhode Island Red • Wyandotte *Note:* Pastured breeds tend to have long bodies, long legs, and smaller breasts for ease of mobility.	**Birth:** Day-old chicks from a reliable local or regional hatchery; managed in a clean brooder for 2 to 3 weeks with minimal loss. Naturally mated if heritage. **Land:** Live continuously on rotational pasture after brooding, depending on time of year; follow cows to manage parasites and enrich soil health; shelter from weather and predators; environmental features that encourage roaming; birds given adequate space to roam, adjusted as they grow **Feed:** Certified organic or chemical-free starter and adult feed; no hormones, antibiotics, or growth enhancers; constant water supply **Life span:** Processed 9 to 10 weeks **Harvest:** Certified humane environment, either farm or processor, depending on quantity	Pastured Chicken Heritage Chicken Animal Welfare Approved certification	Backs Necks Feet Entire carcass (body of the animal after the meat is removed, mainly bones) Whole animal
Turkey	Heritage varieties that thrive outdoors, such as: • Spanish Black • American Bronze • Bourbon Red • Narragansett • White Holland *Note:* Slow-growing varieties tend to have normal bone development that builds wing and leg strength for flying, perching, and roosting—behavior not seen in conventional counterparts.	**Birth:** Day-old poults from a reliable local or regional hatchery; managed in clean brooders for several weeks with minimal loss. Brooders should be temperature-controlled and sized for growth of turkeys. Naturally mated if heritage. **Land:** Live continuously on rotational pasture after brooding; shelter from weather and predators; environmental features that encourage roosting and roaming; birds given adequate space to roam, adjusted as they grow **Feed:** Certified organic or chemical-free starter and adult feed; no hormones, antibiotics, or growth enhancers; nutritive balancer for leg strength and high protein content for overall strength; access to granite grit for gizzard health; constant water supply **Life span:** Processed 4 to 8 months **Harvest:** Certified humane environment, either farm or processor, depending on quantity	Pastured Turkey Heritage Turkey Animal Welfare Approved certification	Backs Necks Feet Entire carcass Whole animal
Duck	Common breeds, such as: • Moulard • Pekin • Muscovy Or rare breeds, including: • Ancona • Saxony	**Birth:** Day-old ducklings from a reliable local or regional hatchery; managed in a clean brooder for 2 to 7 weeks, depending on weather, with minimal loss **Land:** Raised on pasture and without cages; access to creek or pond; shelter from predators and extreme weather **Feed:** Certified organic or chemical-free high-protein starter and adult feed; no hormones, antibiotics, or growth enhancers; access to granite grit for gizzard health; optional fresh greens; constant water supply **Life span:** Typically processed 7 to 8 weeks, when feathers are first mature **Harvest:** Certified humane environment, either farm or processor, depending on quantity	Cage-Free Duck Pastured Duck Animal Welfare Approved certification	Backs Necks Feet Entire carcass Whole animal

TABLE A.2. Sourcing Guidelines for Poultry (*continued*)

Animal	Example Breeds	Farming Practices	Labels to Look For	Bone Types
Rabbit	Medium-weight breeds, such as: • Chinchilla • New Zealand White Or medium-weight heritage breeds, such as: • Silver • Lilac	**Birth:** Young bucks are matched with young does; one doe can manage a litter of seven rabbits **Housing:** Indoor rabbit houses; colonies preferable to cages; or humane enclosures; access to fresh air in warm months **Feed:** Raised on mother's milk for first few weeks; alfalfa and leafy clover hay, or whole-grain pellets; plenty of clean water **Life span:** Processed 10 to 12 weeks **Harvest:** Certified humane environment, either farm or processor, depending on quantity	Fresh Hormone Free Antibiotic Free Legs	Spine Rib Loin Legs Entire carcass Whole animal

TABLE A.3. Sourcing Guidelines for Fish

Fish Type	Example Varieties	Harvesting Practices	Preferred Labels	Bone Types
Cod	Atlantic cod types include: • Codfish • Scrod • True Cod • Whitefish Pacific cod types include: • Alaska • Grey • Treska • True Cod	Select Pacific cod from Alaskan fisheries that use bottom longline methods. Alternatively, select Atlantic cod from recirculating aquaculture systems that use closed tanks. Cod caught using handline methods on both coasts are good alternatives. Avoid other sources due to overfishing and entanglement of other species, including whales.	Certified Sustainable Seafood (Pacific only)	Spine Head
Flounder	Types with healthy stocks from responsible fisheries include: • Alaskan Arrowtooth • California • Flathead • Kamchatka • Starry	Atlantic flounder stocks have been depleted and overfishing still occurs. Look for Summer (handline) or Windowpane (bottom trawl), which are both identified as good alternatives.	Certified Sustainable Seafood (Flathead and Kamchatka only)	Spine Head
Halibut	Types include: • Greenland Turbot • Hirame	Select from Pacific waters using longline methods. Stock is depleted in US Atlantic. Atlantic halibut from recirculating aquaculture systems that use closed tanks, particularly from Canada, are identified as good alternative.	Certified Sustainable Seafood (Pacific only)	Spine Collar

TABLE A.3. Sourcing Guidelines for Fish (*continued*)

Fish Type	Example Varieties	Harvesting Practices	Preferred Labels	Bone Types
Monkfish	Also known as Goosefish. Types include: • Abbot • Allmouth • Angler • Ankimo • Ankoh • Fishing Frog • Lotte • Molligut • Sea-devil	Identified as good alternative. Bottom gillnet or trawl from US Atlantic waters. No longer overfished, but method involves bycatch that threatens protected species. *Due to fishing methods, it is recommended that you eat monkfish occasionally and sparingly.*	No certifications have been identified to date.	Tail
Grouper	Identified as good alternative. Grouper types that are considered acceptable include: • Black • Gag, handline method • Hawaiian • Red	*Due to overexploitation of grouper across the globe, the Sustainable Fisheries Partnership has developed a roundtable of suppliers and buyers to monitor and assess the industry.*	No certifications in the US Atlantic or Pacific have been identified to date.	Spine Collar
Skate	Good alternatives include: • Big • California • Winter	Seek out Longnose Skates caught using longline or bottom trawl methods from the US West Coast. *Due to fishing methods and population uncertainty, it is recommended that you eat skate occasionally and sparingly.*	Certified Sustainable Seafood (U.S. West Coast)	Wing
Snapper	Types with healthy stocks from responsible fisheries include: • Gray, diver-caught in Gulf of Mexico • Mutton Good alternatives include: • Gray, South Atlantic • Jobfish, Hawaii • Oblique-banded • Red, Gulf of Mexico • Ruby • Vermilion • Yellowstripe • Yellowtail, South Atlantic and Gulf of Mexico only	*Due to overexploitation of snapper across the globe, the Sustainable Fisheries Partnership has developed a roundtable of suppliers and buyers to monitor and assess the industry.*	No certifications in the US Atlantic or Pacific have been identified to date.	Spine Head
Sole	Types with healthy stocks from responsible fisheries include: • Dover • English • Flathead • Petrale, California • Rex • Southern Rock, Alaska • Yellowfin	Purchase sole harvested in the United States. Good alternatives come from British Columbia, but are less desirable because they are caught with other over-fished or at-risk species.	Certified Sustainable Seafood	Spine Head

SOURCING GUIDELINES

TABLE A.4. Sourcing Guidelines for Shellfish

Seafood Type	Example Varieties		Harvesting Practices	Preferred Labels	Bone Types
Clams	• Littleneck • Cherrystone • Northern Quahog	• Northern Razor • Razor • Softshell (Steamers)	Farmed and hand-harvested; raked or shoveled is acceptable; avoid dredged clams	Certified Sustainable Seafood	Whole, Live
Lobster	• American • California Spiny • Caribbean Spiny	• European • Rock • Western Red	Traps or pots, sometimes baited, and hoop nets	Certified Sustainable Seafood	Shells, including claws, tail, and body
Mussels	• Blue • California • Chilean	• Mediterranean • New Zealand Green	Farmed on the seafloor or in suspended systems	Certified Sustainable Seafood (New Zealand only)	Whole, Live
Oysters	• Chilean • Kumamoto • Olympia	• Portuguese • Sydney Rock	Farmed on the seafloor or in suspended systems	Certified Sustainable Seafood (Edible and Pacific)	Whole, Live

TABLE A.5. Sourcing Guidelines for Vegetables

Vegetable Type	Example Varieties	Farming Practices	Preferred Labels
Mixed	• Carrots • Celery root • Fennel • Leeks • Onions	Integrated farming systems that strive for sustainability. Some responsible farmers choose not to be certified; speak with them to learn about their methods.	Certified Organic Certified Naturally Grown Food Alliance Certified
Mushrooms	• White button • Cremini • Dried • Wild (morels, porcini, chanterelle, etc.)	Many varieties cultivated year-round on logs outdoors or in indoor systems. Wild mushrooms are foraged seasonally based on climate and location.	Cultivated Foraged (wild) Local
Squash	Summer squash varieties include: • Crookneck Early-Golden • Easy Prolific Straightneck Winter squash varieties include: • Butternut, Waltham variety • Kabocha	Summer squash is easy to find throughout the warm months. Winter squash is available throughout the cold months. It should be properly cured after harvest. Look for locally grown varieties from a responsible farmer.	Certified Organic Certified Naturally Grown Food Alliance Certified
Tomato	Heirloom varieties include: • Brandywine • Cherokee Purple Commonly grown hybrid varieties include: • Roma • Beefsteak	Heirloom tomatoes have been developed through open pollination over many years. Hybrid tomatoes are the result of forced cross-pollination between two varieties. Look for locally grown varieties from a responsible farmer. Avoid GMO varieties often found at the supermarket.	Certified Organic Certified Naturally Grown Food Alliance Certified
Garlic	Softneck varieties include: • Silver Rose • Thermadrone Hardneck varieties include: • Purple Stripe • German White	Heirloom garlic comes from certified organic seed stock and should follow approved methodology from harvest to cleaning to storage. Seek garlic that has been grown within your region. Avoid common garlic from overseas.	Certified Organic Certified Naturally Grown Food Alliance Certified
Seaweed	• Kelp • Kombu	Seasonally hand-harvested and monitored to ensure no product contamination or resource depletion	Local Regional Wild Atlantic OCIA Certified Organic

TABLE A.6. Sourcing Guidelines for Dairy

Dairy Type	Example Varieties	Farming Practices	Preferred Labels
Milk (Cow)	• Whole Milk • Raw Milk • Cultured Buttermilk	Seek locally or regionally produced milk, preferably from cows that are raised on pasture. Excellent breed types for dairy production include: • Jersey • Guernsey • Normande Recent studies show that full-fat milk is better for you than reduced-fat milk. Avoid ultra-high-temperature (UHT) milk when making whey. Raw milk straight from a local farm is preferable.	Raw Organic Pastured Jersey Cow
Cheese (Parmesan)	• Parmigiano-Reggiano	Look for Parmesan cheese that abides by Italian standards of production. There are many false Parmesan cheeses in the United States; some have been identified to contain wood pulp. Avoid labels with cellulose powder, potassium sorbate, and cheese cultures. Buy in blocks, never grated.	Protected Designation of Origin (PDO)

Stock and Broth Quick Guidelines

This section provides specifications about each stock, broth, and base recipe in this book. Use these tables as a quick reference for determining the differences between each stock type—for instance, when bones are blanched or roasted or how a bone broth differs from its stock counterpart. Remember that the total cooking time includes idle activities, such as soaking and simmering. The properties listed are intended as guidelines only; your stocks may vary by flavor, texture, and color, depending on quality of materials and cooking conditions.

TABLE B.1. Guidelines for Meat Stocks and Broths

Type	Distinction	Cook Time	Properties
VEAL: ROSE			
Basic Stock	Bones are blanched; vegetables are raw.	Active Time: 2 hours Total Time: 7 hours	Flavor: Neutral, savory Texture: Gelatinous Color: Light brown
Roasted Stock	Bones and vegetables are roasted and deglazed with red wine.	Active Time: 2 hours Total Time: 10 hours	Flavor: Caramelized, savory Texture: Gelatinous Color: Mahogany
Two-Day Stock	Bones are blanched and simmered in 2 extractions. Both extractions are combined and reduced for the final stock.	Active Time: 3 hours Total Time: 2 days	Flavor: Mellow, savory Texture: Gelatinous, silky Color: Medium brown
Classic Demi-Glace	Roasted veal stock and classic brown sauce are reduced by half. Can also make with beef or poultry stock.	Active Time: ½ hour Total Time: 2 hours	Flavor: Complex, savory Texture: Dense, slippery Color: Dark mahogany
BEEF: GRASS-FED OR PASTURED			
Basic Stock	Bones are blanched; calf's foot optional. Vegetables are raw; parsnips and garlic included.	Active Time: 2 hours Total Time: 9 hours	Flavor: Grassy, complex Texture: Viscous, if foot used. Silky otherwise. Color: Medium brown
Roasted Stock	Bones and vegetables are roasted; calf's foot optional; charred onion added for color.	Active Time: 2 hours Total Time: 10 hours	Flavor: Caramelized, roasted Texture: Viscous, if foot used. Silky otherwise. Color: Mahogany
Bone Broth	Bones and vegetables are roasted; calf's foot required; marrow bones recommended; vinegar soak optional.	Active Time: 3 hours Total Time: 2 days	Flavor: Grassy, complex Texture: Gelatinous, thick Color: Mahogany
LAMB: PASTURED			
Basic Stock	Bones are blanched; calf's foot recommended. Vegetables are sautéed with white wine. Celery root is added; touch of vinegar at end.	Active Time: 2 hours Total Time: 7 hours	Flavor: Grassy, complex Texture: Slightly gelatinous, if foot used. Silky otherwise. Color: Light brown
Roasted Stock	Bones are roasted; calf's foot recommended. Vegetables are raw; tomatoes and tomato paste added for color and texture.	Active Time: 2 hours Total Time: 10 hours	Flavor: Roasted, savory Texture: Slightly gelatinous, if foot used. Silky otherwise. Color: Mahogany
PORK: PASTURED AND/OR HERITAGE BREED			
Basic Stock	Bones are blanched; trotter recommended. Vegetables are raw; parsnips and mushrooms added for flavor.	Active Time: 2 hours Total Time: 7 hours	Flavor: Neutral, Savory Texture: Gelatinous, if trotter used. Silky otherwise. Color: Light brown

TABLE B.1. Guidelines for Meat Stocks and Broths (*continued*)

Type	Distinction	Cook Time	Properties
Roasted Stock	Bones and vegetables are roasted and deglazed with red wine. Trotter is optional.	Active Time: 2 hours Total Time: 10 hours	Flavor: Caramelized, savory Texture: Gelatinous, if trotter used. Silky otherwise. Color: Golden brown
Smoked Stock	Smoked ham hocks are required; trotter is optional. Bones and vegetables are roasted and deglazed with hard apple cider.	Active Time: 2 hours Total Time: 10 hours	Flavor: Salty, smoky, sweet Texture: Gelatinous, if trotter used. Silky otherwise. Color: Golden brown
Bone Broth	Bones and vegetables are roasted; natural ham hocks and trotters required; vinegar soak optional.	Active Time: 3 hours Total Time: 2 days	Flavor: Intense, savory Texture: Very gelatinous Color: Deep golden brown

TABLE B.2. Guidelines for Poultry Stocks and Broths

Type	Distinction	Cook Time	Properties
CHICKEN: PASTURED			
Basic Stock	Bones are washed or blanched; chicken feet optional. Ice cubes added during initial simmer to help remove fat.	Active Time: 2 hours Total Time: 5 to 6 hours	Flavor: Neutral, savory Texture: Gelatinous, if feet used. Silky otherwise. Color: Light brown, golden hue
Roasted Stock	Bones and vegetables are roasted; chicken feet optional.	Active Time: 2 hours Total Time: 6½ hours	Flavor: Caramelized, savory Texture: Gelatinous, if feet used. Silky otherwise. Color: Golden brown
Bone Broth	Whole chicken instead of backs and necks; chicken feet required; vinegar soak optional. Ice cubes added during initial simmer to help remove fat.	Active Time: 2½ hours Total Time: 8 to 12 hours	Flavor: Neutral, savory Texture: Very gelatinous Color: Golden brown
TURKEY: PASTURED AND/OR HERITAGE BREED			
Basic Stock	Bones are washed or blanched, not roasted; chicken feet optional. Ice cubes added during initial simmer to help remove fat. Fennel, apple, and marjoram added for sweetness.	Active Time: 2 hours Total Time: 6 to 7 hours	Flavor: Mild, savory Texture: Gelatinous, if feet used. Silky otherwise. Color: Light brown, golden hue
Roasted Stock	Whole carcass from roasted turkey used. Bones and vegetables are roasted; chicken feet optional. Cognac recommended for deglazing.	Active Time: 2 hours Total Time: 7½ to 8½ hours	Flavor: Caramelized, savory Texture: Gelatinous, if feet used. Silky otherwise. Color: Golden brown

TABLE B.2. Guidelines for Poultry Stocks and Broths (*continued*)

Type	Distinction	Cook Time	Properties
Bone Broth	More bones to same amount of water; chicken feet required; vinegar soak optional. Ice cubes added during initial simmer to help remove fat.	Active Time: 2½ hours Total Time: 10 to 12 hours	Flavor: Intensely savory Texture: Very gelatinous Color: Golden brown
Giblet Stock	Sautéed gizzard and neck are used to make a low-yielding stock intended for gravy. Good to make while turkey is roasting.	Active Time: 2 hours Total Time: 5 hours	Flavor: Mild, savory Texture: Fluid Color: Light brown, golden hue
DUCK: PASTURED OR CAGE FREE			
Basic Stock	Bones are blanched; duck or chicken feet recommended. Ice cubes added during initial simmer to help remove fat. Vegetables are sautéed with white wine. Parsnip is added; touch of vinegar at end.	Active Time: 2 hours Total Time: 6 to 7 hours	Flavor: Mild, savory Texture: Gelatinous, if feet used. Silky otherwise. Color: Golden brown
Roasted Stock	Bones are roasted; duck or chicken feet recommended. Vegetables are raw; tomatoes and tomato paste added for color and texture. Juniper berries for spice.	Active Time: 2 hours Total Time: 8 hours	Flavor: Caramelized, savory Texture: Gelatinous, if feet used. Silky otherwise. Color: Mahogany
RABBIT: HUMANELY RAISED, HORMONE AND ANTIBIOTIC FREE			
Basic Stock	Bones are washed or blanched, not roasted. Ice cubes added during initial simmer to help remove fat.	Active Time: 2 hours Total Time: 5 to 6 hours	Flavor: Neutral, savory Texture: Slightly gelatinous Color: Light brown, golden hue
Roasted Stock	Bones and vegetables are roasted. Tomatoes added for color; dry sherry recommended for deglazing.	Active Time: 2 hours Total Time: 6½ hours	Flavor: Caramelized, savory Texture: Slightly gelatinous Color: Golden brown
Bone Broth	Whole rabbits instead of carcasses; chicken feet recommended; vinegar soak optional. Ice cubes added during initial simmer to help remove fat.	Active Time: 2½ hours Total Time: 8 to 12 hours	Flavor: Mild, savory Texture: Very gelatinous, if feet used. Slightly gelatinous otherwise. Color: Golden brown

STOCK AND BROTH QUICK GUIDELINES

TABLE B.3. Guidelines for Seafood Stocks and Broths

Type	Distinction	Cook Time	Properties
FISH: Consult private interest groups, such as Monterey Bay Aquarium Seafood Watch and Marine Stewardship Council, to determine up-to-date best practices.			
Basic Fumet	White flat or bony fish can be used, if simmered for under an hour. Bones are thoroughly cleaned and leached of blood in water overnight. Vegetables are sautéed with white wine.	Active Time: 2 hours Total Time: 9+ hours	Flavor: Neutral, briny Texture: Silky Color: Light gray
Roasted Stock	White bony fish, such as snapper, grouper, or cod. Heads included. Bones and vegetables are roasted and deglazed with white wine.	Active Time: 2 hours Total Time: 4 hours	Flavor: Caramelized, briny Texture: Slightly gelatinous Color: Light brown
Bone Broth	White bony fish, such as snapper, grouper, or cod. Monkfish tail recommended for mild flavor. Skate wing and fish collars added for cartilage. Vegetables are sautéed and deglazed with vinegar.	Active Time: 2 hours Total Time: 12+ hours	Flavor: Mild, briny Texture: Gelatinous Color: Light gray
SHELLFISH: Seek sustainable aquaculture farmers. Local or regional, when possible. Shellfish should always be freshly harvested and alive when purchased.			
Shellfish Stock	Vegetables are sautéed and deglazed with white wine. Shellfish are added alive and removed after liquor is extracted. Aromatics include saffron and tomato; anise liqueur is added to round flavor.	Active Time: 1 hour Total Time: 2 hours	Flavor: Sweet, briny Texture: Fluid Color: Golden, yellow hue
Mussel Stock	Vegetables are sautéed and deglazed with dry vermouth. Shellfish are added alive and removed after liquor is extracted.	Active Time: 1 hour Total Time: 2 hours	Flavor: Sweet, briny Texture: Fluid Color: Light gray
Clam Liquor	No vegetables are used; only bay leaf to enhance essence. Shellfish are added alive and removed after liquor is extracted.	Active Time: ¾ hour Total Time: 1½ hours	Flavor: Sweet, briny Texture: Fluid Color: Light gray
Oyster Essence	Vegetables are sautéed and deglazed with white wine; celery root added. Shellfish are added alive and removed after liquor is extracted.	Active Time: ¾ hour Total Time: 1 hour	Flavor: Mild, briny Texture: Fluid Color: Light gray
SHELLFISH: Seek responsible lobstering operations that abide by seasonal harvesting rules. Local or regional, when possible.			
Lobster Stock	Cleaned lobster bodies and vegetables are sautéed with white wine. Tarragon is added for subtle anise flavor.	Active Time: 1 hour Total Time: 3 hours	Flavor: Buttery, bright Texture: Fluid Color: Golden, coral hue

TABLE B.4. Guidelines for Vegetable Stocks and Broths

Type	Distinction	Cook Time	Properties
MIXED VEGETABLES: LOCAL FARM; ORGANIC, WHEN POSSIBLE			
Basic Stock	Vegetables are finely chopped, sautéed, and deglazed with white wine.	Active Time: ¾ hour Total Time: 2 hours	Flavor: Neutral, vegetal Texture: Fluid Color: Golden, light yellow hue
Roasted Stock	Vegetables are chopped into small mirepoix and roasted for color and flavor.	Active Time: ½ hour Total Time: 2½ hours	Flavor: Caramelized, earthy Texture: Fluid Color: Light brown
Velvety Stock	Vegetables are finely chopped and kelp is incorporated to increase viscosity, replacing wine. Tamari or light soy sauce can be added at end for depth of flavor.	Active Time: ¾ hour Total Time: 2½ hours	Flavor: Vegetal, briny Texture: Silky Color: Golden, light green hue
MUSHROOM: LOCAL CULTIVATOR			
Basic Stock	Button mushrooms and vegetables are finely chopped, sautéed, and deglazed with white wine. Celery root is included.	Active Time: ¾ hour Total Time: 2 hours	Flavor: Earthy, savory Texture: Fluid Color: Oyster brown
Roasted Stock	Cremini mushrooms and vegetables are chopped into small dice, roasted, and deglazed with dry vermouth. Parsnips are included.	Active Time: ½ hour Total Time: 2½ hours	Flavor: Earthy, savory Texture: Fluid Color: Dark brown
Dried Essence	Dried wild mushrooms are reconstituted and added to stock. Vegetables are chopped finely and sautéed with olive oil. White miso can be added for depth of flavor.	Active Time: 1 hour Total Time: 2 hours	Flavor: Earthy, savory Texture: Fluid Color: Light brown
SQUASH: LOCAL FARM; ORGANIC, WHEN POSSIBLE			
Summer Stock	Yellow crookneck squash and alliums are sautéed in olive oil and butter. Lemon juice is added at end of simmer to brighten dish.	Active Time: ½ hour Total Time: 1¼ hours	Flavor: Buttery, bright Texture: Fluid Color: Bright yellow
Winter Stock	Winter squash is dehydrated to add sweetness and maintain clarity. Vegetables are chopped into small dice and sautéed.	Active Time: 1 hour Total Time: 10 hours	Flavor: Slightly sweet, salty Texture: Fluid Color: Yellow hue
TOMATO: LOCAL FARM; ORGANIC AND HEIRLOOM, WHEN POSSIBLE			
Basic Stock	Thin-skinned tomatoes are simmered with sautéed vegetables. Anchovies can be added at end for depth of flavor.	Active Time: ½ hour Total Time: 1½ hours	Flavor: Sweet, slightly acidic Texture: Fluid Color: Light red hue
Green Tomato	Unripe tomatoes are simmered with roasted garlic and sautéed vegetables. Pancetta can be incorporated for cured flavor.	Active Time: ¾ hour Total Time: 2¼ hours	Flavor: Slightly sweet and sour; balanced salinity with pancetta Texture: Fluid Color: Light green hue

TABLE B.4. Guidelines for Vegetable Stocks and Broths (*continued*)

Type	Distinction	Cook Time	Properties
Fire-Roasted Tomato	Roma tomatoes and onions are grilled and simmered with sautéed vegetables. Anchovies can be added at end for depth of flavor.	Active Time: 1 hour Total Time: 2 hours	Flavor: Caramelized, slightly acidic Texture: Fluid Color: Dark red hue
ONION: LOCAL FARM; ORGANIC, WHEN POSSIBLE			
Buttery Leek	Dark green leek tops are simmered with sautéed vegetables and deglazed with dry sherry and white wine.	Active Time: ½ hour Total Time: 1½ hours	Flavor: Buttery, sweet, balanced Texture: Fluid Color: Golden
Caramelized Onion	Slowly caramelized onions are simmered with sautéed vegetables and deglazed with white wine. Balsamic vinegar and cayenne pepper balance sweetness from onions.	Active Time: ½ hour Total Time: 2 hours	Flavor: Caramelized, sweet, complex Texture: Fluid Color: Dark brown
Ramp Stock	Seasonal wild onion bulbs are simmered with sautéed vegetables and deglazed with dry vermouth.	Active Time: ¾ hour Total Time: 2 hours	Flavor: Garlicky, bright Texture: Fluid Color: Golden
GARLIC: LOCAL FARM; ORGANIC, WHEN POSSIBLE			
Garlic Scape	Young garlic scape stalks with closed buds are lightly simmered with basic herbs and spices.	Active Time: ½ hour Total Time: 1¼ hours	Flavor: Clean, bright Texture: Fluid Color: Golden
Green Garlic	Young green garlic is crushed, sautéed with vegetables, and deglazed with white wine.	Active Time: ½ hour Total Time: 1½ hours	Flavor: Clean, bright Texture: Fluid Color: Golden
Aged Garlic	Black garlic is simmered with roasted vegetables. Tamari or light soy sauce can be added at end for depth of flavor.	Active Time: ½ hour Total Time: 2 hours	Flavor: Sweet, complex Texture: Fluid Color: Light brown
Roasted Garlic	Whole heads of garlic are roasted, simmered with sautéed vegetables, and deglazed with red wine.	Active Time: ½ hour Total Time: 2 hours	Flavor: Mild, sweet Texture: Fluid Color: Deep amber
Garlic Confit	Peeled garlic cloves are infused in oil, strained, sautéed with vegetables, and deglazed with white wine.	Active Time: 1 hour Total Time: 2½ hours	Flavor: Rich, sweet Texture: Fluid Color: Golden
SEAWEED: REGIONAL FARM, WHEN POSSIBLE. Look for kelp or kombu that is yellowish brown instead of dark brown or black.			
Kelp Stock	Kelp is steeped in cold water overnight and strained for clarity.	Active Time: ½ hour Total Time: 8 hours	Flavor: Briny, sweet Texture: Silky Color: Light green
Dashi	High-quality bonito flakes are lightly simmered with kelp stock and strained for clarity.	Active Time: ½ hour Total Time: ¾ hour	Flavor: Briny, complex Texture: Silky Color: Light green

TABLE B.5. Guidelines for Dairy Stocks and Broths

Type	Distinction	Cook Time	Properties
WHEY: Seek producers that follow humane animal practices and follow organic standards. Local or regional, when possible.			
Basic	Pasteurized milk and lemon juice are simmered until curds separate from whey and are strained. Do not use ultra-high-temperature (UHT) pasteurized milk. Separation will not occur.	Active Time: ½ hour Total Time: 1 hour	Flavor: Nutty, tangy Texture: Fluid Color: Cloudy white
Buttermilk	Pasteurized milk and buttermilk are simmered until curds separate from whey and are strained. Cream can be added for more flavor. Do not use ultra-high-temperature (UHT) pasteurized milk. Separation will not occur.	Active Time: ½ hour Total Time: 1 hour	Flavor: Nutty, tangy, creamy Texture: Fluid Color: Cloudy white
Raw	Fresh raw milk is left at room temperature, undisturbed, until separation occurs and curds are strained out.	Active Time: ½ hour Total Time: 2 to 3 days	Flavor: Nutty, tangy, grassy Texture: Fluid Color: Cloudy white
Yogurt	Full-fat yogurt is left at room temperature, undisturbed, until separation occurs and curds are strained out.	Active Time: ½ hour Total Time: 2 to 3 days	Flavor: Nutty, tangy Texture: Fluid Color: Cloudy white
CHEESE			
Parmesan	Parmesan rinds are simmered with sautéed vegetables.	Active Time: ½ hour Total Time: 2½ hours	Flavor: Nutty, tangy Texture: Fluid Color: Golden

NOTES

INTRODUCTION

1. Thomas Keller, *The French Laundry Cookbook* (New York: Artisan, 1999).
2. Nicolette Hahn Niman, *Defending Beef: The Case for Sustainable Meat Production* (White River Junction, VT: Chelsea Green Publishing, 2014).
3. Adam Danforth, http://www.adamdanforth.com.
4. Animal Welfare Approved, August 3, 2010, http://animalwelfareapproved.us/2010/08/03/clinton-mezvinsky-wedding-featured-animal-welfare-approved-short-ribs-from-grazin-angus-acres.
5. Patricia Leigh Brown, "For Local Fisheries, a Line of Hope," *New York Times*, October 1, 2012.
6. John Wymer, *The Paleolithic Age* (London: Croom Helm, 1982).
7. James Owen, "Bone Flute Is Oldest Instrument, Study Says," *National Geographic News*, June 24, 2009.
8. Victor H. Mair, "The Case of the Wayward Oracle Bone," *Expedition* 43, no. 2 (2001): 41–45.
9. Edward Allworthy Armstrong, *The Folklore of Birds: An Enquiry into the Origins and Distribution of Some Magico-Religious Traditions* (New York: Dover Publications, 1970).
10. Gerard C. Wertkin, *Encyclopedia of American Folk Art* (London: Routledge, 2004).
11. Endymion Porter Wilkinson, *Chinese History: A New Manual*, 4th ed. (Cambridge, MA: Harvard University Asia Center, 2015).
12. USDA, "Compliance Guides Index," Food Safety and Inspecion Service, last modified June 1, 2016, http://www.fsis.usda.gov/wps/portal/fsis/topics/regulatory-compliance/compliance-guides-index.
13. John Fawell, *Fluoride in Drinking-Water* (Geneva: Worldwide Health Organization, 2006).
14. Purevsuren Barnasan, Budeebazar Avid, T. Gerelmaa, Davaajav Yadamsuren, Trevor J. Morgan, A. A. Herod, and R. Kandiyoti, "The Characterisation of Tar from the Pyrolysis of Animal Bones," *Fuel* 83, no. 7–8 (May 2004): 799–805.
15. Mike Callicrate, "Bone Char: From Farm to Phosphorous," Callicrate Cattle Co., accessed March 2016, http://www.callicratecattleco.com/soilproducts.htm.
16. Susan Mussi, "Bone Ash—Manufacture," *Ceramic-Pottery Dictionary*, accessed March 2016, http://ceramicdictionary.com/en/b/4031/bone-ash-manufacture.
17. Hugh Merwin, "Hot Hot Hot: Could High-End Charcoal Become a Thing?," *Grub Street*, January 12, 2012, http://www.grubstreet.com/2012/01/chefs-using-custom-high-end-charcoal.html.
18. Alanna Petroff, "The World Wastes $400 Billion in Food Every Year," *CNN Money*, February 26, 2015, http://money.cnn.com/2015/02/26/news/economy/food-waste.
19. Sally Fallon Morell, "Broth Is Beautiful," The Weston A. Price Foundation, January 1, 2000, http://www.westonaprice.org/health-topics/broth-is-beautiful.

CHAPTER ONE: THE IMPORTANCE OF STOCKS AND BROTHS

1. Sally Fallon Morell, "Broth Is Beautiful," The Weston A. Price Foundation, January 1, 2000, http://www.westonaprice.org/health-topics/broth-is-beautiful.
2. "The State of the Specialty Food Industry 2016," Specialty Food Association, March 30, 2016, https://www.specialtyfood.com/news/article/state-specialty-food-industry-2016.

3. Harold McGee, *On Food and Cooking: The Science and Lore of the Kitchen* (New York: Scribner, 2004).

4. Auguste Escoffier, *Escoffier: Le Guide Culinaire, Revised* (New Jersey: Wiley, 2011).

5. McGee, *On Food and Cooking*.

6. Sally Fallon Morell and Kaayla T. Daniel, *Nourishing Broth: An Old-Fashioned Remedy for the Modern World* (New York: Grand Central Life & Style, 2014).

7. Kate Shannon, "The Truth About Beef Broth," *Cook's Illustrated*, January 1, 2016, https://www .cooksillustrated.com/articles/149-the-truth -about-beef-broth.

8. Jill Tieman, "Store Bought Beef Broth or Stock— Not the Real Deal," Real Food Forager, accessed April 2016, http://realfoodforager.com/store -bought-beef-broth-or-stock-not-the-real-deal.

9. Amélie A. Walker, "Oldest Glue Discovered," *Archaeology*, May 21, 1998, http://archive .archaeology.org/online/news/glue.html.

10. Robert H. Bogue, "Conditions Affecting the Hydrolysis of Collagen to Gelatin," *Industrial and Engineering Chemistry* 15, no. 11 (November 1923): 1154–59.

11. TreeHouse Foods, "Knox History," Knox Gelatine, accessed April 2016, http://www.knoxgelatine .com/history.htm.

12. "Natural Health Products Ingredients Database: Hydrolyzed Collagen," Government of Canada, Health Canada, Health Products and Food Branch, Natural Health Products Directorate, June 12, 2013.

13. "National Organic Standards Board Technical Advisory Panel Review: Gelatin Processing," accessed April 2016, Organic Materials Review Institute.

14. A. G. Ward and A. Courts, *The Science and Technology of Gelatin* (New York: Academic Press, 1977).

15. Joseph B Michaelson and David J. Huntsman, "New Aspects of the Effects of Gelatin on Fingernails," *Journal of the Society of Cosmetics Chemists* 14, no. 9 (August 1963): 443–54; Maryam Borumand and Sara Sibilla, "Daily Consumption of the Collagen Supplement Pure Gold Collagen® Reduces Visible Signs of Aging," *Clinical Interventions in Aging* 9 (October 13, 2014): 1747–58.

16. "Natural Health Products Ingredients Database: Hydrolyzed Collagen."

CHAPTER TWO: THE FUNDAMENTALS OF STOCKS AND BROTHS

1. Bernd Lindemann, Yoko Ogiwara, and Yuzo Ninomiya, "The Discovery of Umami," *Chemical Senses* 27, no. 9 (November 1, 2002): 843–44, doi:10.1093/chemse/27.9.843.

2. "Seonnong dan," *Doosan Encyclopedia*.

3. Laura Kelley, *The Silk Road Gourmet*: vol. 1: *Western and Southern Asia* (Indiana: iUniverse, 2009).

4. Cuong Huynh, "The History and Evolution of Pho: A Hundred Years' Journey," LovingPho, April 8, 2009, http://www.lovingpho.com/pho -opinion-editorial/history-and-evolution-of -vietnamese-pho.

CHAPTER THREE: A BRIEF HISTORY OF STOCKS AND BROTHS

1. Xiaohong Wu, Chi Zhang, Paul Goldberg, David Cohen, Yan Pan, Trina Arpin, and Ofer Bar-Yosef, "Early Pottery at 20,000 Years Ago in Xianrendong Cave, China," *Science* 336, no. 6089 (June 29, 2012): 1969–1700, doi:10.1126/science.1218643.

2. Jake Page, "Hot-Rock Cooking Party," *Smithsonian Magazine*, November 1997, http://www .smithsonianmag.com/science-nature/hot-rock -cooking-party-145917013.

3. Amanda G. Henry, Alison S. Brooks, and Dolores R. Piperno, "Microfossils in Calculus Demonstrate Consumption of Plants and Cooked Foods in Neanderthal Diets (Shanidar III, Iraq; Spy I and II, Belgium)," *Proceedings of the National Academy of Sciences of the United States* 108, no. 2 (November 12, 2010): 486–91, doi:10.1073/pnas.1016868108.

4. Sarah Zielinski, "Stone Age Stew? Soup Making May Be Older than We Thought," *NPR: The Salt*, February 6, 2013, http://www.npr.org/sections /thesalt/2013/02/06/171104410/stone-age-stew -soup-making-may-be-older-than-wed-thought.

5. Rod Benson, "Montana Earth Science," Montana's Earth Science Pictures, accessed May 2016, http://formontana.net/boiling.html.

6. Barbara Flower and Elisabeth Rosenbaum, trans., *The Roman Cookery Book: A Critical Translation of The Art of Cooking by Apicius, for Use in the Study and the Kitchen* (London: Harrap, 1958).

7. Apicius, trans. Joseph Dommers Vehling, *Cookery and Dining in Imperial Rome* (Chicago: Hill, 1936). Available at Project Gutenberg, accessed May 2016, http://www.gutenberg.org/files/29728/29728-h/29728-h.htm.

8. James Grout, "Garum," *Encyclopædia Romana*, accessed May 2016, http://penelope.uchicago.edu/~grout/encyclopaedia_romana/wine/garum.html.

9. Sally Grainger, "Garum, Liquamen and Muria: A New Approach to the Problem of Definition," accessed May 2016, http://www.academia.edu/5850522/Garum_liquamen_and_muria_a_new_approach_to_the_problem_of_definition.

10. Deena Prichep, "Fish Sauce: An Ancient Roman Condiment Rises Again," *NPR: The Salt,* October 26, 2013, http://www.npr.org/sections/thesalt/2013/10/26/240237774/fish-sauce-an-ancient-roman-condiment-rises-again.

11. Apicius, *Cookery and Dining in Imperial Rome.*

12. Anthony Di Renzo, *Bitter Greens: Essays on Food, Politics, and Ethnicity from the Imperial Kitchen* (Albany, NY: Excelsior Editions, 2010).

13. Malcom Thick, *Sir Hugh Plat: The Search for Useful Knowledge in Early Modern London* (Totnes, Devon: Prospect Books, 2010).

14. Hannah Glasse, *The Art of Cookery Made Plain and Easy: The Revolutionary 1805 Classic* (Mineola, NY: Dover Publications, 2015).

15. Kevin Joel Berland, ed., *The Dividing Line Histories of William Byrd II of Westover* (Chapel Hill, NC: University of North Carolina Press, 2013).

16. Sylvanus Urban, *The Gentleman's Magazine, and Historical Chronicle*, vol. 59, part 1 (London: St. John's Gate, 1789).

17. Rebecca Rupp, "The Luke-Warm, Gluey, History of Portable Soup," *National Geographic*, September 25, 2014, http://theplate.nationalgeographic.com/2014/09/25/the-luke-warm-gluey-history-of-portable-soup.

18. Victoria R. Rumble, *Soup through the Ages: A Culinary History with Period Recipes* (Jefferson, NC: McFarland & Co., 2009).

19. Leandra Zim Holland, *Feasting and Fasting with Lewis and Clark: A Food and Social History of the Early 1800s* (Emigrant, MT: Old Yellowstone Publishing, 2003).

20. E. C. Spary, *Eating the Enlightenment: Food and the Sciences in France, 1670–1760* (Chicago: University of Chicago Press, 2012).

21. Richard D. Semba, *The Vitamin A Story: Lifting the Shadow of Death* (Basel: Karger, 2012).

22. Dana Simmons, *Vital Minimum: Need, Science, and Politics in Modern France* (Chicago: University of Chicago Press, 2015).

23. James H. Collins, *The Story of Canned Foods* (New York: E. P. Dutton, 1924).

24. John D. Post, *The Last Great Subsistence Crisis in the Western World* (Baltimore: Johns Hopkins University Press, 1977).

25. Harold McGee, *Keys to Good Cooking: A Guide to the Best of Foods and Recipes* (New York: Penguin Books, 2010).

26. Clay Cansler, "Where's the Beef?," *Distillations*, Fall 2013 / Winter 2014, accessed May 2016, https://www.chemheritage.org/distillations/article/where's-beef.

27. William H. Brock, *Justus von Liebig: The Chemical Gatekeeper* (Cambridge, U.K.: Cambridge University Press, 1997).

28. F. C. Cook, "Bouillon Cubes," *Journal of Industrial & Engineering Chemistry* 5, no. 12 (December 1913): 989–90, doi:10.1021/ie50060a009.

29. Prosper Montagné, *Larousse Gastronomique* (New York: Clarkson Potter, 2001, originally published in 1938).

30. Marie-Noël Rio, *The Food of Paris: Authentic Recipes from Parisian Bistros and Restaurants* (Singapore: Periplus, 2002).

31. Maguelonne Toussaint-Samat, trans. Anthea Bell, *A History of Food* (Cambridge, MA: Blackwell Reference, 1993).

32. Jules Gouffé, trans. Alphonse Gouffé, *The Royal Cookery Book (Le Livre de Cuisine)* (London: Sampson Low, Son, and Marston, 1869).

33. Harold Brubaker, "Campbell Soup Shares Fall on Sales Decline," *Philadelphia Inquirer*, May 20, 2016.

CHAPTER FOUR: THE COMPOSITION OF STOCKS AND BROTHS

1. Brendon Hong, "China Is Brewing Wine from Tiger Bones," *Daily Beast*, July 22, 2014, http://www.thedailybeast.com/articles/2014/07/22/china-is-brewing-wine-from-tiger-bones.html.

2. Sharon Guynup, "Tigers in Traditional Chinese Medicine: A Universal Apothecary," *National Geographic*, April 29, 2014, http://voices.nationalgeographic.com/2014/04/29/tigers-in-traditional-chinese-medicine-a-universal-apothecary.

3. Amy Blaszyk, "Taking Stock of Bone Broth: Sorry, No Cure-All Here," *NPR: The Salt*, February 10, 2015, http://www.npr.org/sections/thesalt/2015/02/10/384948585/taking-stock-of-bone-broth-sorry-no-cure-all-here.

4. R. A. McCance, W. Sheldon, and E. M. Widdowson, "Bone and Vegetable Broth," *Archives of Disease in Childhood* 9, no. 52 (August 1934): 251–58, http://www.ncbi.nlm.nih.gov/pmc/articles/PMC1975347.

5. USDA, "Broth," USDA Food Composition Databases, United States Department of Agriculture Agricultural Research Service, accessed May 2016.

6. Kristina Bravo, "12 Surprising Foods with More Sugar than a Krispy Kreme Doughnut," *Takepart*, April 17, 2014, http://www.takepart.com/photos/shocking-sugar-stats.

7. Kiera Butler, "Enough Already with the Bone Broth Hype," *Mother Jones*, November 9, 2015, http://www.motherjones.com/environment/2015/11/truth-about-bone-broth.

8. E. C. Spary, *Eating the Enlightenment: Food and the Sciences in France, 1670–1760* (Chicago: University of Chicago Press, 2012).

9. Amy Christine Brown, *Understanding Food: Principles and Preparation*, 5th ed. (Stamford, CT: Cengage Learning, 2015).

10. V. R. Young and P. L. Pellett, "Plant Proteins in Relation to Human Protein and Amino Acid Nutrition," *American Journal of Clinical Nutrition* 59, no. 5 (May 1994): 1203s–12.

11. Blaszyk, "Taking Stock of Bone Broth: Sorry, No Cure-All Here."

12. Joseph B Michaelson and David J. Huntsman, "New Aspects of the Effects of Gelatin on Fingernails," *Journal of the Society of Cosmetics Chemists* 14, no. 9 (August 1963): 443–54.

13. Michael G. Mulinos and Ellen D. Kadison, "Effect of Gelatin on the Vascularity of the Finger," *Angiology* 16 (April 1965): 170–76.

14. Maryam Borumand and Sara Sibilla, "Daily Consumption of the Collagen Supplement Pure Gold Collagen® Reduces Visible Signs of Aging," *Clinical Interventions in Aging* 9 (October 13, 2014): 1747–58.

15. D. E. Trentham, R. A. Dynesius-Trentham, E. J. Orav, D. Combitchi, C. Lorenzo, K. L. Sewell, D. A. Hafler, and H. L. Weiner, "Effects of Oral Administration of Type II Collagen on Rheumatoid Arthritis," *Science* 261, no. 5129 (September 24, 1993): 1727–30.

16. Alexander G. Schauss, Jerome Stenehjem, Joosang Park, John R. Endres, and Amy Clewell, "Effect of the Novel Low Molecular Weight Hydrolyzed Chicken Sternal Cartilage Extract, BioCell Collagen, on Improving Osteoarthritis-Related Symptoms: A Randomized, Double-Blind, Placebo-Controlled Trial," *Journal of Agricultural and Food Chemistry* 60, no. 16 (April 2012): 4096–101, doi:10.1021/jf205295u.

17. European Food Safety Authority, "Scientific Opinion on the Substantiation of a Health Claim Related to Collagen Hydrolysate and Maintenance of Joints Pursuant to Article 13(5) of Regulation (EC) No 1924/2006," *EFSA Journal* 9, no. 7 (July 20, 2011): 2291–301.

18. Joseph Stromberg, "Why Asparagus Makes Your Urine Smell," *Smithsonian Magazine*, May 3, 2013,

http://www.smithsonianmag.com/science-nature
/why-asparagus-makes-your-urine-smell-49961252.

19. Barbara O. Rennard, Ronald F. Ertl, Gail L. Goss-
man, Richard A. Robbins, and Stephen I. Rennard,
"Chicken Soup Inhibits Neutrophil Chemotaxis
in Vitro," *Chest Journal* 118, no. 4 (October 2000):
1150–57.

20. K. Saketkhoo, A. Januszkiewicz, and M. A.
Sackner, "Effects of Drinking Hot Water, Cold
Water, and Chicken Soup on Nasal Mucus Velocity
and Nasal Airflow Resistance," *Chest Journal* 74,
no. 4 (October 1978): 408–10.

21. Joseph Stromberg, "A Hot Drink on a Hot Day
Can Cool You Down," *Smithsonian Magazine*,
July 10, 2012, http://www.smithsonianmag.com
/science-nature/a-hot-drink-on-a-hot-day-can
-cool-you-down-1338875.

22. Allan Savory and Jody Butterfield, *Holistic Management: A New Framework for Decision Making*, 2nd
ed. (Washington, DC: Island Press, 1998).

23. Orville Schell, *Modern Meat: Antibiotics,
Hormones, and the Pharmaceutical Farm* (New
York: Random House, 1984).

24. "Facts about Antibiotic Resistance," Infectious
Disease Society of America, last updated April
2001, http://www.idsociety.org/AR_Facts.

25. "Not Just the Cows: Pastured Pork and Poultry,"
Paleo Leap, accessed May 2016, http://paleoleap
.com/just-cows-pastured-pork-poultry.

26. Cynthia Daley, Amber Abbott, Patrick S. Doyle,
Glenn A. Nader, and Stephanie Larson, "A Review
of Fatty Acid Profiles and Antioxidant Content in
Grass-Fed and Grain-Fed Beef," *Nutrition Journal* 9
(March 10, 2010): 10.

27. Chris Kresser, "Grass-Fed vs. Conventional Meat:
It's Not Black or White," January 4, 2011, http://
chriskresser.com/grass-fed-vs-conventional-meat
-its-not-black-or-white.

28. Heather Pickett, "Nutritional Benefits of Higher
Welfare Animal Products," Compassion in World
Farming, July 2012, http://ciwf.org/nutrition.

29. "Slow Growth Means Higher Welfare for
Chickens," The Poultry Site, July 1, 2013, http://
www.thepoultrysite.com/poultrynews/29349
/slow-growth-means-higher-welfare-for-chickens.

30. Butler, "Enough Already with the Bone Broth Hype."

31. Cristiana Miglio, Emma Chiavaro, Attilio Visconti,
Vincenzo Fogliano, and Nicoletta Pellegrini,
"Effects of Different Cooking Methods on
Nutritional and Physiochemical Characteristics of
Selected Vegetables," *Journal of Agricultural and
Food Chemistry* 56, no. 1 (February 2008): 139–47.

32. Tara Parker-Pope, "Ask Well: Does Boiling or
Baking Vegetables Destroy Their Vitamins?," *Well*
(*New York Times* blog), October 18, 2013.

33. Blaszyk, "Taking Stock of Bone Broth: Sorry, No
Cure-All Here."

34. Albert E. Purcell and William M. Walter Jr., "Stability of Amino Acids During Cooking and Processing
of Sweet Potatoes," *Journal of Agricultural Food
Chemistry* 30, no. 3 (May 1982): 443–44.

35. Mark Krasnow, Tucker Bunch, Charles Shoemaker,
and Christopher R. Loss, "Effects of Cooking
Temperature on the Physiochemical Properties and
Consumer Acceptance of Chicken Stock," *Journal
of Food Science* 77, no. 1 (January 2012): s19–23.

36. Jean A. Monro, R. Leon, and Basant K. Puri, "The
Risk of Lead Contamination in Bone Broth Diets,"
Medical Hypotheses 80, no. 4 (January 2013).

37. Chris Kresser, "Bone Broth and Lead Toxicity:
Should You Be Concerned?," February 8, 2013,
https://chriskresser.com/bone-broth-and-lead-
toxicity-should-you-be-concerned.

38. Kaayla Daniels, "Bone Broth and Lead Contamination: A Very Flawed Study in *Medical Hypotheses*,"
Weston A. Price Foundation, March 12, 2013,
http://www.westonaprice.org/health-topics/soy
-alert/bone-broth-and-lead-contamination-a-very
-flawed-study-in-medical-hypotheses.

39. Kim Schuette, "Stock vs. Broth: Are You Confused?," Biodynamic Wellness, accessed May 2016,
http://www.biodynamicwellness.com/stock
-vs-broth-confused.

40. Robert J. Taylor, "Nutrition to Fight Lead Poisoning,"
Lead Action News 10, no. 2 (June 2010): http://
www.lead.org.au/lanv10n2/lanv10n2-11.html.

41. Tommaso Iannitti, Daniele Lodi, and Beniamino Palmieri, "Intra-Articular Injections for the Treatment of Osteoarthritis," *Drugs in R&D* 11, no. 1 (March 2011): 13–27, doi:10.2165/11539760 -000000000-00000.

42. R. A. McCance, W. Sheldon, and E. M. Widdowson, "Bone and Vegetable Broth," *Archives of Disease in Childhood* 9, no. 25 (August 1934): 251–58, http://www.ncbi.nlm.nih.gov/pmc /articles/PMC1975347.

43. Maria Christensen, "Benefits of Seaweed and Kelp," last updated March 12, 2014, Livestrong.com, http://www.livestrong.com/article/156593 -benefits-of-seaweed-kelp.

CHAPTER FIVE: THE SIGNIFICANCE OF QUALITY SOURCING

1. Erin Zimmer, "Meet Your Farmers: Jen Small and Mike Yezzi, Flying Pigs Farm in New York," *Serious Eats*, October 12, 2009, http://www.seriouseats .com/2009/10/farmers-jen-small-and-mike-yezzi -flying-pigs-farm-nyc-greenmarkets.html.

2. "Questions to Ask a Beef Farmer," *Sustainable Table*, GRACE Communications Foundation, accessed May 2016, http://www.sustainabletable .org/2224/questions-to-ask#Beef_Farmer.

3. Roberto A. Ferdman, "The Shrimp You're Buying Isn't Always What It Claims to Be," *Washington Post*, October 31, 2014, https://www.washingtonpost .com/news/wonk/wp/2014/10/31/the-shrimp -youre-buying-isnt-always-what-it-claims-to-be.

4. "Questions to Ask a Produce Farmer," *Sustainable Table*, GRACE Communications Foundation,

accessed May 2016, http://www.sustainabletable .org/2224/questions-to-ask#Produce_Farmer.

5. Akiko Katayama, "A Kombu Primer," *Lucky Peach*, August 10, 2015, http://luckypeach.com/a -kombu-primer.

CHAPTER SIX: SETTING UP YOUR KITCHEN FOR MAKING STOCKS AND BROTHS

1. "Water Quality and Testing," Centers for Disease Control and Prevention, last updated April 2009, https://www.cdc.gov/healthywater/drinking /public/water_quality.html.

CHAPTER SEVEN: THE BASIC SCIENCE OF A GOOD FOUNDATION

1. Harold McGee, "A Hot-Water Bath for Thawing Meats," *New York Times*, June 6, 2011, http://www .nytimes.com/2011/06/08/dining/a-hot-water -bath-for-thawing-meats-the-curious-cook.html

2. R. A. McCance, W. Sheldon, and E. M. Widdowson, "Bone and Vegetable Broth," *Archives of Disease in Childhood* 9, no. 52 (August 1934): 251–58, http:// www.ncbi.nlm.nih.gov/pmc/articles/PMC1975347.

3. "Food Code 2013," US Food and Drug Administration, last updated July 2, 2015, http://www.fda .gov/Food/GuidanceRegulation/RetailFood Protection/FoodCode/ucm374275.htm.

4. Harold McGee, "The Essence of Nearly Anything, Drop by Limpid Drop," *New York Times*, September 5, 2007, http://www.nytimes.com/2007/09 /05/dining/05curi.html.

GLOSSARY

A

À la nage. A French term that means "while swimming" and refers to poaching delicate food in court bouillon.

Agar-agar. A gelatinous thickening agent derived from algae.

Aged garlic. White garlic that has been slowly caramelized to yield sweet black cloves; often used in Asian cuisine. Also known as black garlic.

Allec. The secondary extraction of garum; a thick concentrate considered to be lesser quality than the first extraction.

Aromatics. Any ingredient—vegetable, herb, or spice—that is used to enhance flavor in food or drinks. Aromatics are commonly used to enhance the color and flavor of stocks and broths.

Aspic. A clear jelly made from animal or fish stocks. Aspic can also be made by adding gelatin to vegetable stocks. See also Meat Jelly.

Autolyzed yeast extract. A substance that occurs when enzymes in yeast are used to break down proteins into simpler compounds. It is a natural source of free glutamic acid and often listed as an ingredient in highly processed foods.

B

Baste. A slow-cooking technique that produces a succulent texture in roasted meat or vegetables by moistening with stock, pan juices, or melted fat.

Beef extract. A paste made from the soluble elements of beef. According to the USDA, beef extract is a mixture made from boiling consecutive batches of meat in the same cooking liquid until it yields 75 percent solids to 25 percent moisture.

Beef fat. The USDA term for concentrated meat stock made from beef. Not tallow. See also Meat Extract.

Biochar. A charcoal made through pyrolysis used for agricultural purposes.

Blast chiller. A commercial appliance that rapidly cools hot liquids to a safe temperature, typically within ninety minutes.

Bloom scale. The grading system for assessing the molecular weight of gelatin.

Boil. The state when liquid reaches the temperature at which it turns to vapor. In water (at sea level) the boiling point is 212°F (100°C).

Bone ash. The white ash that results from calcination of bones; often used for fertilizer and to make bone china. See also Bone China.

Bone black. A black pigment used for artistic applications. Also known as ivory black.

Bone broth. An animal stock that uses collagen-rich bones and simmers for an extended time to maximize gelatin extraction into the liquid.

Bone carvings. Artifacts made from bone that were used for religious ceremonies and made into jewelry.

Bone char. The product of burning bones in a low-oxygen vessel to render activated carbon.

Bone china. The white porcelain made from bone ash. See also Bone Ash.

Bone flute. The oldest known instrument made from the wing bones of a vulture and a mute swan, and ivory from the woolly mammoth.

Bone meal. Ground animal bones used as fertilizer and a nutritional supplement for animals.

Bonito flakes. The dried, smoked shavings of a type of tuna used in Japanese cuisine. Also known as *katsuobushi*.

Bony fish. Fish from the dominant vertebrate order, including snapper, grouper, and cod.

Bouillabaisse. A traditional fish stew from Marseille made with fish, shellfish, tomatoes, and saffron, and garnished with rouille.

Bouilli. The braised meat in pot au feu. See also Pot au Feu.

Bouillon. A liquid broth made by simmering meat, fish, or vegetables in water.

Bouillon cube. A dehydrated form of bouillon. Commercial varieties are heavily processed.

Bouillons de tablettes. An early literary reference to consommé in tablet form or portable soup.

Bourride. A Provençal fish stew typically thickened with aioli.

Bouquet garni. A bundle of herbs often wrapped in a green leek top and secured with butcher's twine. It is added to a soup pot to enhance flavor and packaged for easy removal.

Braise. A slow-cooking method that uses moist and dry heat to break down tough cuts of meat, fish, or vegetables.

Brew. A liquid infusion by soaking, boiling, and fermentation or by steeping in hot water.

Brine. A curing agent produced by saturating water with salt.

Brodo. An Italian term that refers to a broth that is the base for a finished dish (e.g., tortellini en brodo).

Brown stock. A dark cooking liquid made by roasting bones and vegetables before simmering in water. Also known as fond brun.

Broth. A substance prepared by boiling; often a stock enhanced with meat, vegetables, and/or starches to yield a finished dish.

Brunoise. A fine dice of vegetables used to enhance the flavor and texture of finished dishes.

C

Cartilage. Connective tissue found in skeleton structure that converts to bone with maturation.

Caul fat. The thin, lacy membrane that surrounds internal organs of some animals, such as cows, pigs, and sheep.

Cheesecloth. A lightweight, loosely woven cotton fabric used to filter liquids, wrap cheese, and for other methods of food preparation.

China cap. A metal conical strainer with holes that are larger than those on a chinois. It is ideal for filtering bones from stocks and broths before running the liquid through a fine-mesh strainer.

Chinois. A fine-mesh strainer that appears as a conical sieve; it is used to produce a fine texture in purées, sauces, and custards.

Coddle. A technique where food is cooked slowly in liquid held just below the boiling point.

Collagen. The structural protein found in connective tissue of animals; it renders into gelatin when simmered.

Community Supported Agriculture. A food production and distribution system where growers and consumers share the risks and benefits of farming vegetables and livestock often within a regenerative landscape.

Community Supported Fisheries. A food production and distribution system where fishermen and consumers share the risks and benefits of harvesting fish and seafood in a sustainable manner.

Compound stock. A stock or broth made from a another batch of stock or broth. Also known as double stock.

Confit. A preservation technique that involves cooking meat in its own fat.

Consommé. A clear, flavorful broth made from a clarified concentrated stock.

Cooling ice paddle. An industrial tool for rapidly chilling hot liquids to a safe temperature. Ice paddles are made of thick food-grade plastic that withstands heat when full of frozen water.

D

Dashi. A fundamental broth in Japanese cuisine made from dried bonito and dried kelp.

Degustation. A meal devised of small dishes to highlight a chef's talent in the kitchen; a tasting menu.

Dehydrator. An appliance that removes moisture from food for concentrated flavor and long-term storage.

Demi-glace. A concentrated reduction of brown stock and brown sauce that yields a rich, dense glaze; commonly flavored with red wine. Also known as half glaze.

Deviled. A term used to describe foods that are cooked with hot spices or condiments.

Diffusion. The spreading of molecules of one substance through those of another substance, caused by thermal agitation.

Digester. A high-pressure steam cooker that dissolves bones into gelatin. Also known as Papin's Digester.

Dippel's Oil. The dark oil that remains as a toxic by-product from the distillation of bones. Also known as bone oil.

Double consommé. A clear, flavorful broth made from a clarified concentrated stock reduced by half.

Dragon bones. A divination tool commonly made from ox bones in ancient China. Also known as oracle bones.

Dry-aging. The process of hanging animal carcasses in refrigeration and at a certain humidity to encourage enzymatic changes that improves texture and develop flavor.

F

Farce. A French term that refers to forcemeat stuffing.

Fat (animal). The greasy material that acts as insulation under the skin or around certain organs; when harvested, animal fats can be rendered and used as a cooking agent or for cosmetics.

Fermentation. A metabolic process that transforms and preserves the sugars and starches of organic materials. Beer, wine, kimchi, and yogurt are examples of fermented foods. See also Lacto-Fermentation.

Fine-mesh strainer. A bowl-shaped metal sieve that is used to drain liquids from solids and to refine the texture of sauces.

Fish sauce. A liquid condiment typically made from fermented anchovies and salt, common to Thailand, Vietnam, and Korea.

Flatfish. A spiny fish that has a flat body and swims with its eyes on the upper side. Flatfish include halibut, flounder, and sole.

Fond. A French term referring to the base or foundation of cuisine; also refers to the browned crust that develops on the bottom of a pan while cooking.

Food waste. The loss of organic material throughout its consumptive life, often due to faults in production and distribution; food that is discarded, spoiled, expired, or uneaten.

Fumet. A classic stock commonly made from cooking fish, meat, or vegetables and used to enhance sauces.

G

Garum. A fermented fish sauce heavily used as a condiment in ancient Greece, Rome, and Byzantium. See also Liquamen.

Gelatin. A tacky substance made by simmering animal tissue in water.

Gelatin-filtered consommé. A modern clarifying technique that removes fat and solid particles from a concentrated stock. See also Ice Filtration.

Gelometer. An apparatus used to measure the strength of gelatin.

Glace de viande. A meat glaze made by reducing unsalted meat stock to about 20 percent of its original volume. Also known as meat glass.

Glaze. The flavorful coating that appears on food as it cooks; also, the syrup that develops from reducing a stock.

Glutamate. A salt or ester of glutamic acid. Also known as monosodium glutamate.

Grass-fed beef. Cattle that are raised on grass from birth through harvest; these animals are never fed grain.

Gribenes. A Yiddish term that refers to the crispy poultry skin that develops when rendering schmaltz; similar to cracklings.

H

Herb sachet. A small packet of herbs and spices wrapped in cheesecloth that is added to simmering liquid and allows for easy removal.

Heritage breed. Traditional livestock breeds that were raised by farmers before the introduction of industrial agriculture.

Humane slaughter. A method of killing an animal by stunning it prior to death; a means of ensuring the animal does not suffer.

Hydrogarum. A fish sauce that is diluted with water; common to ancient Greece, Rome, and Byzantium.

Hydrolysis. A chemical reaction where water is used to break down a compound.

I

Ice filtration. A method of extracting solid particles from a liquid to achieve clarity; a technique for making consommé. See also Gelatin-Filtered Consommé.

Isinglass. A type of gelatin obtained from the air bladders of certain fish, such as sturgeon.

Ivory black. See Bone Black.

K

Kelp. Large, brown, cold-water seaweed from the family Laminariaceae. See also Kombu.

Kombu. A type of edible kelp that is widely used in East Asian cuisine. See also Kelp.

L

Lacto-fermentation. A microbial process where starches and sugars convert to lactic acid when beneficial bacteria are introduced to an anaerobic environment. See also Fermentation.

Lard. Fat from a hog that can be rendered and clarified for cooking and crafting.

Leaf gelatin. A colorless, odorless, brittle gelling agent derived from collagen and produced in sheets.

Leaky gut syndrome. A medical condition that some practitioners believe is the cause of serious chronic disease, such as diabetes and multiple sclerosis.

Liaison. A binding agent in cooking, such as flour or cornstarch; also refers to the use of cream and egg yolks to thicken soup and sauce.

Liquamen. A fermented fish sauce similar to and often synonymous with garum in ancient Greece, Rome, and Byzantium. See also Garum.

Liquor (shellfish). The natural brine contained within shellfish, such as clams and oysters.

M

Master stock. A Chinese stock that is repeatedly used to poach and braise meats.

Marrow. The nutrient-dense connective tissue that fills the cavities of bones.

Meat extract. A highly concentrated beef stock invented by Baron Justus von Liebig in the nineteenth century. See also Beef Fat.

Meat jelly. A clear jelly made from animal or fish stocks. See also Aspic.

Mellogarum. A fish sauce that is mixed with honey; common to ancient Greece, Rome, and Byzantium.

Merguez. A spicy sausage typically made from lamb and/or beef and seasoned with red pepper; of Moroccan origin.

Mise en place. A French culinary phrase that refers to having ingredients at hand before starting the cooking process.

Mirepoix. A finely diced mixture of vegetables, typically sautéed to enhance a dish.

Moisture-Protein Ratio (MPR). An USDA indicator of shelf stability—or the ratio of fat, moisture, and protein—in retail meat products.

Monosodium glutamate. See Glutamate.

Mother sauces. The five basic sauces that form the foundation of cooking in French cuisine: béchamel, Espagnole, hollandaise, tomate, velouté.

O

Oenogarum. A fish sauce that is mixed with wine; common to ancient Greece, Rome, and Byzantium.

Oracle bones. See Dragon Bones.

Oxygarum. A fish sauce that is mixed with vinegar; common to ancient Greece, Rome, and Byzantium.

P

Pastured beef. Cattle that are raised on grass and finished on grain.

Pastured poultry. Chickens, turkeys, and/or ducks that are raised with access to land for foraging and indoor protection from predators at night.

Pemmican. A concentrated, preserved food made of dried, pulverized meat, animal fat, and fruits or berries; commonly used by North American Indians.

Permaculture. Agricultural methods that endeavor to be self-sufficient and symbiotic with natural surroundings.

Pho. A popular Vietnamese soup made with beef stock, aromatic spices, and rice noodles.

Pit oven. An ancient cooking mechanism made by trapping heat inside the ground to bake, smoke, or steam food.

Poach. A culinary method that cooks food in simmering liquid.

Portable soup. A dehydrated food that was used on early expeditions and served as a precursor to meat extract and bouillon cubes. Also known as pocket soup or veal glew (glue).

Pot au feu. A classic French stew made of beef and vegetables cooked in one pot.

Pot-pourri. The French term for a Spanish stew specific to the town of Burgos; translates to "rotten pot."

Pottage. A thick soup or stew from the Middle Ages that is made with vegetables and grains, as well as fish or meat when available.

Poule au pot. A French dish that involves cooking an entire chicken with broth and vegetables in a stockpot.

Pressure canner. A device used to preserve food in sealed jars by pressurizing the contents for a period of time.

Pressure cooker. An airtight cooking apparatus that applies steam pressure to cook food.

Q

Quick sauce. A sauce that begins with a brown stock and is iteratively reduced and clarified until the proper texture and flavor are achieved.

R

Raft. A traditional technique of simmering egg whites, eggshells, and/or ground meat in a stock to gather impurities and form a consommé.

Ramps. A rare wild onion found in eastern North America; noted by its delicate flat leaves, pinkish white bulbs, and pungent flavor.

Raw milk. Dairy milk from a mammal that has not been pasteurized for consumption.

Rare breed. A livestock breed that is uncommon to large-scale commercial farming; typically selected for traits that fit its habitat.

Reduction. The culinary process of thickening a liquid to intensify flavor and concentrate texture.

Rejuvelac. A tangy non-alcoholic fermented beverage made from sprouting grains.

Remouillage. A French term that refers to the re-wetting of bones to yield a second stock extraction. Also known as second stock.

Restaurant. An establishment where one goes to consume food and beverage; originally a reference to a fortifying broth that was served in French establishments of the same name.

Reverse osmosis water. A water filtration system where water pressure is pushed through a semi-permeable membrane to filter solids from a solution.

Rille. An Old French word that refers to a slice of pork, particularly the appearance of rails that develop as it cooks.

Rillettes. A preparation of highly spiced meat that is slowly cooked in animal fat to render a consistency similar to pâté.

Rishiri. A type of aged kelp that is used for making dashi.

Rose veal. Calves raised on farms under humane conditions; the meat is slightly pink in color due to a later harvesting age than factory-farmed calves.

Rouille. A sauce that typically accompanies bouillabaisse—made by combining garlic, bread crumbs, and red peppers with stock and olive oil.

Rotational grazing. A holistic land management strategy that raises livestock on subdivided pastures to enrich soil and grass conditions.

S

Saucier. A cook or chef who prepares sauces.

GLOSSARY

Schmaltz. A Yiddish term that refers to rendered animal fat, most often chicken.

Scrimshaw. An outdated craft that uses whalebone, ivory, or shells as a material for elaborate carvings.

Second stock. See Remouillage.

Slow cooker. An electric appliance that cooks food slowly in one large pot.

Slurry. A mixture of starch and water used as a thickening agent for cooking.

Soccarat. The crispy caramelized layer of rice that develops on the bottom of the pan when making paella.

Sofrito. A sautéed mixture of finely chopped vegetables commonly used as a base in Spanish, Caribbean, and Latin American cooking.

Solar evaporation. An extraction method where wind and sun assist salt collection from shallow pools of seawater. All sea salt is gathered in this manner.

Solution mining. An extraction method that injects fresh well water into salt beds to dissolve the salt, after which the brine is pumped out and delivered to plants for evaporation. Examples of salt mined in this way include common table salt and kosher salt.

Sop. A term used to describe dipping a piece of bread or toast in liquid, commonly referred to in medieval cookery.

Spatchcock. A technique of removing the backbone from poultry or game to butterfly the bird before cooking.

Sprouting. The process of germinating seeds of grains, legumes, and nuts to activate beneficial enzymes and ease digestibility.

Steam-jacketed kettle. An industrial pot used to prepare large quantities of food in a commercial kitchen.

Stew. A culinary dish comprising meat and/or vegetables cooked in liquid, such as stock, wine, or beer, to develop a thick gravy.

Stock. A culinary foundation prepared by simmering animal bones and/or vegetables and spices in water to develop a flavorful base for cooking.

Stockpot. A large pot intended for making long-simmering stock, broth, and soup.

T

Tallow. The rendered animal fat from cattle or sheep, used for cooking or making soap, candles, and cosmetics.

Terroir. The characteristic flavor imparted to food and wine from its origin environment.

Traiteur. An historical French term to describe the keeper and cook of an early restaurant.

U

Ugly produce. A colloquial phrase that refers to fruits and vegetables that are rejected by retailers because of their inconsistent appearance or bruised state.

Unrefined sea salt. A type of salt produced from the evaporation of seawater that maintains its mineral composition.

V

Veal glew. A veal glaze, or glace de viande, that is preserved through dehydration. See also Portable Soup.

W

Whey. The cloudy part of milk that separates from the curds when making cheese.

White stock. A light cooking liquid made by blanching and simmering unroasted bones and/or vegetables in water. Also known as fond blanc.

Y

Yeast extract. See Autolyzed Yeast Extract.

BIBLIOGRAPHY

Apicius, trans. Barbara Flower and Elisabeth Rosenbaum. *The Roman Cookery Book: A Critical Translation of the Art of Cooking by Apicius for Use in the Study and the Kitchen*. London: Harrap, 1958.

Apicius, trans. Joseph Dommers Vehling. *Cookery and Dining in Imperial Rome* (1936). Accessed May 2016, http://www.gutenberg.org/files/29728 /29728-h/29728-h.htm.

Appert, Nicolas. *The Art of Preserving All Kinds of Animal and Vegetable Substances for Several Years* (1811). Montana: Kessinger Publishing, 2010.

Barber, Dan. *The Third Plate: Field Notes on the Future of Food*. New York: Penguin Press, 2014.

Berland, Kevin, ed. *The Dividing Line Histories of William Byrd II of Westover*. North Carolina: University of North Carolina, 2013.

Bittman, Mark. *How to Cook Everything: 2,000 Simple Recipes for Great Food* (10th ed.). Massachusetts: Houghton Mifflin Harcourt, 2008.

Blencowe, Ann. *The Receipt Book of Mrs. Ann Blencowe (1694)*. London: Adelphi Guy Chapman, 1925.

"*Corpus Inscriptionum Latinarum*." Berlin-Brandenburg Academy of Sciences and Humanities. Retrieved November 2009, http://cil.bbaw.de/cil_en/index _en.html.

Danforth, Adam. *Butchering Poultry, Rabbit, Lamb, Goat, and Pork*. Massachusetts: Storey Publishing, 2014.

Davidson, Alan, edited by Tom Jaine. *The Oxford Companion to Food* (3rd ed.). Oxford, U.K.: Oxford University Press, 2014.

Escoffier, Auguste, edited by H. L. Cracknell and R. J. Kaufmann. *Escoffier: Le Guide Culinaire, Revised*. New Jersey: Wiley, 2011.

Escoffier, Auguste. *The Escoffier Cookbook and Guide to the Fine Art of Cookery*. New York: Crown Publishers, 1989.

Furetière, Antoine. *Essais d'un dictionnaire universel (1690)*. Accessed May 2016, http://www.gutenberg .org/files/47459/47459-h/47459-h.htm.

Glasse, Hannah. *The Art of Cookery Made Plain and Easy (1747)*. New York: Dover Publications, 2015.

Gouffé, Jules, and Alphonse Gouffé. *The Royal Cookery Book: (Le Livre de Cuisine) (1869)*. South Carolina: Nabu Press, 2014.

Greenaway, Twilight. "Protein: The Lay of the Lamb." *Grist*. February 2, 2012, http://grist.org/food /protein-the-lay-of-the-lamb.

Hill, Kate. *Cassoulet: A French Obsession*. France: Camont Press, 2015.

Keller, Thomas. *The French Laundry Cookbook*. New York: Artisan, 1999.

Kelly, Ian. *Cooking for Kings: The Life of Antonin Carême, the First Celebrity Chef*. London: Walker Books, 2009.

La Varenne, Francois Pierre. *The French Cook: Englished by I.D.G. (1653)*. United Kingdom: Equinox Publishing, 2001.

Liebig, Justus von. *Chemistry in Its Application to Agriculture and Physiology (1843)*. Massachusetts: Adamant Media Corp., 2002.

López-Alt, J. Kenji. *The Food Lab: Better Home-Cooking Through Science*. New York: W. W. Norton & Company, 2015.

McGee, Harold. *Keys to Good Cooking: A Guide to the Best of Foods and Recipes*. London: Penguin Publishing, 2010.

McGee, Harold. *On Food and Cooking: The Science and Lore of the Kitchen*. New York: Scribner, 2004.

Montagne, Prosper. *Larousse Gastronomique (1938)*. New York: Clarkson Potter, 2001.

Morell, Sally Fallon, and Kaayla T. Daniel. *Nourishing Broth: An Old-Fashioned Remedy for the Modern World*. New York: Grand Central Life & Style, 2014.

Morell, Sally Fallon, and Mary G. Enig. *Nourishing Traditions: The Cookbook That Challenges Politically Correct Nutrition and Diet Dictocrats* (2nd ed.). Maryland: New Trends Publishing, 2001.

Niman, Nicolette Hahn. *Defending Beef: The Case for Sustainable Meat Production*. Vermont: Chelsea Green Publishing, 2014.

O'Brian, Patrick. *The Far Side of the World* (book 10, Aubrey/Maturin novels). New York: W. W. Norton & Co., 1992.

Owen, Thomas, trans. *Geōponika: Agricultural Pursuits* (vol. 2). London: J. White, 1806.

Pollan, Michael. *The Omnivore's Dilemma: A Natural History of Four Meals*. London: Bloomsbury Publishing, 2011.

Rio, Marie-Noël. *The Food of Paris: Delicious Recipes from Parisian Bistros and Restaurants*. Singapore: Perplus Editions, 2002.

Robbins, Chandler S., Bertel Bruun, and Herbert S. Zim. *Birds of North America: A Guide to Field Identification* (2nd ed.). New York: St. Martin's Press, 2001.

Skutecki, Kathy. "Praise the Lard, Again." *Stresscake: Exploring the Bake & Release Theory*. Accessed April 2016, https://stresscake.wordpress.com/2013/05/17/praise-the-lard-again-chocolate-lard-bourbon-cake.

Salatin, Joel. *Folks, This Ain't Normal: A Farmer's Advice for Happier Hens, Healthier People, and a Better World*. New York: Center Street, 2011.

Smith, Andrew F. *A Critique of the Moral Defense of Vegetarianism* (eBook ed.). London: Palgrave Macmillan, 2016.

Spary, E. C. *Eating the Enlightenment: Food and the Sciences in France, 1670–1760*. Chicago: University of Chicago, 2012.

Spang, Rebecca L. *The Invention of the Restaurant: Paris and Modern Gastronomic Culture* (Harvard historical studies). Massachusetts: Harvard University Press, 2001.

Spong, Matthew. *Household Cyclopedia of 1881*. Indiana: Repressed Publishing, 2012.

Thick, Malcom. *Sir Hugh Plat: The Search for Useful Knowledge in Early Modern England*. London: Prospect Books, 2010.

White, Joyce. "Sobaheg Stew: A Wampanoag Inspired Thanksgiving Recipe." *A Taste of History with Joyce White*. Accessed May 2016, http://atasteofhistorywithjoycewhite.blogspot.com/2014/11/sobaheg-stew-wampanoag-inspired.html.

Wolfert, Paula. *The Food of Morocco*. New York: Ecco Press, 2009.

RECENT INDEX

INDEX

Note: Page numbers in **bold** refer to recipe instructions. Page numbers followed by *t* refer to tables.

INDEX

INDEX

INDEX

INDEX

ABOUT THE AUTHOR

RACHAEL S. MAMANE is the chef and founder of Brooklyn Bouillon, a culinary stock company that endeavors to minimize agricultural food waste while making staple products for home cooks. Her work in reducing consumptive waste streams has been featured by the *New York Times*, *Modern Farmer*, *The Splendid Table*, *Forbes*, and *Food Curated*. Her project participation with Feeding the 5000 was supported by the United Nations Environmental Program. She has exhibited at Harvard Law School and participated in early food incubators at Stanford University and Babson College.

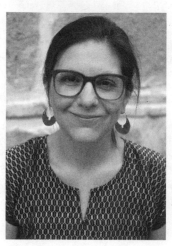

SCOTT MARC BECKER

Rachael brings a rich personal history to the cooking experience, influenced by a lost heritage, guided by a science degree, and taken in by professionals who share a passion for good, healthy food. She is unafraid to spend nights with slow-roasting animals and is genuinely excited about eating carrot tops.